Here May Bee
Perfect Health For
You And Your Family!

While Health
Isn't Everything,
Without Health,
Nothing Else
Matters!

THE WORLD'S ONLY
PERFECT FOOD BOOK
The Bee Pollen Bible

THE WORLD'S ONLY PERFECT FOOD BOOK

The Bee Pollen Bible

Featuring

The Perfect Miracle Foods from the Beehive

HONEYBEE POLLEN - ROYAL JELLY - PROPOLIS

Scientifically-Documented

The Comprehensive All-Encompassing Book
on the Bee

By

Royden Brown

Publisher
Hohm Press
P.O. Box 2501
Prescott, AZ 86302

THE WORLD'S ONLY PERFECT FOOD BOOK
The Bee Pollen Bible

ISBN: 0-934252-31-9

Library of Congress Catalog Number: 92 054951

Printed in the United States of America

Published by Hohm Press, P.O. Box 2501, Prescott, Arizona 86302

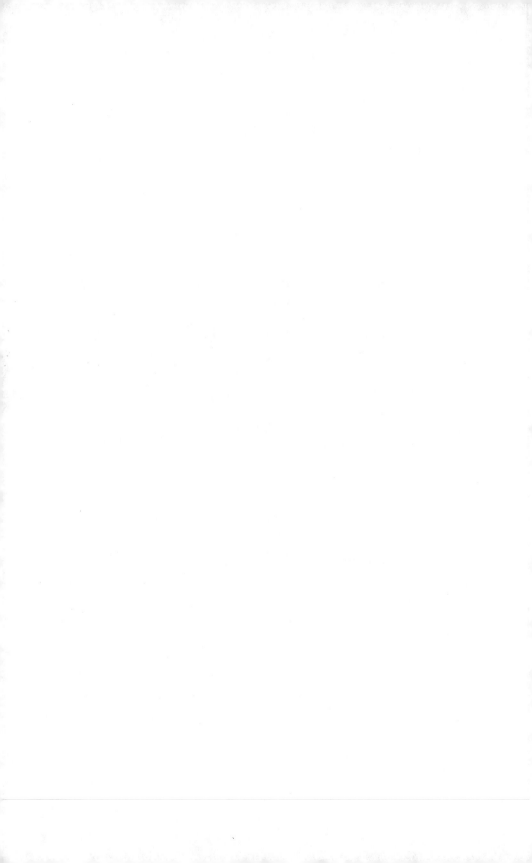

DEDICATION

We fondly dedicate *The Bee Pollen Bible* to the humans who share the earth with the quite remarkable honeybee. This book is a joyous celebration of the life of Apis Mellifera, the little critters who work so hard to provide mankind with the mysterious and powerful products of the beehive.

FOREWORD

Since antiquity, man has been a consumer of bee pollen as an ingestible dietary supplement, unfailingly expressing the conviction that pollen improves health, vigor, and vitality. While such historical practices and empirical observations cannot be accepted as proof positive, they have been at least partially responsible for attracting a diverse and persistent scientific community who have provided facts and analysis, deduced from research, which has consistently shown a beneficial effect when bee pollen is ingested by man. The research data, compiled and culled from highly respected sources and ranging in content from archeological studies of pollen shell markings and genetics, which reflect historical weather patterns and channels of population and food migration, to exhaustive analyses of the chemical composition and function of various substances found in pollen.

From my perspective as a physician, I have reviewed the scientific inquiry and considered the clinical and nutritional findings published throughout the world by respected authorities, which invariably identify pollen as of high nutritive value and composed of identifiable and measurable metabolically-active substances of variable concentrations of protein, free amino acids, and a balanced array of metabolically-active substates, enzymes, co-enzymes, vitamins, minerals and trace elements, sterols, and hormones. Pollens differ, for example, in that the highest nutritive values derived from fruit trees, palms, willows, corn, white clover, etc., while the stimulus to the increased strength and endurance effect appears to arise from the specific actions and high concentration of enzymes, which provide energy for attaching, splitting, transferring or transporting biochemical elements; carotenoids, highly reactive energy sources which bind and hold the elements together; lipids and phospholipids; and particular elements, vitamin-C and amino acids, lysine and valine.

The anti-infective properties of beehive propolis and royal jelly against colds, open wounds, and chronic prostatitis has been shown to result from the antimicrobial activity of specific agents, which have been identified and tested against bacteria and fungi. These subjects and numerous other characteristics and attributes of pollen and beehive related products are covered in this text. Given the limitations in producing qualitative and quantitative provable attributes, accessing the enormous body of literature, and the necessity of categorizing and relating personal experiences of scores of professional scientists, nutritionists, athletes, physical fitness experts and lay-witness consumers of pollen provides testimony to the rather profound effect that pollen exerts on the human body.

This text is extremely helpful and informative to laypersons and professionals alike, since the author has extracted, synthesized and summarized worldwide investigative findings in terms freed from scientific jargon, intertwined with personal experiences and collected knowledge.

Herbert B. Avery, M.D.
Los Angeles, CA

An Open Letter from Albert Earl Carter

Dear Folks,

I am happy to add my voice to the many who are praising this book. As a comprehensive overview on the life and lore of the bee, it is a fascinating glimpse into the community of the hive. For that reason alone, you will find the material instructive and entertaining.

But my main reason for writing this letter to you is because of the huge mass of research Royden Brown presents here concerning the properties of the products of the bee's industry. I believe in the dynamic benefits of all the products of the beehive, but especially bee pollen. I am very impressed with the thoroughness of this presentation. The scientific documentation is impeccable.

Those of you who have heard me lecture, who have attended one of my Reboundology Seminars, or who have read my books already know me as the originator of The Healthy Cell Concept, published initially in *The Cancer Answer*, closely followed by *The New Miracles of Rebound Exercise*. In *The Cancer Answer*, I converse with my coauther, Larry Lymphocyte, a killer T-Cell of the immune system. Larry is a figment of my imagination, an outspoken wiseguy who delights in shooting down medical myths, and Larry is an advocate of The Healthy Cell Concept.

In brief, The Healthy Cell Concept is a regimen which is broken down into four parts: Cell Food, Cell Environment, Cell Exercise and Cell Communication. When you provide the cells of your body with the best of these four essentials, you insure the health of each and every one of the 75 trillion cells that make up the human body, including the immune system defense forces of the body that keep us well. When all the cells of your body are functioning in perfect harmony with each other, you enjoy the best of health.

If Larry Lymphocyte, a commander of an army of immune system cells, had the ability to do the grocery shopping, you would find nothing but whole Cell Foods in his shopping cart. As nature's most perfect whole food, bee pollen is the best Cell Food of all. Bee pollen is the one unvarying component in the Cell Food category of my Healthy Cell Concept. Because High Desert is the best bee pollen I know, you will find High Desert mentioned by name in my books.

I think it's important that you know my endorsement of this book is not a case of 'one hand washing the other.' I have no financial interest in this book, nor in the High Desert products of the beehive; Royden Brown has no financial interest in my work. But there is a common bond between us, as you will see when you read this book.

Just like Royden Brown, I insist on the best of everything. In the words of the popular commercial, "I'm worth it." So are you.

To your very good health,

Albert Earl Carter, President
National Institute of Reboundology & Health, Inc.

TABLE OF CONTENTS

DISCLAIMER

This book is informational only and should not be considered a substitute for consultation with a duly licensed medical doctor. Any attempt to diagnose and treat an illness should come under the direction of a physician. The author is not a medical doctor and does not purport to offer medical advice, make diagnoses, prescribe remedies for specific medical conditions, or substitute for medical consultation.

When actual persons are referred to herein, the names have been altered and/or initials have been used to protect the privacy of the individuals involved.

Unique among all God's creatures,
only the honeybee improves the environment
and preys not on any other species.

CHAPTER 1

IN THE BEGINNING . . .

She was very special, but then they were all very special. The tiny Apis Mellifera egg was just one of more than 2,000 tucked neatly into her very own spanking-clean brood cell that day by the Queen Mother. Oblivious to her destiny, the little egg nested cozily inside her hexagonal waxen nursery as her nucleus greedily absorbed the special nutriments surrounding her. As a developing embryo, she was soon exhibiting tiny buds of tissue, which would be her antennae and mandibles, and the small lobes which would be her two pairs of maxillae. She would not need her antennae for some time yet, but her mandibles and maxillae, her feeding organs, were going to be very important very soon.

When she emerged as a larva, she was still a helpless baby without legs or wings. The nurse bees tended to her needs carefully, just as they cared for all the other tiny newly-hatched baby honeybees. Her little body, less than a quarter of an inch long, was an eating factory. As a young larva, her inner organs were not yet completely formed. It was but a short route from her mouth to an enormous food repository, her stomach. Her intestines were shut off from her stomach, and her excretory organs were slender tubules, not the full tubes they would become as she matured.

The nurse bees fed her sips of diluted royal jelly mixed with honey for three days only, the one time in her life she was to be allowed even a taste of the royal milk, normally reserved exclusively for the Queen. Her main nutriment was bits of bee bread, the incredibly nutritious pollen her older sisters had harvested from flowers and stored in the hive as food for the colony, plus some rich raw honey, itself, cloudy with pollen particles taken from the comb. Still in her brood chamber, she ate contentedly and almost constantly and steadily developed until she was literally full almost to bursting.

Like all her sisters, she was 'toilet trained' without being taught. It was unthinkable that her nursery cell be fouled with excrement. As a richly well-fed and rapidly maturing larva, she was ready to spin her cocoon, moult for the final time, wait for her sisters to cap her cell snugly with wax, and settle down until she emerged as a pupa. As the time came, the contents of her stomach were finally processed and discharged into her intestines and allowed to exit her anus into the bottom end of her cell. She remained clean and pristine and 'above it all' in her newly-spun pupal cocoon. Once she became a fully-formed pupa, she threw off the shell of her larval cuticle and, still tucked into her cocoon, took on the appearance of the adult bee she was close to becoming. Her special larval tissues were breaking down into food for her still-maturing adult tissues.

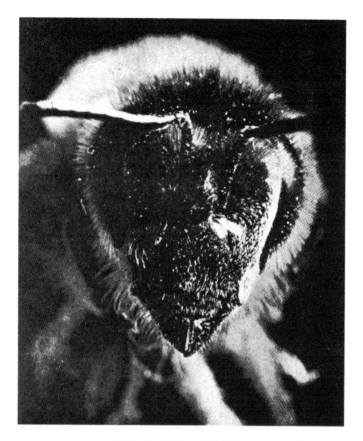

Portrait of The Little Bee

When her final metamorphosis was complete, she split open her fragile pupal shell and stepped daintily forth as a half-inch long adult bee ready to undertake her duties in the communal society of the hive. Like all worker bees, she had jaws that bite inward, special smell-sensors in her antennae (with more than 2,000 sense-plates), and jewel-bright eyes color-blind to red, but which can detect ultra-violet rays invisible to man. It is this ability which enables the bee to make its way in the darkness of the hive.

She was not conscious of the ancient genetic programming that dictated her behavior. She couldn't know that her ancestral sisters had been revered by Pharoahs, or that her species had been immortalized in paintings and carvings ordered to adorn fabulous tombs, rich with the beaten gold and obsidian and lapis of ancient Egypt. She had no way of knowing that her story had been told and retold since the beginning of time, in every form and medium and language from cave paintings to rock carvings to hieroglyphs on papyrus scrolls to feathery brushstrokes on rice paper to the writings of many diverse civilizations and religious sects, from ancient to modern.

Her many nannies had not told her, for they themselves did not know, that the products of their industry were (and are) so rare and so unique and so precious that they figure prominently in holy writings. The nectar she was to drink and transform into honey is mentioned 68 times in the Holy Bible . . . the pollen she was to collect and store in the honeycomb she was to manufacture would be recognized as the same honey and pollen-filled comb as that given to the risen Jesus Christ in the early days of the Christian era . . . the resinous sap she was to collect from spruce buds and conifers as the antibiotic disinfectant propolis was so similar to the legendary frankincense and myrrh of Biblical times that many scholars believe they are one and the same . . . the royal jelly she was to produce was the same rejuvenating nutriment prized by ancient oriental potentates as a guarantee of a long and healthy life and as an aid to sexual prowess . . . and candles made from the beeswax she was to secrete are still known, as they always were, as the finest candles of all.

She couldn't know that modern science says it is aerodynamically impossible for a honeybee to fly, that her fragile gossamer wings cannot lift her heavy ungainly body into the air and sustain flight. And she was oblivious to the fact that her species, alone among all others, was perfectly formed and perfectly equipped and perfectly programmed to carry out its work right from their beginnings. The Indians call the coyote, 'God's dog.' Perhaps the bee should be called 'God's bug.' As it was, so it ever shall be. The bee has not evolved one whit since the moment of her creation.

When the little bee emerged as an adult, she took up her responsibilities within the hive immediately. There was no census taker, but her colony averaged around 30,000 worker bees like herself, between 500 to 2,000 drones, and a single ruling Queen Bee. She was too newly hatched to leave home, so her first chore consisted of cleaning up her own brood chamber, as well as some additional cells left littered by some of her sisters.

A day or so after her metamorphosis, the little bee helped the older nurse bees feed developing larvae older than three days. Along with many other 'nannies,' she visited the pantry situated close to the edge of the brood-comb. These pantry-cells were packed with 'bee bread,' the highly nutritious pollen needed for feeding maturing grubs. The nurse bees removed just a bit at a time for ease of transport. If we were to peel the wax from one hexagonal 'pill' of bee pollen from one storage cell, we would see that it looks rather like a miniature layer cake. A tiny pantry-cell can contain eight or more layers of different colored pollens packed tightly together.

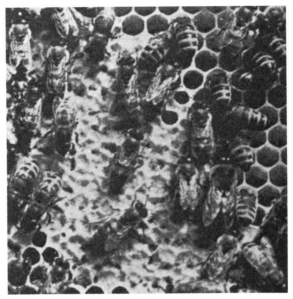

A Trip to the Pantry

She also busied herself with the housekeeping for several more days, a chore shared among many of the sisters. At between six and twelve days of age, the young bee was secreting royal jelly and qualified to feed the fragile very young larvae less than three days old. She had attained the status of fully-fledged nursing bee.

When the majestic Queen came into the vicinity, every worker in the area paid her the deference due royalty, as well as the honor due the Queen Mother. They buzzed excitedly and presented their little faces to her and clustered around her imposing Queen-sized body in a big circle, the little bee among them. Not one dared turn their backside to the Queen bee. They took turns serving the Queen her royal diet of royal jelly and groomed her carefully.

During her third week of life, the little bee took her first 'play' flight near the entrance of the hive. She was afraid to venture far from the security of the colony her first time out. She had graduated from nursery chores by this time and was pitching in and helping with a wider variety of jobs. A few leaves and twigs had somehow blown into the hive when the wind whipped up during the night. She dragged them out and dropped them to the ground. Two aged bees had died in the midst of bringing pollen into the hive. They were too heavy for her to manage alone. She and several sisters joined together in taking them out.

During this period in her life, she took several more important orientation flights outside the hive. She was getting her bearings, but still didn't go far. The little bee instinctively knew what else needed doing. So she joined the 'receiving' bees and helped pack pollen in cells and assisted in ripening a quantity of the nectar brought in by some of the older sisters. She worked as a 'builder' and manufactured wax to repair some damaged comb. She even collected a bit of the special sap, kneaded it into wax flakes she manufactured, and patched up a few small cracks with propolis. She was very busy and never took a minute for herself while she was on duty. There is no day and night inside the hive. The colony buzzes with activity 24 hours a day and the workers snatch a snooze only when they're too tired to continue working.

It came to pass that the little bee was awakened once from a much-needed nap by a tremendous humming and buzzing that vibrated throughout the hive. The colony had grown too large and many of her sisters were preparing to follow the present Queen as she flew forth to find a new home.

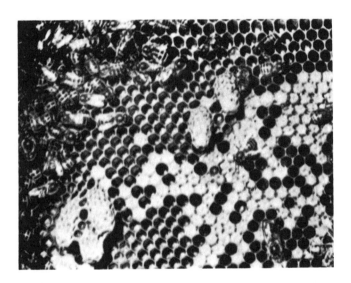

Queen Cells on Comb Amidst Capped Worker Brood Cells

In domesticated hives, the beekeeper regularly slips out an aging queen and substitutes a vibrant young queen to keep the colony strong. Requeening is usually done yearly. In the wild, the bees manage this chore themselves. A queen bee may live for five to six years or even longer, but centuries-old-programming dictates that bees prepare queen cells when the hive becomes too crowded and swarming is necessary, or if their queen is no longer laying sufficient brood. The eggs deposited in the special queen cells, no different in any way from the eggs destined to become the workers of the hive, are groomed to become future queen mothers. From the time they develop into tiny larvae, these royal bees are fed rich royal jelly and choice bits of the richest, most superior bee pollen. It is this special diet alone which transforms these special larvae into queens. The first royal to crawl forth from her brood chamber quickly destroys all the other young queens still in their cells. This is the only time in her life that the queen bee uses her stinger. There can only be one queen.

The real excitement in the hive that day was caused because two new queens were emerging from their large peanut-shaped cells at the same time. The sisters remaining behind took no notice when the old queen exited the hive with a mass of bees trailing behind her. They were all too intent on the drama attending the royal births. As the two young queens squared off to fight to the death, the members of the colony were all frantic with worry. It was possible that both new queens might be serverely injured. They knew instinctively that a colony without a queen cannot survive.

As the royal battle was joined, the bees milled together and watched the spectacle intently. None dared interfere at this point. They hummed and buzzed nervously and danced this way and that, tumbling over one another in their excitement and fear. The advantage seemed first with one, then with the other. When it became clear that one young queen would prevail, though she was still at considerable risk from the other, many of the sisters crowded forward, eager to give their lives to insure the survival of the colony. The weaker queen was stung to death. The victorious new Queen moved purposefully forward and disposed of all the young queens still sleeping in their chambers.

All that remained was for the virgin Queen to take her mating flight from the hive, which she would do when she was three to five days old. This newly crowned Queen instinctively went forth when the sun was at its zenith. The heated air that time of day insured that the drones would be out and about and flying freely. This would be the only time she left the hive, and it would take between ten and thirty minutes for her purpose to be accomplished. Her wings beating the air at 11,400 strokes per minute, she soared upward. Attracted by the heady scent of her pheremones, the male population of the hive followed eagerly as she went higher and higher. One by one, the drones faltered and fell behind.

The Queen flew higher and higher and still higher until just one male, the strongest and mightiest of all, reached her and impregnated her. The male's spermatozoa entered her vagina and passed into her sperm reservoir. It was prevented from flowing out again by the mucous plug which the drone ejaculated immediately after copulation. This single impregnation is sufficient to fertilize all eggs she will lay in her lifetime as ruling Queen of the hive.

Within two or three days after her mating flight, the new

Queen Bee commenced laying brood. As Queen Mother, she will lay upwards of 2,000 eggs daily, the equivalent of more than half her own body weight, for two or three years until her supply of sperm is exhausted. When that happens, the colony will raise a new crop of queens. The curtain will rise and the drama will commence again, just as it has been played out since the beginning of time. In our hive, the little bee and her sisters settled down contentedly under their new queen and the business of the hive resumed as before.

When she turned 21 (days old), our little bee went to work as a guard bee. Along with many of her sisters, she flew patrol around the entrance of the colony. This select group of guards set up a fierce angry buzzing when anything came too close to the hive. An unwary wasp found itself with more than it could handle. After surviving the first few stings, he fell to the ground full of venom. He did not survive the assault for long, but many of the sisters gave their lives in this encounter. The barbs on the end of their stingers insures that the victim cannot pull out the needle-sharp instrument of vengeance. When the bee itself tries to withdraw its stinger, a portion of her abdomen pulls away with it. But the stinger keeps pumping and delivers a full load of venom nonetheless. After using her stinger just once, a honeybee dies.

Somehow a big ugly beetle managed to make its way into the hive unnoticed, probably during the full alert when the wasp was destroyed. Within a millisecond, the intruder was surrounded by a dense cloud of angry buzzing bees, the little bee among them. His time in the hive was short, but this large hard-shell-ed beetle proved impossible to drag out, even when many of the sisters clustered around to help. It was unthinkable that the interior of their home should be fouled by this alien. Some of the sisters quickly buzzed off to tightly-furled nearby leafbuds, a rich source of the necessary propolis, and scurried back, each armed with as much propolis as they could carry. Sooner than you would believe possible, the dead beetle was completly en-cased in a sarcophagus of mother nature's disinfecting propolis. The antiseptic cleanliness of the hive was restored and preserved.

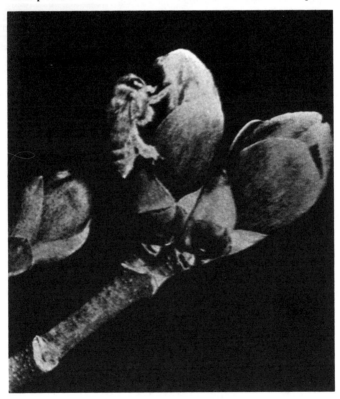

A Hunter Gathering Propolis

Because the temperature of the hive is maintained at a near-constant 94 degrees at all times, the little bee joined her sisters at odd moments in 'air-conditioning' the colony. As the outside temperature climbed over 100 degrees near noon, more and more bees began fanning their stubby wings over droplets of water, sending cool breezes throughout the hive. During the hot weather of summer, the bees engaged in inside chores moved further apart to allow the dispersion of body heat. If it had been a cold blustery winter day, the little bee would have joined her sisters as they clustered together to release the metabolic heat necessary to keep the interior of their home snug and cozy.

One day when she was close to four weeks old, the little bee suddenly felt impelled to become a forager. A sister a little older than she came dancing excitedly into the hive full of tremendous news. This sister had located a source of superior pollen and nectar and enthusiastically transmitted the location to the colony. She performed a half-circle, took a sharp turn, ran in a straight line while wiggling her body sideways, then moved half-circle in the opposite direction. She repeated this dance several times, all the while emitting blips of sound of such low frequency as to be inaudible to human ears. This wag-tail dance was most complicated, but easily deciphered by the sisters.

The little bee flew off excitedly. Her interpretation of the dance was unerring. Even though this was her first real maiden flight from the hive, she was first on the scene. She settled contentedly on one of many sweet-smelling colorful blossoms. As she sucked up the deliciously sweet nectar, her stubby little body became covered with the golden dust of the rich pollen. On her way to the next flower, she quickly brushed the bright gold flecks of pollen into the pollen baskets on her rear legs and tamped it down. She was fairly dizzy with the heady scent and brilliant profusion of the flowers. Her ancient genetic programming led her from blossom to blossom. Even in the excitement of her first foraging expedition, she selected only the most perfect and most superior flowers, pollinating as she went, thus insuring superior growth the following season. Very soon her honey pouch was full, and both her pollen baskets were loaded with tightly--packed kernels of the rich highly-nutritive golden dust.

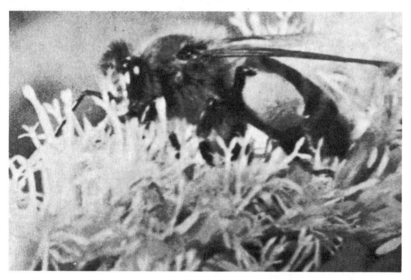

Baskets Loaded With Floral Gold

This little bee lived in a lopsided globe of a nest fastened high in the leafy branches of an old apple tree (see page 15). Her hive was built in the ages-old way and might have graced any other tree down through history. She found her way home instinctively. She knew she was in the right place when she caught the scent of her very own Queen Mother's pheremones.

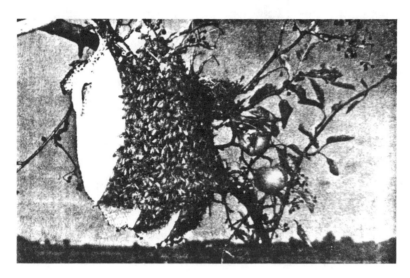

Wild Bee Hive on Apple Tree

Proudly, she entered the nest where many sisters were waiting to help her unpack. If she had been born into a bee-keeper's colony (see Chapter 2), she would have entered the hive by passing through a pollen trap, which would have gently reliev-ed her of a portion of the contents of her pollen baskets. As it was, she accepted the assistance of the 'receiving' sisters and flew right back out again. Barely in her fourth week, she had become a field forager. She made many more trips before darkness fell.

Foraging now dominated her life. It was intoxicating to fly out of the hive in the morning when the sun had warmed the earth. She herself found another important source of pollen and nectar and returned home to dance her news before a crowd of enthusiastic and admiring sisters. She was busy and life was good. For the next two weeks, she feverishly foraged, participated briefly in the communal life of the hive, but was a solitary harvester for the most part. It was what she was born for. The little honeybee asked nothing more.

In the course of just one day's work the little bee, together with all her sisters, visited more than 250,000 blooms. To produce a single pound of honey, the hard-working members of the colony had to make around 37,000 trips to the fields. She was nearing the sixth week of her life when she felt the work becoming harder. She refused to slow down though and continued winging her way to the flower fields every morning, making thousands of trips back and forth every day with her honey pouch bulging and her pollen baskets fully loaded.

But the morning finally came when she crawled to the exit and discovered she couldn't make the flight with her sisters. No matter how hard she tried, her tattered worn-out wings and aging body just wouldn't cooperate. Still trying, she worked her way laboriously to the edge and tumbled lifeless to the ground. She had fulfilled her programming. She had accomplished the grand design set out for her and her species in the dawn of creation. She was gone. But her species, the remarkable honeybee, will continue until the world ends and time is no more. As it was in the beginning, so it ever shall be.

CHAPTER 2

THE BEEKEEPER TODAY

Anywhere Flowers Flourish

Beekeeping Past

The beekeeper of old fashioned hives from a variety of materials. He then sat back and hoped the bees would take up residence, or tried to capture a swarm. These manmade hives ranged from rudely cut logs nailed to a tree, called 'bee gums,' to cylinders shaped from river clay, to tightly-woven straw 'skeps,' which resembled a conical-shaped upside-down straw basket. Depending on the materials available, crude hives such as these are still in use. They can be found in jungle clearings in Africa, dotting the countrysides of many European and Asian countries, and even in the backwoods of America.

Beekeeping was revolutionized in the mid to late 1800s when several important facts came to light. First, the Reverend L.L. Langstroth discovered the significance of bee-space in the interior of the beehive. He found that bees require a ⅜th to ½ inch space for passage. If the space is smaller, the bees can't maneuver. If the space allotted is larger, the bees promptly fill it up with comb. Langstroth designed the movable-comb hive, a rectangular 'bee box' with vertical wooden frames on which the bees could build comb. When the top is lifted off, the frames the bees have obligingly filled with honeycomb can be easily removed for harvest and an empty one slipped in.

Second, Johannes Mehring, a German beekeeper, came up with the idea of giving the bees a headstart by supplying the hive with a beeswax foundation on which to build their comb. He imprinted a thin flat sheet of beeswax with the precise impression of the hexagonal cells of the comb and fastened it to one of the Langstroth's movable frames. His bees took to this idea immediately. All they were required to do was add additional wax and draw the cells out to the proper depth. This is why we have straight uniform honeycomb today, instead of the hodgepodge conglomeration of odd shapes the bees build in the wild.

Third, a beekeeper residing in Italy by the name of Franz Hruschka found an easy way to remove the honey from the comb. Instead of cutting the comb apart and squeezing to separate the liquid honey from the wax, he put centrifugal force to work and the honey-extractor was born. The resulting honey was clear and free of all hive debris. Best of all, after the honey was extracted, the combs were returned to the hive. The bees promptly repaired any broken cell walls and filled them up with honey. And this procedure was continued over and over again.

Beekeeping Present

These three advances in the beekeeper's art heralded the modern age of beekeeping. Because they were so right,

Langstroth's movable-frames with carefully measured bee-space, Mehring's foundation comb, and Hruschka's method of honey extraction are still in use, with one questionable advance. Today, the beekeeper can choose from wax or *plastic* foundation comb.

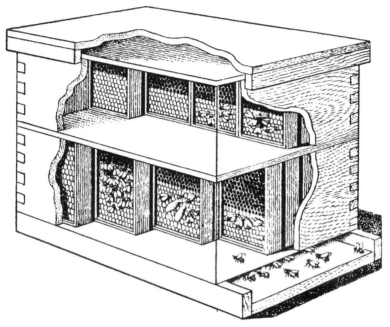

Cut-Away Drawing of a Modern 'Bee Box.'

In this manmade hive, the bees carry on their activities just as in the wild. They enter and leave at the bottom from their own 'landing pad.' Young are raised in the lower level, or brood chamber. Honey and pollen (bee bread) are stored in the upper chamber. Additional sections, called 'supers,' can be added to the top of the hive for still more honey and pollen storage. By lifting off the removable top, the beekeeper can easily remove the honey-filled frames without disturbing the colony.

That's where the matter rested until the *re*discovery of the other valuable products of the hive, bee pollen, propolis, and royal jelly. We stress *re*discovery because the renowned healers of antiquity employed all these products of the beehive. It was when the laboratories of the world community of nations confirmed that bee pollen contains all nutrients necessary in human nutrition that an efficient way to harvest bee pollen for the use of man became a necessity.

In the natural order of things, the pollen-foraging bee fills her honey-sac on her way out of the hive. Once she selects a blossom, she settles herself and scrapes the loose live pollen from the stamen with her jaws and front legs, moistening it with a dab of honey. As she proceeds to the next flower, she uses her pollen-combs to scrape the golden dust covering her stubby little body into her pollen baskets. The honeybee is admirably equipped for her task. (see below)

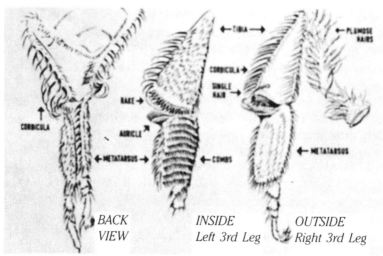

BACK VIEW   *INSIDE Left 3rd Leg*   *OUTSIDE Right 3rd Leg*

The Pollen Gathering Apparatus of the Honeybee

As she flits from flower to flower, the process is repeated over and over again. The pollen dust is tamped down until her baskets are full. In the course of her work, a pollen forager will visit as many as 1,500 blossoms. A single granule of bee pollen contains from five hundred thousand to five million live pollen spores.

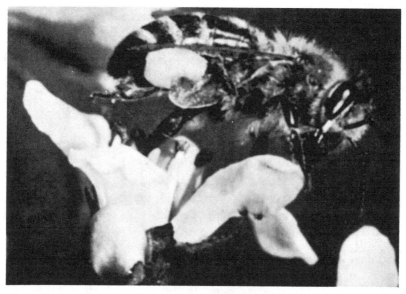

Time to head home.
This weary bee has gathered pollen from as many as
1,500 flowers to fully fill her baskets.

When the pollen-forager returns to the hive, she slips off the pollen kernel and deposits it in the wax comb. Pollen, sometimes called 'bee bread,' is a necessary part of the bees' diet. Pollen and honey are stored in separate groups of cells inside the honeycomb to be used as needed. Although these two foods are not mixed together by the bee, raw honey in the comb is rich with pollen particles and bears little resemblance to the honey you find in the supermarket.

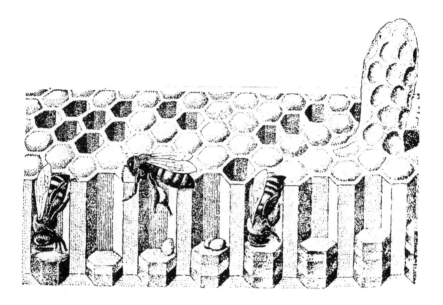

This drawing shows worker bees busily storing away freshly-harvested bee pollen 'balls' and honey (made from fresh flower nectar), in the cells of the hive. After cells are completely filled, they are sealed off with a wax cap in 'pantry cells' to preserve the food until its needed. The peanut-shaped cell at upper right represents the special extra-large cell in which a queen is reared.

Pollen is essential to the life and well being of the hive. In order to gather a portion of this live and potent substance for ourselves, what was needed was a device of some kind which would dislodge a measure of the pollen as the bees enter the hive, while permitting the bees to retain a sufficient portion of the life-giving golden dust for the maintenance of the colony. From 1959 to the present, many different pollen traps have come on the market.

Perhaps the best is the *Universal Super Trap* developed by The C C Pollen Company in 1984. (see below)

Pollen Power

Cut away view of *The Universal Super Trap* in the middle position showing the passage way of the bees, with the pollen drawer open and the top portion of the hive removed.

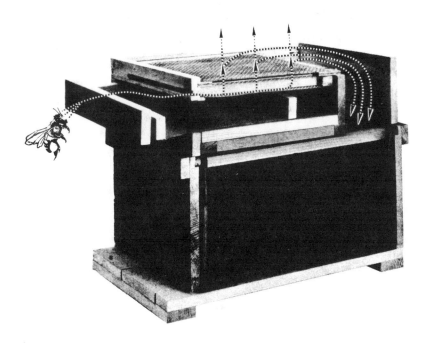

Bee box (hive) with side removed showing the wax foundation panel on which the bees build comb for storing honey and pollen (bee-bread).

This trap consists of a box the same size as a standard bee box, or hive. It is equipped with a series of scientifically-designed wire grids through which the bees must pass to gain entrance to the colony. As they make their way through the grids, approximately sixty percent of the pollen is gently brushed out of their pollen baskets. It falls through a screen into the pollen drawer situated beneath the trap.

The technology of the Universal Super Trap is all-important. It allows sufficient pollen to pass through the grids into the colony for the care and feeding of the hive population, and insures the harvesting of the driest, cleanest pollen possible. Moisture-laden wet pollen from low-lying humid areas ferments quickly, or develops mold. This type of pollen must be heat-treated immediately to preserve it for use. But high heat processing kills the enzymes and reduces the nutrient value considerably, transforming the pollen into a dead food.

When bee pollen is improperly stored and handled, it will lose up to 76 percent of its nutritive value within twelve months. The only satisfactory method of preserving fresh, live bee pollen is flash-freezing at zero degrees to maintain hive-freshness indefinitely and to preserve all vitamins, minerals, and other nutrients intact. Allowing pollen to remain in the trap for as little as ten days results in nutrient loss or worse. Beekeepers who harvest for The C C Pollen Company are required to gather bee pollen two times per week. Each maintains a large chest-type freezer right alongside their honey extractors in the bee house.

The C C Pollen Company mandates that all freshly gathered pollen be immediately flash-frozen in small batches.

Compared to our ancestors, those of us who prize the products of the beehive have it easy today. If your aim is to supply the family table, it's easy to tuck a hive or two behind the garage or the barn. Bees forage wherever flowers grow, including the side of the road where clover and weeds abound. Honeybees have a flight range of twelve square miles and are masters at seeking out sources of pollen and nectar.

The population of your hive will consist of one queen, approximately 20 to 100 thousand workers, and a few hundred drones. These male bees do not engage in foraging of any kind and are totally dependent for their living on the generosity of their sisters. The number of drones in the hive varies according to the time of the year. As winter aproaches, the worker bees drive the drones from the hive. Stored food is too precious to share during the cold months if the colony is to survive.

The worker bees are sexless underdeveloped females, but they do all the work that is done in the hive. They feed and rear brood, tend to the queen, secrete the wax, build comb, ventilate the hive, gather pollen and honey, and fight all the battles necessary to defend the hive. They are the smallest in size, but they hold the power and regulate the ongoing work of the colony.

The queen is the only perfect fully-evolved female in the hive. She is larger than the workers, but her wings are proportionately shorter. Her abdomen tapers to a point to facilitate the deposit of eggs in brood cells.

The drone is shorter, thicker and has more bulk to his body than the queen. His wings reach the entire length of his abdomen; they are much larger and clumsier than the worker's wings. In flight, the buzzing drone is louder and differs in sound from the workers. He has no sting, and no equipment for gathering honey or secreting wax, and no pollen baskets. The only purpose of the drone is to mate with the newly-born young queen.

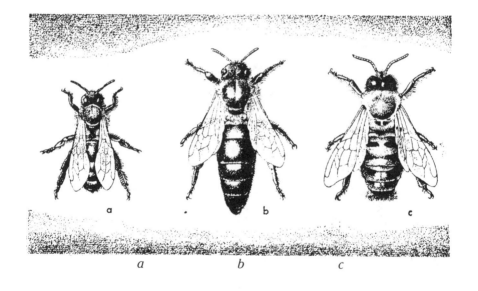

The Three Bees

a) Worker; b) Queen; c) Drone

However, because modern beekeepers requeen their hives every year by purchasing a young fertile fully-impregnated queen, the drones are out of a job. Requeening a hive is a touchy business. The hive is filled with the resident-queen's pheremones. This is the scent that identifies 'home' to all her children, and the workers of the hive will protect their queen mother with their lives. Even after the beekeeper plucks out the old queen, the scent lingers.

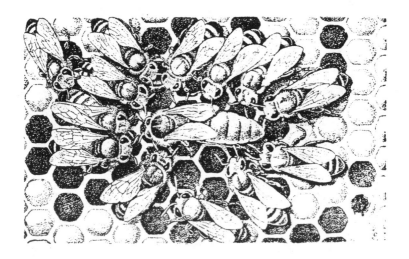

Surrounded By Her Court, The Queen Bee Lays Eggs Endlessly

The new queen arrives in a little wooden box, which the beekeeper places strategically inside the hive. If a new queen should be placed in the hive without this protection, the loyal sisterhood would quickly sting her to death. Therefore, the entrance to the royal traveling case is securely plugged with a sugary 'bee candy.' By the time the workers nibble through the candy, the new queen pheremones have permeated the hive and she

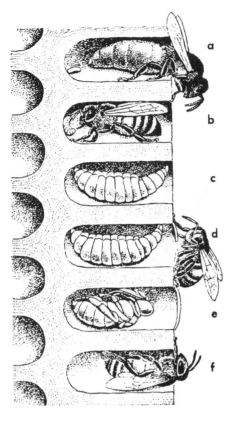

Life Cycle of Worker Bee

is eagerly accepted by her stepchildren. Within eight weeks, all the stepchildren will have joined the dear departed, having worn themselves out with hard work. Their absence will not be noticed. Emerging young bees laid by the old queen will give their allegiance to the new queen. The drawing (see left) shows the life cycle of the worker bee. a) Queen depositing an egg in a prepared cell; b) The tiny newly-hatched larva is fed by a 'nurse bee' until it reaches: c) mature larval size; d) shows a worker capping the cell with wax; e) pupa evolves into adult form; f) young adult bee emerges to take up its life work. All the while, the new young queen has been laying up to 2000 eggs per day since her arrival. No matter where she is in the hive, the queen is always surrounded by her court. The queen is meticulously cleaned and groomed by her ladies-in-waiting and is fed royal jelly by her royal entourage. The workers also tidy up the brood cells and line them with propolis ready for the royal deposit of eggs. The only function of the queen is to lay eggs, a most important job. And so the entire population of the hive renews itself again and again.

Beekeeping As Big Business

There are many bee farms in the U.S. which are maintained only for their honey production. Much of this honey ends up in the supermarkets as a refined liquid sweet with all the bits of pollen and propolis strained out. Unfortunately, only a true unrefined raw honey can be classified as a nutritive food. This type of honey is getting harder and harder to find. A few unrefined honeys still find their way into supermarkets, but health food stores are the place to be certain of finding this unrefined liquid gold, cloudy and rich with suspended bee pollen.

There are very few giant beehive harvesters in the U.S. Without coming right out and naming names, suffice it to say that The C C Pollen Company maintains the standard of excellence in this area. The *High Desert Products of the Beehive* are recognized worldwide as the finest obtainable. For example, The C C Pollen Company offers multiblended bee pollen harvested in environmentally-clean areas where man has not intruded with harmful chemicals, or polluted the surrounding countryside with the byproducts of civilization, such as car exhaust and worse. (see Chapter 13) for more on this subject).

Because of its awesome powers of pollination, the honeybee is partner in many areas of agriculture. Giant bee farms maintain thousands of colonies for the single purpose of fertilizing various crops. They are known as migrating beekeepers in the trade. Farmers contract with such beekeepers for the services of their bees. Hives are carefully loaded as high as twelve-deep on trucks and are transported to various sites around the country, where they are placed near the fields of crops. Because it would be a disaster of huge proportions if the population of their hives were exposed to some of the dangerous agribusiness chemicals, migrating beekeepers are extremely careful to place their hives with farmers who use only harmless chemicals which pose no danger to the bees. The experts say the difference in yields in fields pollinated by the bees can amount to hundreds of millions of dollars per year across the U.S.

Beekeeping As An Absorbing Hobby

If you're interested in keeping a hive or two, it's easy to get started. Any library has books of instruction for the first-time beekeeper. Read up on the subject. It's easier than you think. And bees are really friendly little critters, if they are not provoked.

Once you are familiar with the equipment, you need to consider the population. You can always revert to the old ways and try to track down and capture a swarm. But, unless you really know what you're doing, this is risky business. If you know a friendly neighborhood beekeeper, inquire about the possibility of purchasing a colony. If you aren't acquainted with one, check the yellow pages. Beekeeping is usually a major heading.

However, the easiest and most efficient way to set yourself

up as a beekeeper is to purchase a strong colony and the necessary equipment from the people in the business. Dadant & Sons in Hamilton, Illinois or A.I. Root in Medina, Ohio are both excellent and highly-reputable firms. Each of these companies have published extensively on the honeybee and are very knowledgeable.

You might inquire about literature and the possibility of purchasing a hobby kit. Such a kit will contain everything you need, except the bees themselves. These firms can also provide you with a complete bee colony. The worker bees will be young, well bred, and eager to work, the queen will be an active layer, and you will receive few drones. The best time to establish your beehive population is in the spring.

Oldtime beekeepers grow lyrical about the pleasures of beekeeping. They tell of delights most of us will never experience, of enjoying a piece of fresh comb dripping with honey, of scooping up a handful of bee pollen to munch as they tend the hive, of nipping off a piece of waxy propolis warm from the hive to chew on. And their eyes grow soft as they talk of the soothing buzz of a busy colony on a hot summer day. Some call this hum the finest accompaniment to a drowse in the shade the good Lord ever devised.

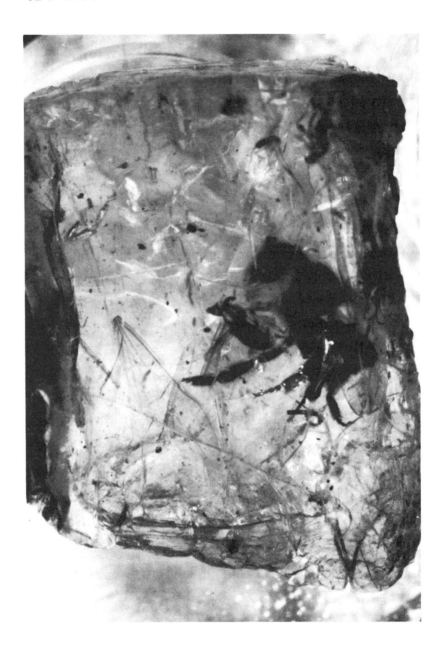

The Oldest Preserved Bee In The World
David Grimaldi, American Museum of Natural History

CHAPTER 3

THE INDUSTRIOUS HONEYBEE

Fact & Fiction

How Old Is The Bee?

To haughty ladies of past centuries, amber ornaments and toiletry articles were as highly prized (and costly) as those fashioned of gold. To David Grimaldi, assistant curator at the American Museum of Natural History in New York, a certain walnut-sized piece of translucent amber containing the fossilized remains of what Grimaldi calls "the oldest bee known" is beyond price. (see page 32) This bit of amber itself has been dated at 80 million years, but the bee preserved inside it may be much older than that. Chemical analysis indicates that the resin components which produced this amber actually came from a family of early conifers which proliferated in the Cretaceous period, from 135 million to 65 million years ago. The grand sequoia of today is a relative of those early pines.

Propolis is often called 'bee-glue.' Bees, then as now, collect propolis, take it back to the hive, mix it with wax flakes they secrete, and use it to chink up stray holes. Because propolis is the strongest natural antibiotic and disinfectant known, the bees also use it to insure that the interior of the hive remains hospital-clean. If a foreign object too large for the housekeeping bees to move contaminates the hive, it is coated with propolis and sealed off. This little bee was undoubtedly on a propolis-gathering mission when she was caught and held fast in the sticky resinous sap of some ancient leafbud.

Prior to this stunning discovery, the oldest preserved bee in existence was only about 45 million years old. However, the experts have long theorized that bees came into being at least 125 million years ago when flowering plants began blossoming in profusion. Bees and flowers are so dependent on one another for their very existence that the experts say they must have 'invented' one other. Many plants depend on the bees for the pollination they require. Bees must have the carbohydrates they glean from the nectar present in the hearts of blossoms, as well as the proteins they require from the pollen they collect. Fossilized remains of pollen, leaves, and even flowers have been dated back to when dinosaurs ruled the land, more than 125 million years ago.

It had already been determined some time back that bees have changed very little in the past 80 million years. Now that finding has been revised. Entomologists who have examined Grimaldi's fossilized bee discovered that the wings and legs of this ancient bee were remarkably 'modern' in design. The scientists point out that the structure of the hind legs show that this ancient bee carried pollen in exactly the same way our bees do today. And they are still mystified that these little critters can fly. It has been scientifically established that it is 'aerodynamically impossible' for those fragile gossamer wings, the same today as yesterday, to lift that heavy ungainly body off the ground and sustain flight. Fortunately for those of us who prize the products of the beehive, the bee herself doesn't know that.

The honeybee has been fulfilling its genetic programming since well before man first appeared on earth. And somewhere back in the long forgotten misty recesses of time some early human had an irresistible taste of honey. How did it happen? Maybe a hive had grown to such great size that the branch of the tree where it was fastened gave way. Perhaps the frightened colony swarmed elsewhere when their waxen metropolis cracked open as it crashed to the ground. But what inspired that first human to actually pick up a piece of comb, poke in a finger, take that first taste, and then greedily suck the comb clean?

However it may have happened, we do know that primitive man not only fought the bees for their honey, but also feasted royally on the bee pollen stored in the comb and even ate the eggs and larvae. Aboriginal tribes still feast on bee grubs and still regard bee pollen and honey as well worth the price of a few stings.

Myths & Mysteries

There are many fanciful stories surrounding the origin of

the honeybee. Some say the gods transformed the goddess Melissa into a bee and bestowed upon her the ability to reproduce without a mate. The ancient Greeks say bees are a result of a mystical marriage between hornets and the sun, a joining which was ordained and blessed by the gods on Mt. Olympus.

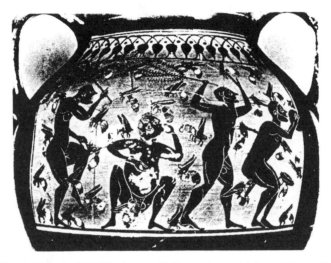

Greek Vase c 540 BC shows Melissa's bees driving off intruders threatening the Infant Zeus lay.

Down through the ages, mankind has revered the bee. Greek legends relate that the infant god Zeus was hidden from the wrath of his father to protect his life. Safe in the cave where he was taken, Zeus was well nourished on goat's milk and raw honey provided by Melissa's bees. The tale tells that when four men came upon the cave where the baby Zeus lay hidden, their leather armor mysteriously fell away and left them unprotected. Thereupon Melissa's bees ferociously attacked the naked men and drove them away, thus preserving the life of the great god

Zeus. A Greek vase c 540 BC (see page 36), currently on display in the British museum, immortalizes this mythical encounter for posterity. The legend concludes by saying that after this selfless service to Zeus, bees were able to reproduce without the mating of male and female. This tale is one of the earliest attempts to explain what the ancients regarded as the mystifying lifestyle of the bees.

Truth Revealed . . . Almost

Because no one had ever seen a bee mating, it was long widely believed that bees were sexless and that baby bees somehow originated in flowers. Much later, it was acknowledged that worker bees were born in the hive, but most people still believed that drones, at least, came from the flowers. This odd explanation didn't satisfy Aristotle, however. Four hundred years before the birth of Christ, Aristotle discarded all the outmoded theories and came up with some explanations of his own. He was almost right.

Artistotle's observations finally revealed why a hive was populated exclusively by drones when the colony was lacking a 'ruler.' When the 'ruler' was in residence, the society was fully populated with both workers and drones. And it wasn't because drones were born in flowers either. The conclusion was obvious: 'Rulers' bred other rulers and workers. When the 'ruler' was absent, workers produced drones. Drones, which were not recognized as males, did not breed. And the large and well formed 'ruler' of the hive had to be the bee 'king.' Because of the patriarchial and chauvinistic nature of the times, it was unthinkable that a 'ruler' of anything should be female. And there the matter rested for the next 200 years.

The Deified Bee

Still, mixed up in all the misrepresentations and legends, one fact stands out clearly. Almost without exception, every age has regarded the bee as a benefactor of mankind and accords this little creature almost holy status.

The Bible, the Talmud, the Torah, the Koran (the Code of Islam), along with the scrolls of the Orient, the writings of ancient Greece and Rome, the legends of the Russian and Slavic people, even the relatively recent Book of Mormon (1830), all praise the industrious honeybee and her highly nutritious and healing products of the beehive.

We need to remember that in times past, all honey was taken in the comb and was therefore rich with bee pollen and propolis. It bore no resemblance to the strained (and sometimes diluted) honeys of today. For example, we are told that DBSH (pronounced 'davash'), a favored Hebrew sweet of centuries ago, was a sticky, thick syrupy combination of honey and bee pollen.

Hebrew scholars of the Torah, the Old Testament of the Christian Bible, say that early translators mistakenly used 'honey' in many scriptures in place of the more accurate phrase 'products of the beehive.'

The experts of today explain that the Hebrew and Aramaic languages used by the original authors of certain of our holy books was lengthy and cumbersome. Because those first translators of so long ago were most familiar with honey, the thinking is that the phrase 'products of the beehive' was shortened to 'honey' in accordance with their personal experience and in the interest of what they no doubt regarded as accuracy. Today's modern linguists also question the interpretation of 'seed' in certain scriptures, insisting that a more accurate translation equates to 'pollen' in some instances.

In light of these revelations, some familiar scriptures take on a whole new meaning. For example:

Genesis 1:29 . . . *And God said, Behold, I have given you every herb bearing seed which is upon the face of all earth, and every tree, in which is the fruit of a tree yielding pollen; to you it shall be for food.*

The Lord God gave man pollen for his food.

Genesis 43:11 . . . *And their father Israel said unto them, If it must be so, now do this; take of the best fruits in the land in your vessels and carry down the man a present, a little balm, and a little honeycomb, spices and myrrh, nuts and almonds.*

The first exchange of gifts between nations recorded in the Bible were the gifts Jacob (Israel) ordered carried to his son Joseph in Egypt when he sent his other sons forth to purchase food to alleviate the severe famine in Israel. These precious gifts included honeycomb and myrrh, which some modern authorities liken to propolis.

Exodus 16:1-36 . . . *And the children of Israel did eat manna for 40 years until they came to a land inhabited: They did eat manna until they came into the borders of Canaan.*

It is written "the taste of it (manna) was like wafers made of honey." The experts of today say manna was pollen of the Tamarisk tree. God counseled the Israelites to eat manna fresh. Science teaches that the hot desert sun would have melted the pollen and caused it to lose nutrients as it aged. Those ancient tribes of Israel survived 40 years of wandering in the desert in perfect health, because they ate the perfect food, manna, the pollen of the Tamarisk tree.

Luke 24:41-43 . . . *Jesus said unto them, "Have ye any food?" And they gave Him a honeycomb and a piece of broiled fish. And He took it and did eat before them.*

The first food the risen Jesus Christ ate after His resurrection was honey and bee pollen in the comb.

Numbers 13:27 . . . *We came unto the land whither Thou sentest us, and surely it floweth with milk and honey and this is the fruit of it.*

In correct translation, this scripture reads: *"We came unto the land whither Thou sentest us, and surely it floweth with milk and all the products of the beehive and pollen is the fruit of it."*

The Church of Jesus Christ of Latter Day Saints, more familiarly known as the Mormons, still holds the honeybee in very high regard today. In fact, if Brigham Young, second president of the LDS church, had had his way, the state of Utah would today carry the name *Deseret*, a term for 'honeybee' from their sacred *Book of Mormon,* which signifies industry. When Young led Mormon pioneers into Utah to escape the persecution church members suffered for their practice of polygamy, the settlement around the Great Salt Lake was named Deseret, in honor of the hard-working honeybee. As governor of the territory, Brigham Young applied for statehood in 1849 under the name of Deseret, but the application was denied. However, a beehive appears on the Great Seal of Utah, and many Mormon industries of today are honored by the name Deseret.

Traveling further backward in time, we find that the holy book of the Hindu's, *The Rig-Veda,* penned in Sanskrit between 2000 and 3000 BC, talks of bees almost with awe. Vishnu, the powerful Preserver & Protector of the Hindu trinity of gods, is often symbolized as a blue bee on a lotus flower. The east Indian god of love, Kama, wields a bow with the string made of an entwined chain of bees. In cultures worshipping a goddess of fertility, variously called Venus, Diana, Ceres, Cybele, or Iris, bees were invariably considered sacred and were minor deities in their own right.

Spring fertility rites often used the bee as a symbol for the festivities. It's easy to understand why. Bees are seldom out and about during seasons of dormancy when growth is scant and blossoms nonexistent. But in the spring, when the sun-warmed earth sends forth fragrant flowers full of nectar and pollen, the bees reappear and joyously go about their tasks. The mysterious dance of the scout bees which signals the location of rich sources of food and sustenance to the rest of the hive was mirrored in the frantic dancing of those long-ago celebrants welcoming the arrival of spring.

The Roman god Bacchus, known to the Greeks as Dionysius, is one of the major deities credited with introducing beekeeping to man. Although this happy god, sacrificed to by the best known party-goers of any century, the Romans, is most often associated with a touch of the grape, there's more reason to think that the drink this legendary god would personally have favored was mead, or honey wine.

Another story purporting to explain how mankind came to keep bees credits Aristaeus, son of Apollo and Cyrene, with bringing the knowledge to mortal man. Aristaeus was supposedly educated by the Muses, the nine Greek goddesses who were patrons of the arts. Perhaps it was this mythical relationship which led to bees being called the 'Birds of the Muses.' It was long believed that if a bee touched a child's lips, he would have magical abilities in the arts. Legend has it that bees kissed Sophocles, Plato, and the renowned Roman poet, Virgil, while they were yet in their cradles. The patron saint of beekeepers, St. Ambrose, was said to have been so blessed by the bees as well. In fact, though we seldom give it a thought, all mankind has been blessed by the bees.

Man & Bee — Together Forever

We have a mysterious kinship with the honeybee that cannot be denied. What the bee does instinctively, we imitate poorly at best. Are not man and bee pleasured by the very same things? Do we not seek sweets for our table, as the bee seeks nectar in the hearts of flowers? Do we not take pleasure in sweet-smelling perfumes, as the bee is attracted to the heady scent of blossoms? Do we not select pleasing colors for our garments and surroundings, as the bee works in the fields of flowers? And, in this dog-eat-dog modern world, who among us does not wish for the God-given ability to live in perfect harmony with all other species?

The world of the bee is rich with the myriad colors and sweet perfumes of the flowers and blossoms where she lives and works. She keeps her house in an orderly manner and maintains absolute antiseptic cleanliness within the hive. Each member of bee society lives in perfect harmony with every other. The bee does not prey on any other species for her livelihood. She harvests and stores the food the colony needs to survive. Alone in the animal kingdom, only the bee has vital work to do. Without her ability to carry the pollen that fertilizes the plants and flowers, many species would fail to survive. The bee truly improves the environment and enriches her corner of the world with her presence.

It's impossible to accurately determine just how long man has prized the hard-working honeybee. In fact, if bees and flowers 'invented' one another, what is the true relationship between man and bee? The ecologists of today reckon that over 100,000 species of plants would die out and become extinct without the pollinating work of the bee. Without these plants, life as we know it, perhaps all life, would become impossible. Early man could not have known that, of course. All the ancients cared about was securing a potful of honey and a bowlful of bee pollen for the table.

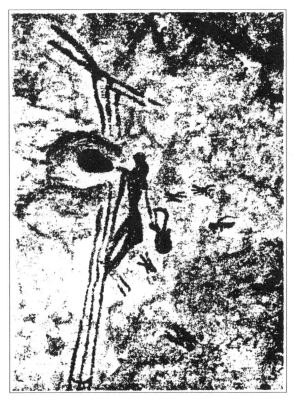

An ancient rock painting, discovered near Valencia, Spain deep inside what has come to be known as *Cueva de la Arana* (Cave of the Spiders), shows a woman mounting a primitive ladder to gather honey from the waxen city a colony of honeybees have tucked into a hole in the side of a cliff. (see left)

Rock painting, dating back to Mesolithic Era, discovered in a cave near Valencia, Spain shows ancient woman gathering honey.

The experts say this cave painting dates back to the Mesolithic Era (c 10,000/8,000 - 3000 BC). A watercolor copy of the original, painted by F. Benitez Mellado, hangs in the Museo de Prehistoria in Valencia. Another rock painting still visible in the Arana Cave depicts early tribesmen robbing wild bees. The homemade dyes fashioned by the unknown artists so long ago are faded with time, but the scenes are unmistakable.

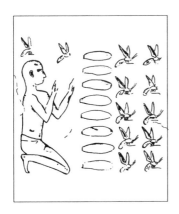

Painting in the tomb of Pa-Bu-Sa (Thebes, Egypt 620 BC) depicts ancient beekeeper.

In Egypt, with its highly advanced culture, the honeybee and the products of the hive were held in the highest esteem. As early as 3500 BC, Egyptians chiseled a likeness of the honeybee on their monuments, painted scenes of beekeepers tending bees on the walls of their tombs (see left), and recorded the life and times of this hard-working little creature in holy hieroglyphics inscribed on papyrus scrolls.

Writings over 2000 years old reveal that Egyptian physicians called honey the "universal healer." In ancient China, honey was used to treat the victims of smallpox. The sticky stuff was smoothed over the entire body of the infected person. According to old records, this very contagious and disfiguring disease was stopped in its tracks and no pitting or scarring ensued.

In light of present day scientific studies by the U.S. Bureau of Entomology showing that typhoid germs are destroyed in 48 hours and dysentery bacteria killed in less than 10 hours, when these bacteria strains are placed in a lab dish with a bit of raw honey, those oldtime healers were onto something big. Raw honey is rich with the bee pollen particles we now know are the true source of honey's remarkable healing powers. Not so very long ago, British researchers at England's Norfolk & Norwich Hospital tried raw honey to treat infected wounds with notable success. In days of old, raw honey was often the treatment of choice for dressing battle wounds.

Down through the ages, honey, that delectable sweet treat from the beehive, was sought after and relished. If they could afford it, those long-ago Egyptians of 3000 BC gladly paid the 3 drachmas per quart that strained honey cost back then. In fact, honey was the main sweet of the world for eons. It was in the 4th century BC that a general under the command of Alexander the Great wrote an accounting of a "wonderous reed (sugar cane) which produces honey without the aid of bees." It was Christopher Columbus who brought sugar cane to the Americas. Today, many authorities name refined sugar a threat to health and are calling for a return to honey as a healthy natural sweet.

Fact or Fancy?

Man has always been fascinated by the buzzing society of the hive. Because they didn't know the facts, they invented fanciful stories to explain the mysteries of the beehive. Northern Europeans believed the bees were the souls of the dead, either returning to earth or passing by on their way to the next world. An early German legend insists that the bees were a gift to mankind by the Lord. This story says the life work of the bee is to provide wax for the immense number of candles needed to light the churches and cathedrals of the world for the glory of God.

An early Christian legend relates that the tears shed by Christ on the Cross turned into bees which flew away, bringing wholesome sweetness to mankind. A French tale involving Jesus Christ explains it still another way. When the Lord bathed in the River Jordan, the drops which fell from His body as he arose from the waters turned into bees. As the little bees were about to fly away, Christ bid them stay together and work for the benefit of mankind. Honeybees have been obeying this holy commandment ever since. Perhaps this lovely legend does contain a modicum of truth after all.

CHAPTER 4

HERE'S WHAT THEY TELL US

From The C C Pollen Company Files

It's impossible to report on the incredible benefits which have been experienced by regular consumers of bee pollen, poured out in heartfelt letters of gratitude or expressed in happy telephone calls, without emphasizing the fact that the individuals we will be introducing to you all have one very important thing in common: They all take *only* High Desert® Honeybee PollenS™ from The C C Pollen Company of Phoenix, Arizona.

The reason we must emphasize this fact as of paramount importance is because only truly superior High Desert Honeybee PollenS (see Chapter 8) deliver the full health-promoting benefits that bring such dramatic results. Be aware that you can't expect such remarkable turn-arounds if you experiment with less expensive and inferior brands.

To protect the privacy of the individuals involved, we have changed most names. However, every single one of the people you're about to meet comes from conversation or correspondence you're about to meet comes from conversation or correspondence with a living, breathing human being. These stories are not made up. The actual letters are on file at The C C Pollen Company.

Keith Carpenter

This handsome young man of twenty-one was embarrassed to go out and about in public because of a long-term case of disfiguring acne. The pimples and pustules he suffered for over five years kept him from a fulfilling relationship with a pretty member of the opposite sex. Rather than risk a look of distaste when anyone glanced his way, he kept to himself. He went to work, came home, and lived a solitary existence. Then he discovered honeybee pollen. Keith tells what happened:

"I am very pleased with your product. I had a problem with acne for about five years and spent hundreds of dollars on doctors, prescriptions, and over-the-counter acne products. I was told to take vitamins, so I tried that for a while. The doctor put me on antibiotics, which I'd rather not take. I got tired of taking handfuls of pills every day. Besides, my face stayed red and I broke out even worse. I could tell that I was going to be scarred really bad if I didn't do something soon. I was already scarred some.

"My brother was taking raw granules of your bee pollen, so I tried some. In just three days of 3,000 mg a day, the redness was almost gone and I could see a big difference. After three days on bee pollen, my skin was 500 percent better! I can't believe all the money I spent on prescriptions and stuff that didn't work. Bee pollen beats the 'heck' out of everything else. My nerves got better. I quit worrying about my complexion. I will continue taking this product forever. It's good for almost anything. I know lots of people who need to take bee pollen. I feel great and I don't need as much sleep. It has made me more alert, too.

"Whoever discovered bee pollen, thanks a million!"

Everett McClean

Like many others, this middle-aged man began taking honeybee pollen as a powerful all-natural vitamin/mineral supplement. He got the surprise of his life when this mighty medicinal accomplished something he thought was impossible.

When Everett McClean phoned The C C Pollen Company, he got to talking to the friendly and concerned voice on the other end of the line. McClean expressed absolute amazement (along with pure joy and undisguised enthusiasm) on discovering that the honeybee pollen he had been taking for just a short time seemed to be clearing up a long-standing condition that had defied his doctor's best efforts for a period of seven years. Here's what he told us:

"My personal experience is certainly a true testimonial to the properties of your bee pollen. I have had San Joaquin Valley Fever for seven years. I have tried everything and investigated all avenues, doctors and otherwise, to eliminate this condition without success.

"I started eating your bee pollen approximately three months ago. I can't believe it, but my San Joaquin Valley Fever has started to disappear! I estimate that my condition is a least 50 percent cured or 50 percent gone. I estimate that in another three months, it will disappear completely and I will not have this dreadful condition.

"I am writing this letter to you and ask that you circularize and publicize it for the benefit of others who have this Fever, or one like it. I urge you to use this letter to encourage others to take advantage of the curative properties of your bee pollen. Thanks again."

Sarah Barnett

Mrs. Barnett says gratefully that High-Desert Bee Pollen changed her life. This forty year old woman suffered for years with serious depression of such magnitude that she could barely function. Mrs. Barnett is also very enthusiastic about one of the side effects she experienced as a result of her bee pollen regimen. We'll let her tell it:

"I had been sleeping ten hours a night and waking up tired. After a week or so of taking your fresh granules, I noticed I didn't feel sleepy so early in the evening, so I gradually started staying up later.

"For years I had suffered from depression so bad that I could hardly drag myself out of bed to face another day. After taking your bee pollen granules for about two months, I woke up one morning and actually looked forward to getting out of bed. What a heavenly day that was! After working all day, I now come home and take a long walk of five miles or more, and still have enough energy left over to do my housework.

"After taking the granules for about a year, I found I had lost twenty-five pounds of unwanted weight without making any effort at all. I didn't take bee pollen to lose the weight. It was an unexpected good effect of taking pollen.

"I tell everybody that High-Desert Bee Pollen is the best thing that ever happened for me."

Frank T. Johnston

Frank Johnston touched our hearts. This young man of twenty-eight says, in part, "Bee pollen is something I had actually been praying for. I believe bee pollen is a revelation Jesus Christ wanted me to experience."

Before he was led to try bee pollen, Frank was overweight by 67 pounds and became overtired very quickly. He tells us he had been fighting obesity all his life, but this was the heaviest he had ever been. His doctor advised a healthy diet and regular exercise and monitored his condition. Then the help he prayed for was revealed to him:

"One night I called home and my mother shared the revolutionary news with me about the bee pollen she had been taking. I read all the information possible on the subject. I was quite impressed.

"My job, which I enjoyed, left me very tired at the end of the day, so I took no exercise. Then I started taking High-Desert Bee Pollen before I ate. After about four months, I started losing two to three pounds per week. I was no longer too tired to exercise and I began playing tennis again. I really started noticing some changes in myself physically. I also noticed changes in my personality. I was more outgoing and had more self-confidence. One of the biggest changes I experienced was an increase in mental alertness. And I was no longer feeling physically or mentally fatigued.

"A lot of this was a result of my personal commitment to Jesus Christ as my personal Savior and my growth in walking with Christ. Bee pollen is something I had actually been praying for. I believe Jesus Christ has brought meaning to my life and that's why I feel so good.

"Bee pollen is a revelation Jesus Christ wanted me to experience. I've never felt this healthy in my life. When I get the common cold or flu, like we all do, people marvel at how fast I recover. I'm thirty now, but I feel like eighteen. I've lost more than 50 pounds. I work hard, but I don't get run down or tired any more. I really believe bee pollen has caused healing to take place in my body.

"My best wishes to all of you."

Jack Argula

Here's an oldie, but a goodie:

"I have been feeling great ever since I started taking High-Desert Bee Pollen. About four years ago, I started taking one-quarter teaspoon of your fresh granules and kept adding a bit every day. I began feeling better and better as time went on. I now take one teaspoonful every morning. I will be seventy-six years old soon and I feel wonderful. I work every day. I take your bee pollen as a complete vitamin and mineral supplement and for the added energy and stamina it gives me. I will be ordering more bee pollen from you soon. I am almost out. Bee pollen keeps me going strong."

Melody Pike

We'll let this young woman of twenty-four set the stage herself on this one:

"Before I found out for myself what was wrong, I suffered (really suffered) from hypoglycemia (low blood sugar). My doctor said my problem was caused by too much stress, overworking. He thought I had something else wrong with me, not hypoglycemia, and put me on all kinds of medication, which I found only made me worse. So I stopped taking them completely. I will never go back to another doctor, unless it's for a strict emergency. I am now healthier than I have ever been following my own nutritional knowledge."

Melody herself explains what happened:

"Two years ago, I wasn't very healthy. I was feeling weak and just not myself. I had developed some female problems after going off birth control pills, which I had taken for two years. I didn't know it back then, but I was really starving from a nutritional deficiency, mainly B vitamins. I went to several doctors, but each one told me I had a different condition. All they did was confuse me more.

"My symptoms were disorientation, heart palpitations, sweaty palms, twitching eyes, a faint feeling that made it hard to breathe at times, pain in my temples, sore stomach, dry mouth, moodiness (I cried for no reason), and a feeling of weakness all over. I just had no energy at all. The doctors prescribed medication for my heart to stop the palpitations, tranquilizers to stabilize my moods, even antibiotics, you name it. I stopped taking all these medications after about two weeks when I figured my condition out for myself by reading many books.

"My condition turned out to be low blood sugar. The book that really helped me was *Hypoglycemia — A New Approach* by Paavo Airola. I immediately switched to an all-vegetarian diet and eliminated all types of sugars, including honey. I had to be extremely careful with my diet, eating at certain times of the day, and I began taking bee pollen with my breakfast every morning.

"After two weeks, I really noticed a drastic improvement. All those symptoms went away! I was more alert and felt I was stronger and healthier. Sometimes I felt really euphoric. This came about with eating lots of bee pollen, raw fruits and veggies, whole grains, and seeds and nuts. I also got lots of sun, fresh air, and exercise. But, if I skipped a meal or forgot my bee pollen, the symptoms returned. If I went an entire day without bee pollen, my lightheadedness came back.

"Today I am healthier than ever. I own my own lawn-care company and have six employees. I compete in jet-ski racing, run a hectic business schedule, and feel terrific! I also recommend drinking wheatgrass juice with the bee pollen for a real energetic rush! After seeing what my regimen does for me, my husband eats this way, too. But that's another story!"

Marvin J. O'Malley

At 257 pounds, Mr. O'Malley was considerably overweight. This forty-seven year old man, a diabetic who had been taking insulin for five years, also took prescription medication for high blood pressure (hypertension), plus drugs to relieve his arthritis, still more medication to soothe an ulcer, and another to counteract gout. After reading an article on bee pollen, Mr. O'Malley decided to give it a try. Today, after several years of taking this 'miracle' from the bees, he reports enthusiastically:

"At present, after taking insulin for five years, I have not taken any in five months. I am now taking medication for my high blood pressure and gout only. I have not needed any arthritis or ulcer medicine in the last year. I attribute my good health now to bee pollen, bee stings, honey, and daily walks of at least five miles.

"When I was on insulin, I was taking 40 units every day. I slowly decreased the dosage until I am now not taking any insulin at all. My blood sugar has stabilized and is checked daily with a glucometer. I have not changed my diet in any way.

"I still visit my doctor regularly. He tells me to continue exactly what I am doing now and to have others take notice. As of yesterday at the doctor's office, my weight was down to 199 pounds! I take my bee pollen only in the morning now because I find that taking it later in the day gives me so much energy I don't sleep. I think the bees and their products are lifesavers!"

Louise Brock

Mrs. Brock, who operates *The Vitamin Store*, a very fine health-food store, writes that she recommends High-Desert Bee Pollen to many of her customers, based on her personal experience. Here's what she wrote us:

"After taking two *Pollenergy* capsules every day at breakfast for two months, the bee pollen totally stopped both my husband's and my snoring and cleared up a long-standing sinus condition for me. The doctor had thought my snoring was caused by polyps.

"One customer's colon infection was cured after taking six caps per day for about four weeks. She had been doctoring for approximately six months and the doctors could not kill the bacteria strain in her colon that was giving her such problems and making her miserable. It is a real miracle.

"I feel bee pollen takes us back to the Lord's feet. It's a natural creation of His. We will never begin to imagine what He has created for us until we meet Him face-to-face."

I. Stephen Freemont, M.D.

The C C Pollen Company had been shipping quantities of High-Desert products to Dr. Freemont for a lengthy period when a letter arrived announcing that he was moving his practice to the Bahamas. This medical doctor knew he would require large shipments of bee pollen on a continuing basis and wanted a guarantee that he would be able to supply his patients with the powerful golden granules. Dr. Freemont says:

"This letter is to certify that I have been using High-Desert Honeybee Pollen from The C C Pollen Company in Phoenix, Arizona and recommend it very highly. It is the best source of bee pollen I have ever used and I hope I will never have to practice medicine without it. I will be moving to the Bahamas shortly and want to continue purchasing directly from you to insure freshness.

"I give this honeybee pollen to all my patients. It is an excellent product. I certainly recommend it to my fellow physicians as the best of its kind."

Joseph Barabas

Although he had been under a doctor's care continually, Mr. Barabas told The C C Pollen Company his health had been seriously deteriorating for three years. This 52-year old man had "hardening of the arteries" (atherosclerosis), suffered a blockage in the heart chamber his doctor deemed "inoperable," and was recovering from a debilitating stroke. His physical activity was restricted, and he was on five different prescription drugs. Then he discovered honeybee pollen, mother nature's wonder worker, and began taking "one healthy teaspoonful" every day. From then on, his progress was rapid. Mr. Barabas says:

"After experiencing a stroke, I could not think very well. After taking your bee pollen, my thinking improved, and so did my overall health. I believe your bee pollen played a big part in my progress.

"I still follow my doctor's advice, and I follow *my* bee pollen plan. I have great faith in your bee pollen. Other than what I have read, I don't know much about it, but I sure know what it does for me. I live by the word "bee pollen" and I talk about it whenever I can. The people I have given bee pollen say they can tell it gives extra energy. I have come a long way."

Nancy Martin

This pretty and articulate young woman in her late twenties had a lot to say. In her own words, here is Nancy Martin's very special story:

"First of all, I'd like to say that my story on honeybee pollen is not yet finished. After taking your bee pollen for one and a half years and receiving many benefits from it, I still feel there are many more good things coming my way from the continuing use of your pollen.

"Secondly, as a little history, I would like to mention that there have been two situations in my life which I feel put abnormal stress on my health. One situation was a car accident in high school. The other was a bite problem which had given me severe headaches for several years. I recently finished three years of periodontal work having this problem corrected.

"By the time I was 22, I was experiencing numerous health problems. I had stopped menstruating; I was losing more hair than normal; I also experienced frequent headaches and backaches; suffered from fatigue, and had a sensitivity to certain cosmetics.

"After seeing several gynecologists and other doctors and

having innumerable tests taken, the only solution I was given was to take female hormones. As far as I was concerned, that was no solution at all. The female hormones did not make me feel better.

"It was at this time that I became interested in food supplements and watched my diet. I avoided sugar, salt, and chemical food additives, and began exercising regularly. I also began seeing a chiropractor regularly. I was satisfied with my chiropractor, but I was not satisfied with the food supplements I was taking. I spent a few years trying dozens of products, but never stayed with any. Some products gave me rashes because of the compounds involved in making the tablets, while other supplements sometimes made me feel either 'hyper' or sleepy. A lot of products, including spirulina, bothered my stomach. I had even tried several other brands of pollen, but could not tolerate the fumigants or other chemicals on the pollen. Eventually, I stopped taking food supplements altogether, but my other health problems remained and I was left feeling very weak.

"It was at this time in my life that I began using your High-Desert Bee Pollen. From the first time I tried it, I knew it was different from all other supplements I had taken. I could tell it was *pure* in the true sense of the word, not just by legal definition. I knew your product was something I could take indefinintely, as no chemicals, additives, or fumigants that could be a problem in my system were present. Almost immediately, I had a more relaxed feeling in my body. In just a few days, I found I was sleeping much better. My husband commented I seemed happier, too.

After taking your pollen for about eight months, I began having regular menstrual periods for the first time in seven years.

"The following is a list of benefits I have received since I have been taking your bee pollen regularly:

1. A general increase in strength.
2. Much sounder sleep.
3. Regular menstrual periods, for the first time in seven years.
4. A more cheerful disposition.
5. Thicker and healthier hair.
6. No more problems with chills.

"I am grateful that your company believes enough in its product to make it available in a completely unaltered and unadulterated state. I am a life-time consumer of your nitrogen-canned pollen."

Evelyn Davidow

At age thirty-eight, Mrs. Davidow was 20 pounds overweight, had been diagnosed as having hypoglycemia (low blood sugar), and, in her words, "felt very sluggish." She tells us she made some healthy changes in her diet, but it was after taking two High-Desert Honeybee Pollen tablets every day for a week that she started noticing some wonderful changes in her life. Mrs. Davidow explains:

"Along with dropping junk food, I started to take your bee pollen because a friend told me it would help clear up the constant infections I had in my ears and throat.

"I personally feel that bee pollen has done a lot for me. My mental attitude has changed from constant fear and depression to a calm cheerfulness. I have energy that won't quit. My friends ask me how I can work, keep up a giant flower garden and a separate vegetable garden at home, work in the city flowerbeds, play raquetball, swim, go to aerobics, and still keep a halfway decent house.

"I will never stop taking High-Desert bee pollen. It gives me wonderful super-energy, without awful side-effects. I have painlessly dropped excess pounds and my overall health has never been better. Oh, yes! I recommend High-Desert to anyone who will listen."

Norma F. Swanson

Mrs. Swanson began taking High-Desert bee pollen at age seventy-two when a friend presented her with a pound bag of fresh granules. She suffered great pain from arthritis in her knees, feet, hands, and back, complicated by osteomyelitis of her right hip, which left her with one leg shorter than the other. In spite of all these problems, this spunky septuagenarian said she was in generally good health, but expressed a desire to lose fifteen pounds! After nibbling on bee pollen granules for a month, Mrs. Swanson reported:

"After I had taken a teaspoonful of bee pollen granules before meals every day for thirty days, I discovered I had more energy than I had had in a long, long time. And, hallelujah, I even experienced a small weight loss! Since I am handicapped, exercise is difficult, but my bee pollen regimen did make moving around easier."

At age seventy-five, Mrs. Swanson wrote:

"I've found that if I stop taking pollen for a period of a week, I simply *do not* have energy. I experience more pain and everything becomes an effort. When I take your bee pollen regularly, I certainly feel better, have scads of energy and much less pain. A recent physical found me in excellent health with, as the doctor put it, 'text-book perfect blood pressure and an excellent blood analysis.' To me, High-Desert is the source of feeling really good and being able, at age seventy-five, to live a fuller more active life in spite of my one short leg. I'll never be without it."

Tick "TT" Taylor

At age fifty-five, "TT" told us he was dissatisfied with the progress he was making under his doctor's care. In spite of prescribed medication taken over a period of fourteen years, he had experienced no relief at all from the psoriasis which covered much of his body and was suffering with psoriatic arthritis. This story is open-ended. We are awaiting more good news from Mr. Taylor. In the meantime, here's an interim report from "TT" — a man of few words:

"I took one or two heaping teaspoons of granules straight. After a few months, I noticed a reduction of the areas of psoriasis, especially on my legs. I definitely had more energy and more strength."

Luellen Carstairs

The only complaint Mrs. Carstairs expressed to us was difficulty in finding a reliable source of High-Desert Bee Pollen! This new mother of thirty-two has nothing but praise for The C C Pollen Company. Here's her story:

"After giving birth to my last child, I nursed him for six months. I had very little milk, but it was very rich and my child flourished! Then I started losing weight and got extremely depressed and very moody. The doctor called it 'baby blues' and gave me an antidepressant. I took several of them, but immediately threw them away because they gave me a 'controlled' feeling that I didn't like at all. I finally figured that having my last child had messed up my hormones because my periods were very irregular. The doctor gave me hormones to bring on my periods, which I took occasionally. All doctors want to do is overmedicate. I really wasn't satisfied with my doctor's care.

"Then my sister-in-law told me that after taking hormones for years, and having all kinds of bad side-effects (she had not menstruated in some years), she began taking your bee pollen and started having normal periods. Well, I got your brand of bee pollen, which was what my sister-in-law was taking. Within three months, I started having normal periods and my moods leveled out. Extra bonus: My nails started growing strong and long! They no longer split and chipped off. I started getting compliments constantly of them. I had all kinds of extra energy — and long nails in the bargain!

"When my sister-in-law and I ran out of your bee pollen, we looked *everywhere*, but could not find your brand. We started to *panic* because the other brands just didn't work! My periods had started getting abnormal again and my nails had started breaking. I finally called your company and you were so kind. We had our shipment within a week. We are very grateful! Your product is just so great! I tell everyone about it."

Paul Brenn

Paul Brenn, who acts as a very knowledgeable nutritional consultant to selected clients, is so high on High-Desert Bee Pollen that he not only tells everyone about it, but also takes the time to let us in on some success stories. Paul writes:

"When I got in touch with my former Scoutmaster of sixty-one years ago, now 81, he had a problem which he explained thus: 'I cannot walk alone. I must lean heavily on my wife's arm to walk. Walking past the fronts of just fourteen houses is my absolute limit.'

"Naturally, I immediately sent him some High-Desert Bee Pollen. Two months later I had a note from him which said, 'You'll surely be interested to know that I now walk a MILE, sit and rest, then return home. BUT, I only hold my wife's arm. I do NOT lean on her anymore. I intend to try to walk by myself for the first time next week. I sure give credit to BEE POLLEN!'

"Some days bee pollen amazes US!"

Here's another amazing turn-around from Paul:

"An elderly neighbor of ours had to live with her daughter, as senility had set in. She is now 76. For approximately three years, she had been nearly a 'vegetable.' Let me explain her daily routine. She was helped out of bed, taken to the bathroom, thence to the breakfast table. After eating, with two people helping, one under each arm at the shoulder, she was placed in a chair with side arms, where she soon fell asleep, awakened, slept fitfully again, thus all day long. Nary a word did she speak. Nor did she so much as turn her head if someone passed by. I saw her twice recently and this was her condition.

"Then I had a long talk with her daughter about bee pollen. They started her on ¼ teaspoon of the fresh granules once a day, building up to three level teaspoonfuls per day. After just five days, they reported:

"Grandma is not sleeping all day anymore. Also, she looks as someone passes by." They also noticed other things about her. After ten days on the bee pollen, she began using single words, or even two or three words at a time, in short answers to questions. These are the first words Grandma has spoken in many years!

"I have asked the family to make a written record each day with changes of note as Grandma continues to improve and to save them carefully for me. I'm afraid that in their happiness they might forget some interesting facts if they don't write things down. I hope they will do this. . ."

Needless to say, the family is overjoyed! At this writing, we are awaiting more sensational news about Grandma's progress.

Short & Sweet

The files at The C C Pollen Company are overflowing with unsolicited testimonials and letters expressing delight in the quality of the products and the many healthful benefits derived from the use of High-Desert products of the beehive. If we were to include them all, this book would end up with as many volumes as an enclyclopedia. So, short and sweet, here's a selection for your review:

"Your bee pollen is all you claim it to be. I thought all bee pollen was the same, but there's just no comparison! I have never experienced such energy in my body." LBH

"I'm a senior citizen and thought I felt good before. But I can't tell you how wonderful I feel now. I'm never tired. Best money I ever spent!" VMO

"Hair is growing on the bald spot on my head and I have more energy than I know what to do with! My temper is stable and I have more love for people, more patience. I no longer care to drink beer or other alcoholic beverages either." Dr.FM

"Your bee pollen has helped me a lot. I'm telling my patients that are interested in their health of my personal experience. Keep up the good work!" Dr.GE

"We want to inform you your High-Desert pollen is the best we've ever had. We are recommending it to all our nutritional counseling clients and will continue to do so." DMacL

"I have been fighting radiation sickness for months now, since I'm taking radiation treatments for cancer. After taking your pollen,

I really feel 100 percent better!" JH

"After eating your honeybee pollen with honey, at 81 years old I gave up the glasses I had needed for forty-four years and regained my sexual potency, which had been missing for sixteen years! Wow!!" JJ

"I am having very good results with your bee pollen and so are most of the people I know that have begun to take it. I have personally noticed not only an increased resistance to infection, but also an energy rush and increased stamina." ME

"I feel much more alert mentally and am rarely depressed now, which was a problem before I started taking your bee pollen. Bless you!" CK

"Now I know why I was losing weight and couldn't figure it out. I didn't need to lose, but bee pollen has reshaped my figure and made it better! Please send more order blanks." AA, RN

"Please send High-Desert Bee Pollen, as prescribed for us by Dr. EG. We need this for my husband who has major and critical health problems, as well as for myself." MCR

"After taking High-Desert daily for a year, I have been relieved of severe depression episodes and have higher energy levels. Pollen helped in my weight reduction program also." GH

"Your bee pollen has been most beneficial! Thank you . . . and the bees and flowers!" SMS

"My wife has been fighting cancer for more than three years. High-Desert has very definitely helped her. You may use this statement anywhere people need help. I really believe in bee pollen." DM

"Two skin lesions about the face and head which refused to heal for over six months have now vanished into thin air. I attribute this to taking honeybee pollen. I also have much more endurance and stamina and require much less sleep. My digestion is greatly enhanced, too." JM

"My wife and I were amazed at the 'shot' of energy we received. If anyone wants to get a 'high,' they don't have to take any drugs. All they have to do is take nature's own High-Desert Honeybee Pollen." WEA

"I had major surgery four months ago and made a rapid recovery. I have more energy and keep going all day." FG

"My allergies are much improved and, for the first time in my life, I don't have a problem with irregularity. Plus, I have experienced some weight loss." BLA

"It works! My gray hair is turning back to black! Please send another two pounds of High-Desert pollen, tablets, too!" AS

"I was getting up every two hours to relieve my kidneys and had chronic constipation and was always fatigued. After about eight months taking your pollen, my friends marvel at my ability to do so many things. At 71, I am more capable than I was fifteen years ago. I feel so good!" LK

"I was looking for a staple food to replace animal products in my diet. Your bee pollen fits this requirement. I sleep better and have much less mental fatigue during work." SHB

"At age 77, after taking two heaping teaspoons of your pollen every day for two years, I have reduced my waist measurement by three inches and lost weight. I no longer have an upset stomach all the time and don't have to take antacids regularly any more. My objective is to further reduce my weight to 190 pounds by my 80th birthday. I am confident I will succeed." EAB

"For the past seven years, I had a terrible skin condition on my face. Treatments by four different dermatologists didn't help much. I finally discovered on my own that Benadryl helped. But, after taking your bee pollen for six to eight weeks, my skin is better than it has been for years! I haven't needed Benadryl lately." ML

"I am taking High-Desert Honeybee Pollen and I think it's wonderful. I feel much better *and* my hair doesn't fall out when I shampoo, the way it did before." AWJ

"Your advice on honeybee pollen was 100 percent correct!! Since I started eating your High-Desert Bee Pollen, I have noticed an incredible increase in stamina and drive. Everyone should try this." AEC

"I had such trouble sleeping nights. No more with your honeybee pollen. I've been using it regularly and feel just *great*!" JR

"I have arthritis in my spine, but the pain no longer wears me out. Since I've been taking your bee pollen for ten months, I even still feel good by nightfall and my constant dizziness is gone. It also gives me a good complexion." TLP

"My hair was getting thin, but after fourteen months on High-Desert, it's really thick, lustrous, and jet black (like it used to be). I'm asked if I dye my hair! My allergies are completely mitigated. I have more stamina and strength, too." CJZ

"After just three weeks, it seems I can see an improvement in my husband's breathing and a loosening of mucus. He has emphysema and is on oxygen 24 hours a day. Please rush us ten more pounds." HGH

"Every day I start off, your pollen ignites my flint. Bee to your health! Thanks again and again!!" CNT

"I am truly amazed at the results I've had taking honeybee pollen tablets. I have increased energy, more pep. And the acne I had for fourteen months has disappeared!" CBM

"For a year and a half I suffered with eczema. My fingers were cracked open and bleeding. After taking your pollen for just three weeks, my eczema cleared and healed completely. When I stopped taking bee pollen for only four days, my fingers started breaking out again. As soon as I got back on the pollen, my skin became normal." JS

"Our dog, Duffy, a 4-lb poodle, had deteriorated to the point of being unable to drag himself over a three inch step. Since I began putting one teaspoon of High-Desert in Duffy's food, he no longer has any arthritis." RM

"At age, 73, I feel like I'm about 50 years of age! After two and a half years on your bee pollen, the pains in my legs are gone! I have lost about fifty pounds, I work every day five days a week, and I feel just great!!" NA

"As a dietitian, I have taken bee pollen in many forms from various sources, but I never had the results and benefits received from your High-Desert pollen." AJF

. . . after a year on High-Desert, "The amazing results I have experienced include: lost 50 pounds, have not had the flu or even a cold, no digestive trouble, plus an incredible rejuvenation of · body, mind, and spirit as well!" GWH

"I am placing an order for 100 pounds of High-Desert bee pollen. We have used your product with great success and never hesitate to recommend it to others." EK

"I had an operation on both feet and attribute my super-fast healing to your bee pollen. Pollen takes the place of the medicine I used to take. I now weigh 112 pounds! Pollen keeps me thin and trim, plus well!" EL

"My wife and I (both 72 years) just started taking your bee pollen on the advice of our nutrition-minded M.D. It does seem quite remarkably effective. We were informed you have the very best and want to order." SPO

"I would appreciate another book. I shared my copy with a friend. She liked it so much and was so impressed that I gave her my book. Please send another." LH

"So far, I don't see how your pollen could be better. Please rush shipment as my husband's prescribed intake has been increased by our doctor. Thank you." CHR

"Our friends want to get started right away on your bee pollen as they have noticed how much weight we both have lost — 56 pounds and 20 pounds — and also how we are now full of such energy and walking up to ten miles every day! Your book confirmed all that happened with us." TMcB

"I bought some other pollen, but like yours much, much better and will be using only High-Desert from now on. I will be

81 soon and am in reasonably good health." RDM

"I had arthritis in a very painful state in my left foot to the extent that I was limping quite noticeably. After eating your High-Desert bee pollen, my arthritic pain has completely vanished! I am now able to walk normal." Rev. DAL

"I went to the Department of Weights & Measures when I commenced my pollen and juice fast. They can confirm that I have gone from a size 40 to a 34 inch waist; my blood pressure dropped from 138 over 90 to a healthy 118 over 80. I have experienced the most exceptional energy levels and mental alertness. My appearance is the best advertisement for your pollen. People say I look in my twenties, but I'm 46. This is a tribute to the transforming power of High-Desert Bee Pollen!" JD

"Both my patients and I have been using your High-Desert products and have been very much satisfied indeed. Health improvements have been phenomenal! Thank you." Dr.TT

"We are almost finished eating the ten pounds I last ordered. My husband is breathing more easily and is eating better. In case you don't remember, he suffers from emphysema." AMH

"I have been taking your pollen for forty-one days. It has already taken away bloatedness, and is helping my arthritis. My ultimate goal is to be free of twenty years as a victim of asthma. My blood pressure is some better, but the medication I take for asthma cancels its real effectiveness on that score. High-Desert has helped my insomnia, too. I am sixty-one years old." LLMcC

"I've been taking your pollen for about three months and I'm so full of energy that I get up at 3 a.m. to do my laundry and housework. All day long, I'm on the go, go, go!" GJS

"I really think your pollen is helping me overcome hypogylcemia. The headaches I had in spite of following the diet my doctor had me on have sure let up. I use one half teaspoon every morning now." FMW

"I've been taking your bee pollen and the results have been great in just a few weeks. Amazing. Every person on earth needs honeybee pollen. May this product be on the market for as long as man lives." CAHJ

"I love your honeybee pollen! I've not tried a more delicious bee pollen yet. Yours is soft, clean, and fresh. Boy, am I impressed!" WH

The High-Desert products of the beehive are guaranteed to impress you, too!

CHAPTER 5

Birth: BABY COLLEEN

The Infant Who Failed to Thrive

On August 31, 1982 in a small town in New England, a daughter was born to Emily and Clement A. Cox. With a 5-year old son, Joshua, at home, the Coxes were overjoyed with baby Colleen and felt they now had the perfect family. Joshua was a much-loved rough and tumble boy with an underlying sweetness of character, but the birth of Colleen had Emily Cox looking forward to ruffles, ribbons, and laces, and even further ahead to dancing lessons with tiny white gloves and patent leather 'Mary Janes,' or perhaps satin-laced ballet shoes and pink tutus. Both Clem and Emily were delighted with their little girl.

Following the usual procedure for newborns, Colleen was scored by the Apgar method. Her heart rate, respiratory effect, muscle tone, reflex irritability and color were all rated. Under this medical procedure, each factor is scored from 0 to 2 sixty seconds after birth, and again five minutes later. Of the infants with a score of 2 or less at birth, an estimated 78 percent will not survive the neonatal period. In newborns with a score of 8 or higher, only an estimated one percent will die in their first month of life. Out of a possible ten, Colleen's Apgar score was a very healthy nine.

When Emily and Clem took Colleen home, Joshua reacted with pride as 'big brother' and welcomed the little pink bundle. This was *his* baby. After all, he had talked to her and patted her and felt her wiggle and laughed when she kicked while she was still a mysterious bulge in his mother's middle. Colleen wasn't a stranger at all. She was his baby sister and he loved to see her crooked smile.

From the very beginning, Colleen was a happy baby. She smiled almost from the first day and looked and seemed very healthy. She breast-fed beautifully with no difficulty whatsoever. Although Clem's parents live out-of-state, Emily's parents live nearby and baby-sit and visit often. Colleen was surrounded by a happy, loving family. There was no reason to suspect she might have problems.

However, when she was six-months old, Emily began to wonder why Colleen made no attempt to reach for an object and hadn't yet rolled over. There was nothing concrete that she could pinpoint. But Colleen wasn't gaining the weight she should, her nails didn't grow, her hair was still a sparse fuzz, and she seemed listless and didn't smile as often as she had.

Thinking back to Joshua at six-months didn't help either. The memories were there, of course, but the exact time when he had rolled over and begun reaching for objects was missing, and there were no other babies in the immediate circle of family and friends for comparison. Emily questioned Colleen's pediatrician and was reassured when she was told that all babies progress at their own rate. Emily told herself that there was really no reason to be upset. Nonetheless, a nagging worry remained.

When Colleen reached the eight-month mark and still showed no interest in objects, had not yet rolled over, and made no attempt to sit, Emily and Clem decided they needed some answers. Once again, they confronted Colleen's pediatrician. On his recommendation, they took Colleen to the Pediatric & Neurology Service at Yale-New Haven Hospital on August 11, 1983 for testing and evaluation.

The diagnosis was cruel. It read: "This is a severely developmentally delayed floppy child whose differential includes a structural abnormality in the brain or a genetic abnormality, some of which may be diagnosed by chromosome analysis or genetic screen."

Emily remembers that the attending physician "didn't seem to care." He promised a prognosis which was never received. Emily and Clem were told by the doctor that he had "never seen a CT scan like Colleen's." Emily says, "If I were a doctor, that would make me very curious. I'd want to find the answer. But all he suggested was a brain biopsy, which we refused."

It appeared that medical science had no help for Colleen. Because she was not responding to treatment, on August 19, 1983, Yale-New Haven referred Colleen to the Easter Seals Foundation Rehabilitation Center with this statement: "We wish to refer this unfortunate child with severe developmental delay and hypotonia. Copy of the Pediatric Neurology Clinic notes of August

11, 1983 are enclosed describing our findings and work up to date."

The Easter Seals Rehab Center listed Colleen's rehabilitation problems as: "(1) Severe receptive and expressive speech/language delay; (2) Immature neuromotor functioning; (3) Delay in development of play/cognitive skills; (4) Questionable hearing acuity/perception; (5) Severe delays in all areas of development; and (6) Severe hypotonia." Colleen's prognosis for improvement was charted as: "Guarded due to as yet unclear etiology. Positive prognostic signs, however, include the early age of intervention plus parental support and motivation. Further statements regarding prognosis should be withheld pending results of neurological testing."

To say that Colleen has "parental support and motivation" can be characterized as an understatement. Emily, Clem, and the nearby maternal grandparents are totally loving and supportive of Colleen. Joshua, a bright and caring youngster, not only understands that his baby sister needs extra care, but is equally protective of her.

Easter Seals recommended a twice-weekly program which included speech and language therapy, occupational therapy, and physical therapy. These half-hour sessions were to be augmented by weekly participation in the Infant Stimulation program. Emily and Clem felt as if they were on the right track at last. They entered Colleen in the program on August 29, 1983. Emily committed herself to the long drive from their home to the Rehab Center twice each week.

In total, Colleen received more than 72 treatments under the Infant Stimulation program with little change in her condition. Emily recalls the Easter Seals Rehab Center as having a good program administered by nice, caring people, but says, "Twice a week was not enough for Colleen. We felt she needed a more intense program. Also, Easter Seals is one of the places we are still paying off. I was under the impression that Easter Seals is nonprofit. But the cost of Colleen's therapy ran us between $400 and $600 per month."

Fortunately, the Coxes have an excellent health insurance program which paid much of the cost of Colleen's care. Clem Cox makes good money as a fine cabinetmaker, and his services as an antique-restorer are in demand. Emily Cox works outside the home; her mother cares for Colleen and Joshua. Still, even with the whole family pulling together, by this stage in their search for help for Colleen, the escalating costs were becoming alarming.

In late October of 1983, the Coxes took Colleen back to the Yale-New Haven Hospital for further evaluation. It was determined that Colleen's EEG was "consistent with possible ongoing seizure activity and her CT scan with a severe developmental process of the brain." Colleen's enzymes were sent to Boston for testing. The attending physician recommended a six-week trial on phenobarbital for Colleen, which was implemented.

Colleen scored poorly when her motor and mental skills were subsequently evaluated. Emily Cox now believes this evaluation was a waste of both time and money. She explains,

"The phenobarb put Colleen to sleep and she slept for the whole trip. Naturally, she was groggy and didn't do half of what she was capable of doing. She was tested just an hour and half after a dose of phenobarbital."

In spite of the phenobarbital, which had been prescribed to prevent a possible seizure, Colleen did seizure. She was rushed to a local hospital by her frantic parents. Emily recalls finding Colleen slumped glassy-eyed in her high chair. She is still angry that no one had explained what to expect in case of a seizure, or what to do in that emergency. It was at this point that the Coxes decided it was necessary to have a medical doctor on hand who was familiar with Colleen's case. Her records were requested and transferred to a local neurologist closer to home.

By December of 1983, Colleen was almost a year and half old and the family had tried everything the orthodox medical establishment had to offer. Emily Cox says, "All the doctors went just so far with Colleen. Then they sort of threw their hands up in the air and adopted a 'wait and see' attitude. We didn't agree. We felt there had to be help for Colleen somewhere."

On December 13th, 1983, Emily Cox took Colleen to see Joseph M. O'Reilly, Jr., Ph.D. at the Wholistic Health Center in Brookfield, Connecticut. She says, "We had been going to the Health Center for about four years ourselves and already believed in a nutritional program."

Colleen was put through a battery of tests, including a neuro-optic evaluation, mineral analysis, and an electroacupressure procedure. Colleen's body tissues and metabolic functions all ranged in the poor-to-severe area of weakness. She registered toxic levels in lead, cadmium, arsenic, mercury, alum, nickel and berylium. Her mineral levels were below range in calcium, magnesium, sodium, potassium, zinc, and iron, all of which are essential minerals.

Toxic metal buildup and mineral deficiencies coupled with inadequate assimilation of necessary nutrients are known to cause a multiplicity of problems, including hair loss, loss of weight, lack of muscle tone, nervous-irritability, weakness, disorientation, colic, constipation, and chronic pain in the joints, exactly the symptoms Colleen exhibited.

As a Doctor of Clinical Organic Nutrition, Dr. O'Reilly recommended bee pollen with its active enzymes, hormones, vitamins, minerals, and essential amino acids as the organic nutrient of choice to correct Colleen's body chemistry and metabolic imbalance. He also recommended a special bee pollen/herbal food tablet to cleanse the blood, improve circulation, increase the oxygen-carrying capacity of the blood to the brain and glands, and to improve the efficiency of her assimilation, digestion, and eliminative functions.

High-Desert Bee PollenS and the *Bee-Young* herbal food tablet from The C C Pollen Company of Phoenix, Arizona were recommended by Dr. O'Reilly as the finest and purest obtainable. Upon being informed of Colleen's condition by Dr. O'Reilly, The C C Pollen Company willingly participated in her nutrient regimen by supplying products to the Coxes without charge. The company continues to do so at this writing.

In addition to Colleen's nutrient program, Dr. O'Reilly recommended eliminating all foods containing chemical additives, preservatives, artificial flavorings and colorings from Colleen's diet, and insisted on the exclusive use of spring water, rather than tap water. Emily Cox was advised to implement these recommendations and return with Colleen in two weeks. Emily says, "When I first started giving Colleen the Bee-Young tablets, she had a strong flush from the niacin in the tablet. That scared me. But I told myself it was a natural substance. If I could give my baby phenobarbital, antibiotics, and the like, why not this?"

Colleen was making slow progress when she suffered what Dr. O'Reilly termed a "healing crisis" on March 18, 1984. It began with what looked like an ordinary cold. Colleen ran a low-grade temperature and had a stuffy nose. But by the next morning, her temperature had reached a frightening 104° and a steady discharge of mucus came from her left nostril, her weakest side.

Emily says, "Dr. O'Reilly was away, but he called me back from New Hampshire! That's much more care and concern than we ever got from the M.D.s. Still, sometimes it's hard to wait out these times. My first instinct was to call Colleen's medical doctor for an antibiotic. But Dr. O'Reilly explained that a fever is the body's way of burning off an infection. He suggested we wait three days, watch her closely, and increase her intake of liquids. That is what we did. I've learned not to go rushing off to the M.D.s every time."

On March 21, 1984, Emily took Colleen in to Dr. O'Reilly for evaluation. Dr. O'Reilly's report notes almost full recovery from the healing crisis, with Colleen doing well and continuing to make progress under the bee pollen nutrient program.

Colleen's tongue was pink and healthy. The rings around her eyes were fading and almost gone. Her color was good. Her facial expressions were clear; the dazed look was gone. Her fingernails were growing and she had new hair growth. Her appetite had improved and she was attempting to drink from a cup. She had begun reaching for objects; her physical activity had increased.

The happiest news of all was that Colleen had lost the 'ragdoll' floppiness which had characterized her physical condition just a few months earlier. She now clung to her mother when held, just as a healthy child might. Although Colleen still had a long way to go, Emily says thankfully that even the neighbors noticed how much brighter and more alert she had become.

Two short months later, Dr. O'Reilly's May 5, 1984 progress report on Colleen noted continuing improvement. Colleen was smiling more. She was making more sounds. Her eyes fixed on colorful objects with interest. She was able to scoot her little body forward while sitting on the couch. She had rolled over for the first time. And, although her left hand and arm were not functioning normally, she reached with her right hand to remove articles from her face and head. Her skin color was much healthier and she now was able to drink from a cup without difficulty. The entire family was delighted with Colleen's progress.

By July of 1984, even her physical therapist noticed there was something different about Colleen. She remarked on how splendidly she was doing in accomplishing roll-overs and so on. Dr. O'Reilly's report of this date noted that Colleen's fingernails were growing normally. They required cutting for the first time since she had been born. Her hair growth was excellent and the baby fuzz was completely gone. Her eye contact was good and remained fixed as she followed objects. Colleen was making more and more meaningful sounds. She showed her displeasure by whining, an important breakthrough. She had begun using her left hand and even made an attempt to push a ball with both hands. It was very apparent that the bee pollen nutrient program recommended by Dr. O'Reilly was making a very real difference.

With her family's love and encouragement, Colleen continued to improve. By September 4, 1984, additional progress was noted by Dr. O'Reilly. Her fingernails and toenails had completely lost their yellow tinge and were a normal healthy pink. Her hands and ankles were noticeably stronger. She was now able to pull herself away from the couch, and even lift one leg and hold onto it with her hands. When Colleen clasped both tiny hands over her head like a victorious boxer, the entire family cheered.

Colleen became more and more active. On October 30, 1984, a little over a month and a half later, she was turning her head to watch a person leaving a room. She looked back and forth from person to object and splashed happily in her bath. Her body, nails and hair growth were judged excellent. Emily says of Dr. O'Reilly, "Some of Colleen's other doctors seemed cold. But Dr. O'Reilly really seems to *care* about her. I can tell when he's with Colleen."

The Coxes are understandably grateful to Dr. O'Reilly and the Wholistic Health Center. "Colleen eats the best," Emily says. "We all want to be as healthy as we can be. We have seen what High-Desert bee pollen, Bee-Young, and her wholesome diet regimen have done for Colleen. Even though old diet-habits are hard to break, we try to use Colleen's guidelines now for the whole family."

In the spring of 1985, Emily Cox herself reported of her then two and a half year old daughter, "Colleen seems more alert as each day passes. She has good control of her head, waves bye-bye, and plays peek-a-boo. She's not staying the same or going backward anymore. Something in her brain is working! Colleen used to have a sort of 'blank' look about her. But now we know she understands. When we ask her a question, she replies with sounds we can differentiate as affirmative or negative. These things may seem insignificant to most parents, but after everything Colleen has been through, we never take any of her progress for granted.

"Colleen is very happy, a joy to all wherever we go. She has beautiful clear skin and wonderful smile. And she loves to kiss! We can't wait for another couple of years to pass by to see what she will be like then. Yet we cherish every moment of the present."

All of the foregoing material on the Cox family was tucked away in The C C Pollen Company files. When Dr. O'Reilly moved his practice to another state and was no longer Colleen's physician-of-record, the company lost track of Colleen's progress. But the officers and staff of CCPC never forgot this special little girl. They spoke of her from time to time with concern and wondered how she was faring. In short, they cared.

A long time passed. Finally a letter was dispatched and a joyful response came back from Emily Cox. We learned that in the intervening years, the Cox family had strengthened their already strong commitment to the Lord Jesus Christ and had dedicated their lives to living His principles. As Colleen was taken to many healing services and given over to the Lord, a great peace came upon the whole family.

With a deep and sure happiness, Emily says that the Great Physician is now dealing with Colleen. Colleen is alert and interested in things around her. Given her condition, this fact alone is something the experts call medically impossible. She reports that Colleen's physicians and therapists are astounded at her steady progress. Although Colleen doesn't yet speak in a fully normal manner, she communicates with recognizable baby-talk. She says "ma-ma" and "da-da," and has a pet name for her big brother. She tells Emily when she is hungry and when she hurts.

Colleen today is a sweetly smiling and laughing child of almost six years. She still loves hugs and kisses and trustingly shares her shining radiance with all who come in contact with her. This pretty little girls draws the eyes of strangers, possibly because her innocent beauty remains unmarred by the intrusion of worldly cares. The Lord and His angels watch over special children like Colleen with a special kind of love. Those who are singled out to give birth to one of these 'angel-babies' have the rare privilege of being entrusted with the care of a pure and loving spirit in mortal form. They are enriched. We who are of this world are never closer to the Lord than when in the presence of the unblemished purity of those such as Colleen.

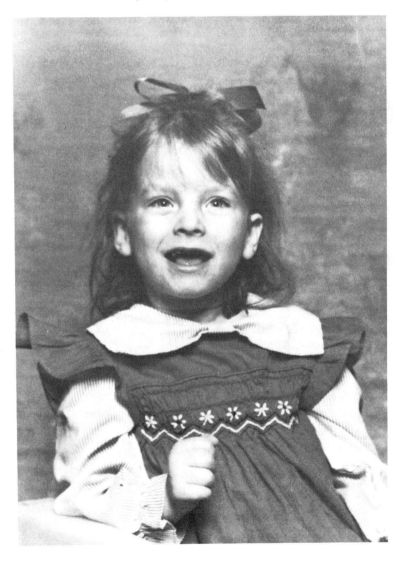

CHAPTER 6

REBIRTH

The Long Life & Fast Times of Noel Johnson

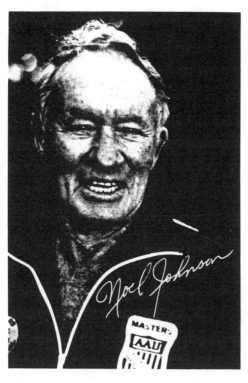

In 1982, Noel Johnson's inspiring autobiography, *A Dud at 70 - A Stud at 80 (and how to do it),* was published by the Plains Corporation of Phoenix, Arizona. You really can't judge a book by its cover after all. A storm of controversy raged over the title, as some misinterpreted its content without having read a line.

Johnson explains why he wrote this book.

"I'm troubled when I read and see and hear of so many people suffering with illness and health-related problems — and too many who die at an early age when they have so much to live for. I don't believe it has to be that way. I believe anyone at any age can reverse the aging process and eliminate poor health. I hope I can serve as a living example of what living the lifestyle the Creator intended can do. I think I've finally got it right. The right attitude, the right nutrition, the right physical conditioning all play a part. But nobody can do it for you. You have to do it for yourself."

In his book, the man his doctors call 'superman' revealed the 'Secrets of Regeneration' that brought him from the edge of the grave back to super health. From birth to rebirth, this is his story.

Noel Johnson was born in the 19th century, July 7th, 1899, in Heron Lake, Minnesota. The third of six children, this small-town boy worked on the family farm and grew strong and healthy on the wholesome home-grown food that graced the family table. Johnson believes that the hard physical work required to maintain the farm contributed to the long life spans achieved by his parents. Johnson's mother died at 70 years of age from a heart attack and his father passed on at 80 from a nerve disorder.

Johnson says that he certainly had no particular genetic advantage and was not born a 'superman.' In fact, although he subsequently served his country, he was so small for his age that all branches of the service turned him down when he tried to enlist at the onset of World War I.

In 1921 after being mustered out of the service, Johnson

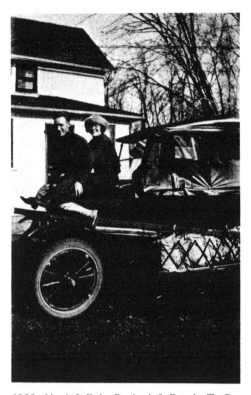

1923: Noel & Zola Packed & Ready To Go

married a Scots lass by the name of Zola Mae Dalzell. He described his red-headed bride as "fiery and talented." After two years of marriage, they were both tired of life on the farm. They bought a shiny new Model T for $350, had the front seats altered so they would recline, arranged a shelf above the back seat for grocery storage and installed a Coleman stove for cooking and heat. Even the running boards served for storage. In November of 1923, they set off for California in this innovative early forerunner of today's RVs. Noel found work quickly. After the bitter winters of Minnesota, they decided early on that they loved the kind climate. And it was fine to be living near the ocean.

Life was very good indeed. Two children were born to the couple. They had many friends and embarked on a round of parties that never stopped, on the beach, at each other's homes, in the jazz clubs of the era, and around and about town. The entire Johnson family was happy and contented. Life progressed in this very pleasant manner for many years.

But a few years after he retired, Noel Johnson was refused life insurance because his heart was seriously damaged. His doctor at the time forbade any physical activity, cautioning him not even to mow the lawn. He warned, "You might not live to trim the border." Visibly fading, Johnson's overall physical condition had become truly alarming.

What was worse, he didn't much care. By this time, his son and daughter were grown and gone and his wife was lost to him. Johnson lived alone. He says, "I shuffled aimlessly around the house eating whatever came to hand and giving no thought to the next day, let alone the next year. I was 35 pounds overweight and suffering from arthritis, bursitis, and gout. I became more and more uncaring and apathetic. I realize now that I was simply waiting for the next and final stop on the journey we call life. Time passed slowly and unproductively. By 1969 when I was 70, I considered I had lived my three-score years and ten. In the traditional and conventional sense, my life was over. Or was it?

"I was worrying my family, living alone and sinking fast, eating improperly and deteriorating daily. My son, Jim, voiced the family's concern with affection. He proposed I go to the hospital for a complete and thorough checkup. It was becoming apparent, he said, that I would soon need someone to look after me. He was right. I certainly wasn't doing a very good job of looking after myself. I had put on even more weight, which put a strain on my already damaged heart, and I couldn't function well.

"The next morning, I looked in the mirror and realized I looked and felt like an old man. For the first 70 years of my life I had lived the good life. The condition I found myself in at 70 years of age was no different than unnumbered others before me. It's 'normal' to be ill and aging at 70. After all, this is merely the natural progression of events — or is it?

"I finally did something I had been carefully avoiding for a long time. I thought. I used the intelligence the Creator had given me. My mind was as rusty and unused as my body. But I persisted and gradually ideas began to form. I was very clear on what I *didn't* want. I didn't want to be a burden to my children. I didn't want to be bedridden and helpless and stuck in a nursing home. I felt it was still my personal responsibility to take charge of my own life and health. I sure didn't want to turn that responsibility over to anyone else.

"First I stripped down and looked in the mirror. All the classic signs of aging and ill health were there. I was overweight, with a bulging gut, lack-lustre eyes, unused muscles hanging slack. I looked defeated. But I used to be a fighter and the thought 'defeated' stirred something in my ego. I remembered back to my days as an amateur boxer. Here I was about to give up and take the count. I decided then and there to beat the bell and come out swinging. They can't count you out when you're trying!

"One of the announcers had hung the name 'Battling Blue Eyes' on me in my early years as a boxer. Well, I had the battle of my life ahead of me to get back in condition. My first enemy was the 40 excess pounds I was carrying around. I suited up and went out to the quarter-mile track near my home. Believe me, I was puffing like a steam engine and I felt every excess pound I was trying to move. Half walking, half shuffling, half jogging, I made it around the track. When I wearily returned home, I sagged down in my easy chair. Ah, the sweet inertia of the easy way."

Reasoning that a clean body full of clean cells cannot support harmful bacteria, Johnson decided to clean up his act. First he eliminated all meat, white flour and refined sugar from his diet, and he gave up his nightly couple of beers. He began eating only natural organic foods, raw whenever possible. He tells us: "If it was green, I ate it, including grass, alfalfa, lemon leaves, and dandelion greens — all right out of the sweet earth. I ate only when I was hungry, not by the clock. I discontinued having those regular meals named breakfast, lunch, and dinner." Instead of snacking on manufactured nibbles like pretzels and potato chips, he munched on sunflower seeds, sesame seeds, raisins and dates. Realizing that exercise would play a vital part in restoring his health, he kept on attacking the track daily.

The comeback trail was long and hard, but Johnson persevered. And he succeeded . . . spectacularly.

Johnson says, "Gradually my arthritis, gout, and bursitis disappeared and it became easier and easier to trot around the track. I had completely forgotten that I was supposed to have a 'heart condition' and never gave my heart a second thought. By 1971, at 72 years of age, my regular regimen included a daily run of eight miles, plus two hours of vigorous calisthenics. Soon

I wanted more of a challenge. I felt mentally alert and stimulated and physically better than I had in many years. I was beginning to get restless."

What happened next determined the exciting title of Johnson's autobiography. We'll let Johnson tell it as it happened:

"I had been living alone for several years with little social life. I wasn't a loner by nature. I had always enjoyed an active social life with many friends and female companionship. But what could I do about it now? Who wants an old man of 72 anyway? After about two years of good nutrition and a lot of running, my body was in quite good condition. I was still an old man, but not a fat old man anymore. I always run without a shirt, so I had quite a healthy tan.

"I was feeling tired one day after a hard run. I passed a massage parlor and thought how relaxing and restful it would be to lie down and have a good hot oil massage. My skin was overdry from being out in the sun and wind so much. In those days, massage parlors didn't have the ugly reputation they have now. So I made an appointment and went in the next day.

"The little girl attendant showed me to a room, asked me to remove my clothes, and told me to lie down on my stomach. She then massaged me from toe to head and I could feel my skin drinking in that hot sweet oil. It was genuinely relaxing. When she asked me to turn over on my back, I felt embarrassed. But she paid no attention to anything but her work and I really began to enjoy the experience. She said I had a much better body than some of the men who came in and asked me what

I did to have such a great tan. I guessed her age to be about thirty. She was divorced, she said, and mentioned that it was hard to get work that paid enough to provide a decent living for herself and her seven-year old daughter. Her name was Linda.

"I made another appointment with Linda for the following week. I was looking forward to lying there again looking up at her as she massaged me. Linda seemed really glad to see me again. She was a very nice looking gal and I found myself liking her quite a lot. I thought how nice it would be if she would lie down with me and I could hold her in my arms while we made love. But I was sure she wouldn't go for that. She was very detached and formal in her work. But I did get up enough nerve to ask her out to dinner. To my surprise and delight, she said 'yes.' We made a date for her day off.

"Boy, how nice she looked that first night! I was so proud to have her with me. During dinner, we talked and talked. After our meal, we drove back to her apartment where I met her little girl and her roommate. We made another date for dinner and the theatre. It was on this date that I asked her if she would come to my place on her days off and give me a massage there. She said she would, but refused payment.

"Being alone in my room, it had to happen. Soon I was massaging her as much as she was massaging me. Of course, the next thing to do was make love. I was surprised when I found I was no good. Although it had been years since I had been with a woman, I always thought I could make love anytime I wanted to. Here was a truly lovely young woman with a beautiful body just waiting for me to make love to her. . . and I was a dud. Linda was patient and understanding, while I was apologetic and embarrassed. She said next time it would be all right. I said I must be out of practice.

"Out of practice! That phrase rang a bell. 'Use it or lose it.' Of course, that was it. To be able to run, you have *to run*. And you have to have the proper nutrition in order to get in condition to run.

"Was it the same with making love? You can't go without sex for a long time and expect to be in condition for it without preparing for it. You need to be tuned up and in good physical condition for running, making love, or any other specific physical activity. I reasoned that the nutrition I needed for the energy to run was not necessarily the food I needed to stimulate the sex glands and get in condition to perform.

"When this calamity hit me, I became determined to find out what food or foods were needed for sexual potency. I read everything I could find — there wasn't much — and studied and thought. Then I came upon a booklet put out by the C C Pollen Company called *The World's Only Perfect Food.* It was subtitled *The Scientific Study on Honeybee Pollen.* It was this little booklet that gave me my answer.

"I learned that one food in all the world has more sex hormones than any other. That food is honeybee pollen. It worked so well that this miraculous substance from the beehive became the cornerstone of my diet. In fact, I believe High Desert Bee Pollen belongs in the forefront of anyone's nutritionally-complete natural diet. I know that bee pollen has been the single largest contributor to my extended lifespan. I believe it is this incredible food that gave me the 'superman' image the doctors were to credit me with a few years in the future. It sustains me yet today.

"Although it took a bit longer than 'next time' for complete success on my part, Linda was wonderfully sympathetic and patient. After a time, there was a definite improvement and finally — full potency. Linda and I shared a warm and intimate companionship for many years.

"I have since enjoyed very satisfying relationships with other women. But a gentleman, even a stud of nearly 90, doesn't provide documented details. Mae West said it best, 'It isn't the men in your life, it's the life in your men that counts.' I have a lot of life in me and I'm not going to lose it again. Although I do give a bit of it away from time to time.

"I have proven to myself that whatever a person wants to do, both body and mind must be in accord. But the physical body cannot perform any and every physical act the mind directs unless the body is in condition to do so. Being mentally and physically in good condition for running, for example, will not guarantee a good performance in bed.

"Total conditioning is the answer. That's why a complete complement of nutrients, along with physical conditioning, is all important. My High Desert Bee Pollen provides me all the necessary nutrients, plus the vital hormones that stimulate and nourish the sex glands of both men and women. I don't think there has ever been one senile old man in this world who was sexually potent. If you can be sexually active, you'll never grow old. Old age and impotence go hand-in-hand."

ON THE COMEBACK TRAIL

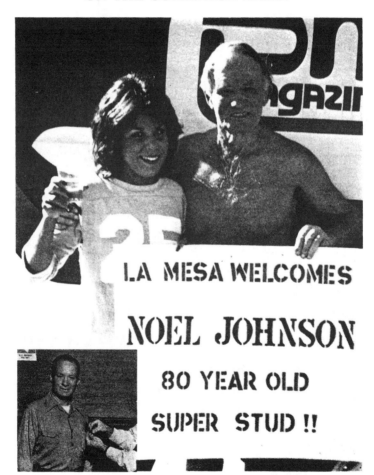

LA MESA WELCOMES

NOEL JOHNSON

80 YEAR OLD

SUPER STUD !!

BEFORE & AFTER
Johnson in 1959 receiving a 20-year award from Convair. He says "My shirt covers slack muscles and an increasing paunch. But I'm not getting older, I'm getting better — as you can see by the welcome I got in La Mesa."

THE SENIOR OLYMPICS

Johnson defeated his 40-year old opponent to win his fifth straight title in the 10th annual Senior Olympics Boxing Championship. Johnson says, "Why can't an 80-year old man fight a 20-year old in the same weight class? I want to show a man of 80 can be as good as the kids of 20."

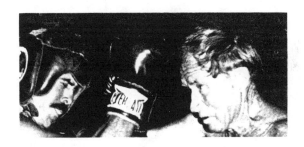

Noel's fight with Leo Pereira in 1979.
Pereira was 40. Johnson was 80.

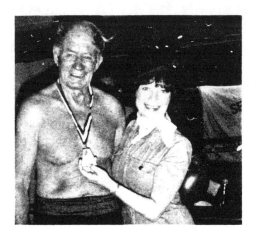

Sybil Jason presenting the gold medal to Johnson after the fight.

HIGHER AND HIGHER...

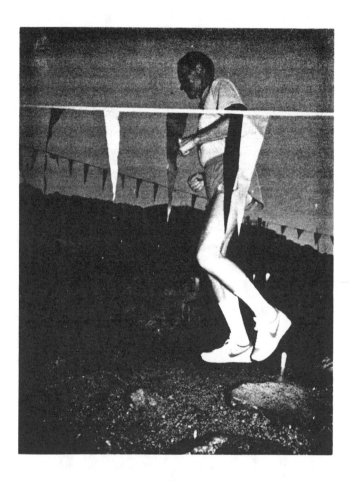

Johnson crossing the finish line of the Pike's Peak Marathon. Most of us couldn't make it. This is the most gruelling run in the world — straight up to an elevation of 14,100 feet!

WHAT COULD TOP THIS?

Don't be surprised if Noel turns out to be the world's oldest space cadet on some future space flight. This intrepid senior's name has been proposed to NASA . . . and it wasn't a joke either.

IN HONOR OF NOEL'S FITNESS LIFESTYLE

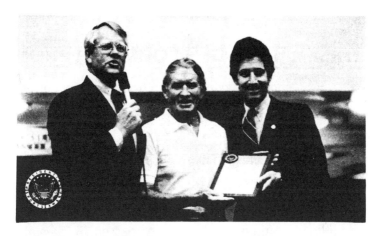

When his incredible accomplishments came to President Reagan's attention, Noel was the proud recipient of a personal letter from the President and was presented with The Presidential Award for Physical Fitness.

Americans have a way of keeping fit.

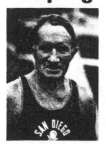

Noel Johnson, 76, holds all records for long distance running (over six miles) in the 70-75 age bracket of the AAU Masters Program. He is the only one in the world his age who runs the 26-mile marathon.

Noel is a member of the "Life Begins at 60" group. In 1974, the group ran a 300-mile relay from Hollywood to Las Vegas in 40 hours and 30 minutes (which certainly shows that people of all ages can remain physically fit).

"Jogging is the best thing I can do for my body. It gets my blood circulating, keeps my heart strong and increases my wind and endurance. I never have to worry about stiffness, arthritis or muscle strain. I have one special exercise I do for stretching my arms, legs, neck and spine. I stand erect, hold my arms out horizontally and twist my upper torso and arms to the right as far as possible. At the same time I kick my right leg in the opposite direction (left). I straighten out and repeat the exercise on the other side.

"Another reason I am so healthy is because I eat well. It's important to eat good, nutritional food."

Noel started his fitness program at 70. "When I started out, I couldn't make it a quarter of a mile around the high school track. I walked part, ran part, until I finally built myself up to where I could run a quarter of a mile. If you set your mind to it, anyone at any age can get himself in good physical shape. It's never too late but you can't do it overnight."

If you are over 40 or have a known health problem, consult your physician before beginning a physical fitness program.

Win the Presidential Sports Award In Your Favorite Sport.

The President's Council on Physical Fitness and Sports offers you the Presidential Sports Award in 39 different sports. For information on how to achieve the award in your sport, write: The Presidential Sports Award, P.O. Box 14, Greene, Rhode Island 02827.

(The above does not constitute endorsement of product.)

In 1977 in their 'Breakfast of Champions' series, five million boxes of Wheaties carried Noel's picture and profile. Johnson was recently approached by the Wheaties people; they want to feature him again.

Noel explains, "I have made High Desert Honeybee Pollen the essential and unvarying foundation of my rejuvenation program. Since I discovered bee pollen at the age of 70, this perfect live food has restored my manhood, brought me to full vigor and sexual potency, and continues to nourish every cell in my body while protecting my health. I am simply never sick. I am now 89 years old and improving in every way. I don't spend five cents on any medication. I am physically able to do whatever I want to do — ballroom dancing, square dancing, long-distance and marathon running, plus championship boxing. You name it and I'll do it — and have — all since I passed 70 years of age.

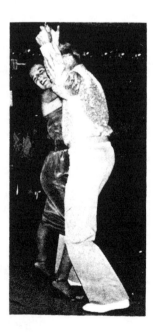 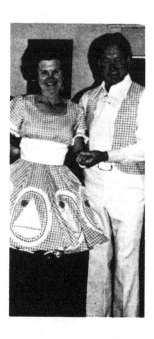

Noel says: "Who wouldn't enjoy dancing with these pretty gals? My partner in the ballroom is Fern. Doreen is my square-dance partner. She even makes our outfits. Two lovely ladies."

"I was dud at 70 and a stud at 80 and I'm still a stud at 89. I know now what you have to do to keep your cells alive and strong. I was not proud of myself at 70 years of age. What did I have to be proud of? What could I do? Now, I'm proud of what I can do on the dance floor, in the ring, on the track — and in bed."

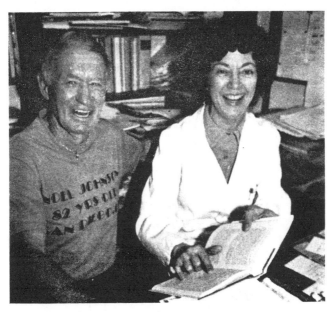

Dr. Lenora Zohman, Mt. Sinai, explaining forthcoming tests to Johnson. Judging by those laughing faces, a good time was had by all.

Noel Johnson has accomplished much that would make anyone proud. That he has seemingly reversed the aging process has been documented in intensive physical tests by a number of admiring doctors. Johnson's initial publicity stemmed from work done by Dr. Jack Wilmore at the University of

California when Dr. Wilmore was researching the difference between biological aging as opposed to social aging. Dr. Wilmore explains, "Social aging refers to the fact that some people become prematurely old because of poor diet and exercise habits. However, the biological changes that take place between birth and death are still poorly defined." Dr. Wilmore pronounced Johnson a "phenomenal man with build and stamina I have never before encountered in a man Johnson's age."

Over the years, other physically stressing tests followed as word of Johnson's accomplishments infiltrated the medical community. Johnson has been examined at the Cardio-Pulmonary Rehabilitation Clinic at Montefiore Hospital in New York, Columbia University, and Mt. Sinai Hospital in Milwaukee. Without exception, the doctors at all these prestigious institutions have expressed amazement at his superb physical (and mental) condition.

Disclaimer

Royden Brown does not advocate, nor promote, sexual intercourse outside of marriage. Royden Brown and the staff of the company where he works believes that all sexual intercourse should be within the confines and under the vows of marriage.

However, in the interest of trying to tell the story the way it was, Royden Brown did not interfere with this part of the true autobiography of Noel Johnson.

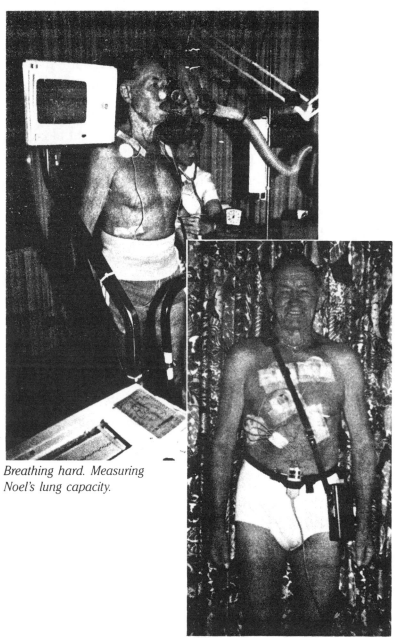

Breathing hard. Measuring Noel's lung capacity.

Wired for 24 hours. A tape ran constantly to record all Johnson's vital signs.

In November of 1987 at age 88, the Ancient Marathoner ran the New York Marathon, just as he has for more than ten years. Although he doesn't quite rate a ticker-tape parade, Noel is such a long-time favorite with the crowds that turn out to encourage the runners that it might seem he brought along his own cheering section. On the day of the race, the Sunday Supplement of the *London Daily Times* carried a feature story on him. and the famous twinkle that prompted one European journalist to dub him 'Maurice Chevalier in running shoes' was much in evidence during his appearance on *David Letterman Late Night.*

New York loves Noel Johnson. And so does London, Australia, Iceland, Sweden, Norway, Finland, Denmark, Hawaii, Japan and everywhere else around the world where this championship runner has competed. No matter where he appears, the media coverage is phenomenal. Noel's 1984 trip to Japan caused quite a stir. We reproduce a translated reprint of just one of the many stories published in the Japanese press. (See page 107.)

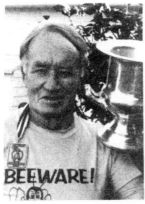

絶倫！84才で30才の女性と…

70才で萎えて、80才で回春。精力絶倫の秘訣は、花粉を食べること！

"A Dud at 70 - A Stud at 80"
UNTIRING 84-YR OLD MAN
ACTIVE WITH 30-YR OLD WOMAN!

Noel Johnson, an American, lost his wife and his health when he was 65 years old. Frightened by the thought of entering a nursing home, he started eating natural foods like bee pollen and tried to regain his strength.

Currently, he is 84 years old and runs over 10 km every day. Surprisingly for an 84-year old, his sexual activity increased. Mr. Johnson met a beautiful masseuse - Linda. They cared for each other and spent time together, but Johnson could not make love.

If he was a Japanese 84-year old, he might have given up. But as a Yankee, he searched and found bee pollen and regained his sexual prowess.

Mr. Johnson not only succeeded in increasing his sexual activity, he ran the New York City Marathon four years in a row and is always the oldest runner, winning the Gold Medal in his Division.

If Popeye eats spinach for health - Mr. Johnson eats bee pollen for health and vigor. Mr. Johnson's bee pollen is from the C C Pollen Company of the U.S. and is sold in Japan through Ohshima Yoko Importing Company.

Would you like to try bee pollen? It is also good for beauty!

Translated Reprint of Japanese Newspaper Articles on Noel Johnson.

Last year, Johnson enjoyed a triumphal tour of Scandinavia, where he won hearts (and gold medals) in races across the continent. The Britic Company of Norway is so enamored of this dynamic senior that his book has been updated and will soon be published in Norwegian. That famous autobiography, which details the lifestyle that transformed him from a worn-out old man with a life-theatening heart condition into a racing (and romancing) machine, has already been published in Japanese and Icelandic and is racking up sky-rocketing sales in both countries. Britic has him under contract to insure his return to Oslo three times every year. The same

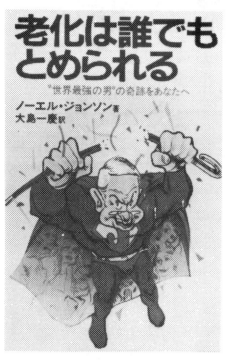

Japanese version of Johnson's auto-biography. Although Noel never needed one, cover shows a revved up bee-pollenized older 'superman' triumphantly breaking a cane.

contract calls for Noel to visit Sydney, Australia twice a year to run for another division of Britic, The C C Pollen Company of Australia, Ltd.

Noel occupies a special place in the hearts of people around the world. Everywhere he travels, he is met with a warm welcome and is given phenomenal press coverage. He was recently offered a Physical Education Director's berth with prestigious cruise ship line. They think this dynamic and charismatic 89-year old dynamo would inspire senior passengers. Nonsense! Why hold him back with an age limit? Noel is an inspiration to all ages. One look at him today, and you know his book has a happy ending. But there's no end in sight for this marathon man; he's still going strong.

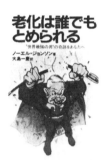
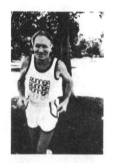
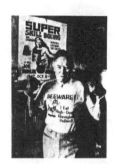

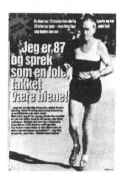
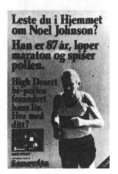
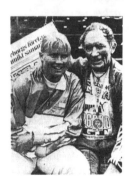

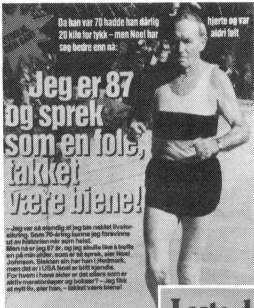

NOEL RUNS
THE WORLD

Cover page of just 2 magazine articles his marathon runs warranted (Norway & Iceland). No matter where he goes, Noel is big news.

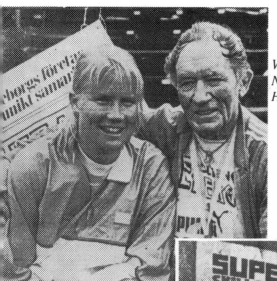

With a pretty Norse admirer, Noel holds local newspaper. He made the first page.

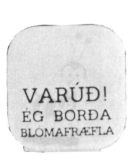

Icelandic Bee Pollen Badge.

When Noel wore his favorite shirt in Iceland (see above), the legend 'Beeware! I Eat High-Desert Honeybee PollenS' caught fire. In Icelandic, that phrase translates to: 'Varud! Eg Borda Blomafraefla.' The Iclandic bee pollen badge is pictured above. A golden-yellow bee appears behind those stirring words, but the camera couldn't pick it up.

Now in what he calls his "second lifetime," Noel says, "I'll be better at the age of 100 than I am today. I know what causes cell deterioration, and I know how to prevent it." Remember, he isn't just a marathon runner either. Noel holds the World's Senior Boxing Championship, often fighting much younger men to keep it, and was the proud recipient of the Presidential Award for Physical Fitness a few years ago. This amazing man certainly seems to know something the rest of us don't.

"How did I do it? It's no secret," says Noel. He credits a natural diet, a daily exercise regimen, and *High-Desert*, his all-time favorite brand of bee pollen, for his dramatic comeback from the edge of the grave.

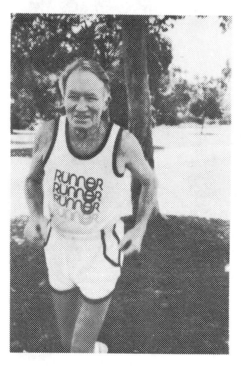

This globe-running senior maintains a schedule that would do in a lesser man. November of 1987 found him in southeast Asia. At the royal invitation of the King, he ran in the Bangkok Marathon and was the only private guest to attend the King's 40th birthday party celebration. Noel's swing through Malaysia culminated in a conversation with the Sultan of Malaysia, who expressed a particular interest in meeting with him. Noel also visited with the richest man in the world, the Sultan of Brunei, in his palace in the tiny Sultanate of Brunei, situated in a corner of northern Borneo. In December, off he went to Sydney, Australia, where he ran yet another marathon.

In the *nineteenth century* when Johnson was born, the life expectancy of the average man was 47 years.

In the *twentieth century,* Johnson turned the odds in life's sweepstakes inside out, grasped the advantage, and intends to keep it.

No matter where he travels, Noel Johnson makes a point of gathering material for his next book, which he confidently plans on publishing in the beginning of the *twenty-first century,* the year 2000.

He already has the title set: *The Living Proof — I Have Found The Fountain of Youth.* At four score years and nine, this incredible man still has miles to run before he sleeps. But who's counting? Certainly not Noel Johnson. He's much too busy.

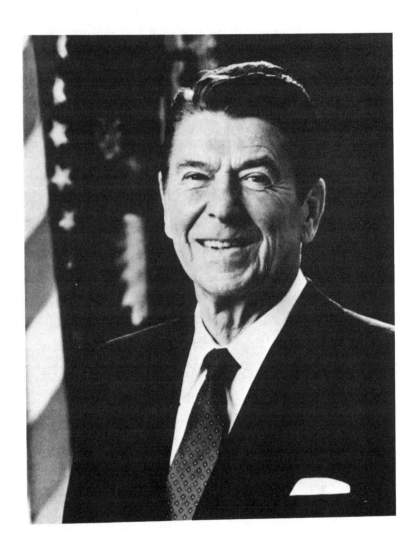

CHAPTER 7

The
REAGAN
WHITE HOUSE

The Most Famous Bee Pollen Fan In The World

"C C Pollen Company. May I help you?"

"This is Air Force One calling. Are you the people who make *The President's Lunch* bars?"

"Ohmigosh. Is this *really* Air Force One? The President's plane?"

"Yes, ma'am. We're trying to reach the company who makes *President's Lunch* bars. I found a crumpled up wrapper from one of these bars. It said 'C C Pollen Company, Scottsdale, Arizona on it, but I'm not sure I have the right number."

"This is C C Pollen. You have the right number. I just can't believe it! Air Force One! Wow! This is so exciting. Are you in mid-air? Are you calling from 35,000 feet?"

Deep chuckle. "No, ma'am. I'm calling from the Steward's Office at Andrews Air Force Base. President Reagan was asking for *President's Lunch* bars on our last flight, but we didn't have any. I want to make sure that never happens again."

"We ship regularly to The White House. I'm sure they would share."

"No, ma'am. That's not how it works. What I want to do is order *President's Lunch* bars from you and have them shipped right here to Air Force One. Can I do that?"

"Yes, sir. You bet! You sure can."

"Uh, ma'am?"

"Yes?"

"I'm not a 'sir,' ma'am. I'm a Master Sergeant in charge of the Presidential plane, Air Force One."

"All right, sergeant. I'll turn you over to someone in sales and they'll be glad to take your order. You just hold on one minute and I'll be quick about it."

"I'll wait, ma'am."

With the intercom wide open and broadcasting to the entire company, The C C Pollen Company receptionist sang out the news:

"Hey, everybody! Air Force One is on line six. The Steward wants to order *President's Lunch* bars. President Reagan asked for one on their last flight, but they didn't have any on board. Is that exciting or what? Who wants to take the order?"

Seventeen extensions clicked into line six all at once. After a bit of flurry, the order was taken.

This conversation occurred shortly after *The President's Lunch* bar was introduced in 1983. Since that time, shipments to Air Force One and Executive One, the First Lady's private plane, have become as commonplace around The C C Pollen Company offices as orders from The White House.

It was in 1961 that Ronald Reagan first learned about the benefits of bee pollen. That was when Marjorie McCormick, author of *The Golden Pollen,* introduced him to the golden granules. Back then, Ronald Reagan was touring the United States on behalf of the U.S. Chamber of Commerce. He traveled the country giving lectures and speeches extolling the virtues of the democratic system.

At the time, Marjorie McCormick was President of the Yakima, Washington Chamber of Commerce. On his swing through the state of Washington, she told Ronald Reagan of the miraculous properties of bee pollen. She gave him a copy of her book and some bee pollen bars. He was obviously impressed by the findings in McCormick's book and the sample bee pollen bars she gave him.

In a handwritten 'thank you' note to McCormick, Reagan said, "I was plowing one of our ranch paddocks and by late in the afternoon, I was exhausted. Then I realized I had one of the bars you sent in my jacket pocket. I ate it and I swear it was not my imagination, but twenty minutes or so later I was definitely conscious that I was no longer fatigued and the chill I'd been feeling was gone." It's certainly clear that President Reagan is personally convinced of the worth of bee pollen. He's been eating it regularly for twenty-seven years.

Because of all the publicity, just about everyone knows of Ronald Reagan's fondness for *High-Desert Honeybee Pollen* and

The Natural Foods Business Journal   JANUARY 1981

WHOLE FOODS™

Presidential Bee Power

In an interview not long ago, comedian Steve Martin was commenting seriously about the physical stress brought on by his demanding schedule. "I went on a vitamin therapy program, but after a while I had to give it up. Oddly enough, the vitamins started turning my hair back to its natural color. So I quit the vitamins because I didn't want people to think I was dying my hair."

While Steve Martin sacrifices to *keep* his grey hair, most people curse its always too early appearance. Grey hair equates to age, and in our youth oriented society advancing age isn't always seen as the most desirable of attributes.'

Thus, when a 69-year-old Ronald Reagan smiles out at us from under a full and youthful looking thatch of dark brown hair, people tend to wonder. At last the wonderings may be giving way to some reasonable answers. In a story run out of Washington by the *Independent News Alliance*, writer Melvina Stephenson reports that, "A physically fit Ronald Reagan fortifies himself with bee pollen."

Since the popular press tends practically to. canonize all new presidents . . . detailing what they eat for breakfast and what their surviving school teachers have to say about them . . . it shouldn't be too long until the 'reading public becomes aware of' president-elect Reagan's active interest in maintaining his own health.

Ms. Stephenson's article continues, " 'He's a great advertisement for clean living,' said daughter Pattie, herself a vegetarian and health food fan. 'He has all those bee pollen bars in the refrigerator.'

"Ed Meese, Reagan's closest

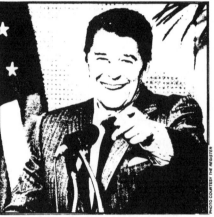

PHOTO COURTESY THE REGISTER

aide, says he has seen (Reagan) munching on the bee bars, but also attributes his physical fitness to regular exercise, proper eating habits and adequate sleep when possible.

"Reagan's apparent vigor and vitality are bound to create great interest and respect for his personal regimen. His reported preference for bee pollen could very well start a run on the market.

"That caused Reagan's son Ron to joke, "If that gets into print, hey'll probably put his picture on the package.'

"Charles W. 'Doc' Turner, trainer at Long Island (New York) University, swears by bee pollen. He

not only advocates it as food supplement, but uses is as a poultice to reduce swelling on injured limbs.

"Author Carlson Wade, another pollen partisan, calls it 'one of the world's oldest youth foods.' "

Every president has some trait that starts a new fad; it's seems to be an ingrained part of the fabric of our national political mystique. Sort of 'Voter see, voter do.' With a final tally of 43,267,489 people casting votes for Ronald Reagan to be our 40th president, that gives the health food industry of America a tremendous potential new audience ready to follow a healthy man's lead into the world of healthy foods.

EDITOR

President's Lunch bars. It was back when Ronald Reagan was still our President-Elect that the first article appeared. In January of 1981, *Whole Foods, The Natural Foods Business Journal.* headlined this kickoff article 'Presidential Bee Power.' (see page 118.) And that was just the beginning.

The fact that the U.S. had a president who followed a healthy lifestyle didn't escape the notice of the American press. Unless it was strictly a hard news story, many of the articles written about Ronald Reagan includes a mention of his bee pollen preference.

Of the tabloids, *Globe* magazine was first with a mention in June of 1981. In part, this blurb says "President Reagan attributes his good health to his honey. No, not the missus, but the bee pollen he's been taking for more than 20 years."

In an interview with Patti Reagan Davis, the January 1982 issue of *Vegetarian Times* brings up the subject of bee pollen. Ms. Davis says, "My father was certainly a good example for healthy living. When I was younger, my Dad used to eat little bars made from bee pollen and honey, or bee pollen and wheat germ. They tasted like hay!" (Editor's Note: The bars discussed in this article predate *The President's Lunch* bars by many years.)

President Ronald Reagan is The C C Pollen Company's most prestigious client. *The President's Lunch* bar was not only named in honor of President Reagan, but was formulated especially to cater to his known penchant for bee pollen bars. These bars were an immediate hit with President Reagan.

The bars were introduced to the public during President

Reagan's visit to Japan in 1983. The *President's Lunch* bars were prominently displayed during a state luncheon in Tokyo, Japan on November 10, 1983. Both President Reagan and Prime Minister Yasuhiro Nakasone munched on bars while the television cameras were rolling, which immediately caught the fancy of the Japanese media. Here's how it happened:

At this state luncheon, President Reagan was asked what his favorite food was. He replied, "The President's Lunch bar," and proceeded to take one from the box of *President's Lunch* bars in front of him. He took out six bars, put five in his coat pocket, unwrapped and ate the other bar in front of the television cameras.

Premier Nakasone, in reply to the same question, said his favorite food was beans. Still, not to be outdone, Premier Nakasone reached into the box of *President's Lunch* bars, took out five bars, put four in his coat pocket, and ate the fifth bar in front of the Japanese national television cameras. The Japanese press was delighted.

Television reports and newspaper articles (see translated sampling of four reprints: pages 121-122) all remarked on President Reagan's fondness for 'the health food, bee pollen.' A report on the newly-formed Japan-U.S. Bee Pollen Association was issued, and it was announced that Oshima Yoko had been awarded the necessary license to bring The C C Pollen Company products into Japan. Today, The C C Pollen Company exports to many countries of the world, including Japan, most of the Asian countries, and the whole of Scandanavia.

REPRESENTATIVE
ARTICLES FROM
THE JAPANESE
PRESS.

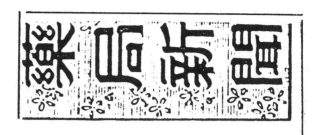

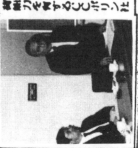

RON AND YASU LOVE HEALTH FOOD!

Ron and Yasu's meeting left questions on defense and trade pending between the U.S. and Japan. It will be interesting for the health-food business to see how this U.S. and Japan balance-of-trade problem will be solved.

At the Hinode-so meeting, there was a conversation about Japanese food and Mr. Reagan and Mr. Nakasone both stated they were very much interested in health food. Mr. Nakasone is a bean lover and Mr. Reagan is a bee pollen lover.

President Reagan is already eating our new product, "The President's Lunch," and these bars started selling in Japan on November 14 with the help of the Japan-U.S. Bee Pollen Association.

BEE POLLEN - THE HEALTH FOOD
6 Different Kinds Imported from U.S.

C C Pollen Company is the biggest pollen collector in the U.S., also biggest wholesaler, and has beekeepers in many states (especially Arizona) and exports to Japan through Ohshima Yoko. Ohshima Yoko was started by the current president, Mr. M. Ohshima, with a capital of 5000000 yen and sales are expected to reach 50000000 yen the first year. It seems the health-food business in Japan will be expanded widely with bee pollen!

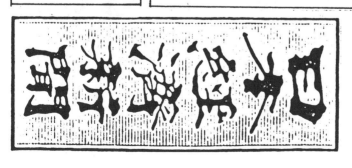

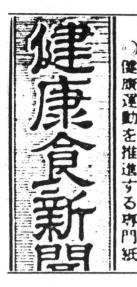

IN HONOR OF U.S. PRESIDENT REAGAN

A new product called "The President's Lunch" is now on the market commemorating the U.S. President's visit to Japan. It is a health bar which contains bee pollen, President Reagan's favorite food.

Ohshima Yoko imports bee pollen from the C C Pollen Company of the U.S. state, Arizona, and three companies, like Uni 8, sell to retailers. Ohshima Yoko is expectiing sales of 50000000 yen the first year.

This new bar is made with bee pollen, oats, honey, nuts and seeds and is compressed. One bar is 380 yen and contains the nutrients necessary for one complete meal.

Since it is imported from the U.S., this bar is called "The President's Lunch," instead of the "Manager's" or "Executive's Lunch."

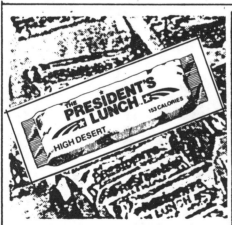

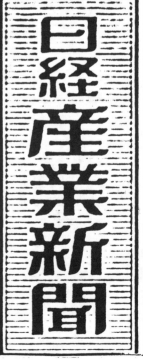

PRESIDENT REAGAN'S FAVORITE FOOD

Ohshima Yoko imports "The President's Lunch" from the C C Pollen Company of Arizona. Bee pollen, which is U.S. President Reagan's favorite food, is being sold widely on the Japanese market.

"The President's Lunch" was introduced in Japan to commemorate the U.S. President's recent historic visit to our country.

By the spring of 1984, President Reagan's fit lifestyle was so well known that *Time Magazine* sent a reporter to C C Pollen Company to check out the facts. Before giving any information to the press about their most famous customer, a C C Pollen Company official phoned the White House for permission to talk with the *Times* reporter. Permission was granted to confirm the fact that the company regularly ships both fresh granules of High-Desert Honeybee Pollen and bars to the First Family. *Time* subsequently ran the article, entitled "Presidential Pollen" in their April 30, 1984 issue. Who says *Time Magazine* doesn't have a sense of humor? The accompanying picture shows a honeybee in place of the usual eagle on the Great Seal of the United States. (see page 124.)

In October of 1984, *The Washington Post* ran a story headlined: "Reagan's Pollen: It's the Bee's Knees." This article reveals that Mrs. Reagan recommended the bars to daughter Maureen Reagan and her husband. The First Lady was quoted as saying, "They're great for taking the edge off your appetite when you're hungry." Mrs. Reagan's svelte figure might be attributed, in part, to the fact that the bars have only 153 calories.

There have been so many, many articles. A Savannah, Georgia *News-Press* release headlined "Pollen Reagan's Secret — Uses Daily" quotes an aide as saying, "He likes it and it's good for you. Mr. Reagan eats bee-pollen snack bars that also contain other natural foods. He eats them all the time."

The *London Sunday Times Magazine* of May 26, 1985 carried a story entitled "Bees In His Bonnet" which shows

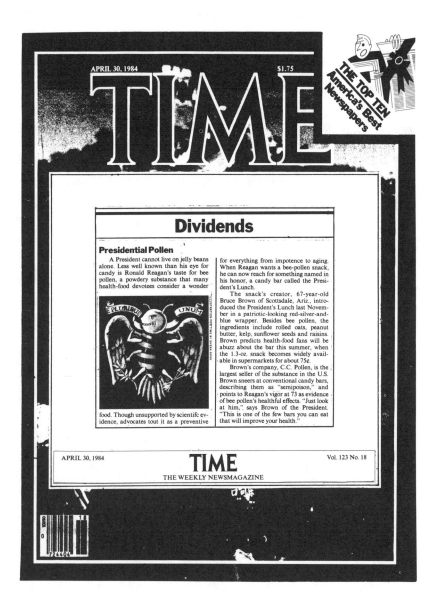

APRIL 30, 1984 $1.75

TIME

Dividends

Presidential Pollen

A President cannot live on jelly beans alone. Less well known than his eye for candy is Ronald Reagan's taste for bee pollen, a powdery substance that many health-food devotees consider a wonder food. Though unsupported by scientifc evidence, advocates tout it as a preventive for everything from impotence to aging. When Reagan wants a bee-pollen snack, he can now reach for something named in his honor, a candy bar called the President's Lunch.

The snack's creator, 67-year-old Bruce Brown of Scottsdale, Ariz., introduced the President's Lunch last November in a patriotic-looking red-silver-and-blue wrapper. Besides bee pollen, the ingredients include rolled oats, peanut butter, kelp, sunflower seeds and raisins. Brown predicts health-food fans will be abuzz about the bar this summer, when the 1.3-oz. snack becomes widely available in supermarkets for about 75¢.

Brown's company, C.C. Pollen, is the largest seller of the substance in the U.S. Brown sneers at conventional candy bars, describing them as "semipoison," and points to Reagan's vigor at 73 as evidence of bee pollen's healthful effects. "Just look at him," says Brown of the President. "This is one of the few bars you can eat that will improve your health."

President Reagan reaching for a *President's Lunch* bar. After stating, "The most powerful men in the western world have not often been celebrated for their eating habits," the story goes on to say, "In 1961, after sampling bee pollen, which is often promoted for its restorative qualities, Reagan was hooked and became a regular user. These days the president takes his pollen in a crunchy snack bar developed by The C C Pollen Company of Phoenix, Arizona, marketed in America as *The President's Lunch*. While Reagan has proved that his auburn tresses are untouched by the dyer's art, millions have wondered about the secret of his youthfulness. Even the President's most ferocious critics must admit he looks darned good for a 74-year old." The article closes with a question, "Could bee pollen propel Mrs. Thatcher to her third government?"

It isn't only President Reagan who likes *President's Lunch* bars either. More and more people have discovered that this is the easy, delicious way to enjoy a daily measure of the best bee pollen in the world. As the general public sought them out in health food stores across the nation, these bars quickly became high volume sellers.

In fact, they became so wildly successful that The C C Pollen Company went into production with the *First Lady's Lunch* bar in 1985. The company reports that Mrs. Reagan was very pleased to have a bee pollen bar named in her honor and gifted company officials with a signed photograph. (see page 126.) The C C Pollen Company records show that these bars, too, are very popular in The White House and are regularly stocked on the First Lady's

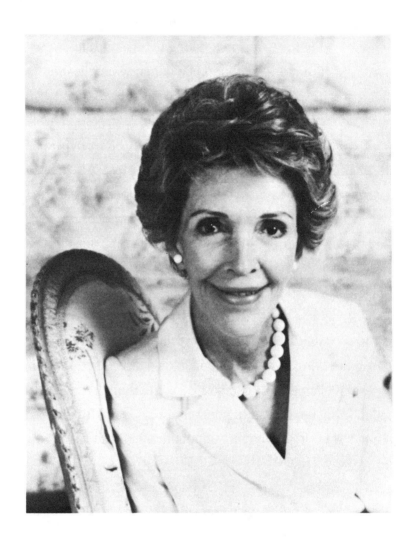

plane, Executive One.

The President's Lunch Bar and the *First Lady's Lunch* Bar may be not only the healthiest "candy bars" available in stores, but they are probably the only bars that will actually build your health, instead of destroying it as ordinary sugar and fat-loaded chocolate candy bars can.

Chocolate is a big offender. Most people don't realize that it takes the human digestive system *fourteen hours* to process and digest just *two tablespoons* of chocolate. The experts say that chocolate is one of the most difficult of all substances to digest and metabolize.

If you want to learn all about the dangers chocolate poses, the book *The Milk of Human Kindness is Not Pasteurized* by Dr. Melvin Davis is an eye-opener. This book elaborates the dangers of chocolate in detail. Dr. Davis also goes into what he claims are the carcinogenic properties of pasteurized and homogenized milk. Dr. Davis calls milk a leading cause of all degenerative diseases.

Ordinary candy bars ultimately stimulate your appetite and end up making you hungrier, but the *President's Lunch* and the *First Lady's Lunch* are very satisfying. I no longer eat these bars between meals because they ruin my appetite. I do, however, eat these bars in place of a meal, especially when I'm on the run and don't have time for a full meal.

The first shipment of 144,000 bars that went to Japan were marketed as a healthy meal replacement for persons who wished to lose weight. Since that first state luncheon when the

President's Lunch was introduced in Japan, our overseas market has grown immensely and now encompasses the world.

Besides President Reagan and First Lady Nancy, the famous people who have enjoyed these bars are legend. Among them are Premier Gorbachev and his wife, Raisa, the Prime Minister of Japan, the King of Thailand, the Mir of Hunza, the Prime Minister of England, the King of Sweden, the Premier of Israel and virtually all the important people who visited President Reagan at the White House.

The development of these energizing, naturally-formulated, delicious, nutritious bars started with *The President's Lunch* bar. And that whole-food bee pollen-spiked recipe catered to President Ronald Reagan's known preference for quality bee pollen bars. We don't have to tell you that The C C Pollen Company is mighty proud to be purveyor to the President.

Whether you are Republican or Democrat, an admirer or detractor; whether you approve of President Reagan's policies or are looking forward to seeing the back of him, doesn't matter one whit. You can't deny that President Reagan remains a fine figure of a man as he left the presidency at the age of 77.

This is the guy who has held down the toughest job in the galaxy for eight years. (Research shows the regular use of bee pollen builds stamina and endurance.) Think about how fast he got back in the Oval Office after being shot in the chest on March 30th, 1981. Remember how quickly he bounced back after undergoing major abdominal surgery on July 13th, 1985. (Studies show that the regular use of bee pollen heightens the body's powers of recovery.) All those nasty rumors that his hair is dyed have been refuted. (There are empirical reports from many delighted regular bee pollen users who have recovered their normal hair color.) And how many photos have you seen of him riding, clearing brush, or chopping wood down on the ranch?

There have been many photographs. The one below was published in *Parade Magazine* December 13, 1987.

P A R A D E ' S   S P E C I A L

Intelligence Report

Because of volume of mail received, Parade regrets it cannot answer queries.

The President's Health Food

t's no earth-shaking matter, but to those of you who have written to this publication asking if President Reagan regularly eats bee pollen, the answer is "yes." He reportedly has been eating the powdery substance since 1961 and says it's an energy restorative.

A supply of bee pollen is kept on hand not only in the White House but also aboard Air Force One, the President's aircraft, and Executive One, the jet which transports Nancy Reagan on her missions throughout the country.

The bee pollen—in the form of a crunchy, 153-calorie snack bar—is manufactured by the CC Pollen Co. of Scottsdale, Ariz., which ships the Reagans a gross from time to time, as well as 5 pounds of the health food in granule form. A spokesman for the company maintains that its bee pollen has rejuvenating properties which help cure fatigue, listlessness and ennui, as well as helping the President retain his natural hair color. No manufacturer of jelly beans, earlier publicized as Ronald Reagan's favorite candy, can equal that claim!

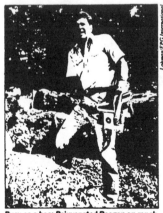

Busy as a bee: Rejuvenated Reagan on ranch

Ronald Reagan is no slouch. In the physical fitness and longevity sweepstakes, research shows that quality bee pollen does make a difference. Ronald Reagan is living proof of that fact.

We close this chapter with best wishes to Ronald Reagan, possibly the greatest of all U.S. Presidents, yes, in our opinion, *the* greatest of the U.S. Presidents, and to our gracious First Lady, Nancy. Although he proved he can mete out stern retribution when such is called for, the Great Communicator prefers dispensing cheer and goodwill. President Reagan not only put a smile on the face of the Soviet Premier, an historic first, he made the rest of us smile, too. Long may he wave.

CHAPTER 8

BEE POLLEN
What It Is and Why We Want It

In spite of all the many books and articles on bee pollen which have been published in the last ten years, there are still some people who aren't sure exactly what bee pollen is. The gal in charge of Consumer Inquiries at The C C Pollen Company calls her desk 'The Weird Letter Office.' She tells us one person wrote the company a serious, otherwise very literate letter, which asked, "Does bee pollen come from outer space?" Another writer queried, "Is bee pollen the poop of the bee?"

And, hard as it may be to believe, a newspaper article published as recently as January 15, 1988 states, in part, "Bee pollen seems to have a little bit of everything that's good for you. And it's yummy. Just don't be put off by the fact that *bee pollen comes from bee excrement.*"

Talk about *mis*information...

What is *Pollen?*

Pollen is the male seed of flowers. It is required to fertilize the plant. The tiny particles consist of 50/1000ths of a millimeter corpuscles, which are formed at the free end of the stamen. Every variety flower in the universe puts forth a dusting of *pollen.* Many orchard fruits and agricultural food crops do, too.

Anemophile Pollens: Anemophile pollens are the wind-carried pollens. As breezes blow, these types of pollen are sent helter-skelter flying through the air. A few varieties of plants depend on the wind to deliver their fertilizing pollens to them. These are the pollens that cause such distress to those who suffer from, for example, hay fever or rose fever. It is the allergens anemophile pollens carry which tickle the nose and trigger sneezing attacks, cause the eyes to swell and itch, and generally make life miserable for those who are allergic to particular seasonal pollens.

Entomophile Pollens: Entomophile pollens hitch a ride on the insects, primarily the honeybees, who forage among their blossoms. These pollens are heavier and of a different variety than anemophile pollens. The plants which produce entomophile pollens must have the help of the bees in order to be sure of fertilization. They never become air-borne and are not the culprits in allergic reactions.

It seems appropriate to add a word of explanation here regarding pollen-induced allergies in order that you not misunderstand.

Bee pollen has been effectively used down through the ages to rid allergy sufferers of their affliction. This technique, called *desensitization,* was developed by St. Mary's Hospital Medical School in London soon after the turn of the century. Treatment consists of administering small amounts of the allergen to stimulate the patient's own immune system to produce antibodies that will eliminate the allergic reaction. It works rather like a vaccination works against childhood diseases. Desensitization is based on the premise that the body will produce antibodies which will cancel out the effects of the offending substance when the next season rolls around and the patient is again exposed to anemophile pollens in the air.

In the not too distant past, honey was administered by great-grandmother as treatment for many minor ills, including allergies, with great success. Modern science has determined that the effective substance in the raw honey fresh from the beehive that great-grandmother used was the microscopic pollen spores suspended in the raw honey.

A British physician rediscovered this old treatment and now successfully treats his hay fever patients with his own unfiltered pollen-laden honey. He reports that during the first year of treatment, attacks are reduced. During the second year of treatment, his patients are entirely free of hay fever symptoms.

Leo Conway, M.D., of Denver, Colorado, went one better. He treated his patients directly with pollen itself by oral ingestion, explaining, "All patients who had taken the antigen (pollen) for three years remained free from all allergy symptoms, no matter where they lived and regardless of diet. Control has been achieved in 100 percent of the earlier cases and the field is ever expanding.

"Since oral feeding of pollen for this use was first perfected in my laboratory, astounding results have been obtained. No ill consequences have resulted. Ninety-four percent of all my patients were completely free from allergy symptoms. Of the other six percent, not one followed directions, but even this small percentage were partially relieved nonetheless. Relief of hay fever, pollen-induced asthma, with ever-increasing control of bronchitis, ulcers of the digestive tract, colitis, migraine headaches and urinary disorders were all totally successful."

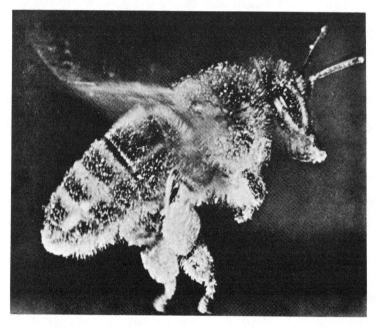

Pollen-foraging bee in flight. Her pollen baskets are fully packed. A portion of the tiny pollen particles covering her body will dust off on the next blossom, and pollination, or fertilization, will be completed.

Unfortunately, this great early pioneer in the field is deceased. Let us now return to the subject at hand.

The honeybees do double-duty. The bees are responsible for the pollination of more than 80 percent of green growing things. In the grand scheme of things, we can conjecture that the bees primary duty is almost certainly to accomplish pollination. They are programmed to gather pollen and carry it back to the hive as food for the colony. As they flit from blossom to blossom, miscroscopic pollen particles coat their stubby little bodies so densely that they sometimes look like little yellow fuzz balls. When they arrive at the next flower, a portion of the golden dust is transferred to that blossom and pollination, or fertilization, is accomplished.

When the Creator wrote out the job description for the bees, their number one responsibility was pollination, which they neatly accomplish in the course of collecting food for the colony. Without the pollen-carrying honeybee, many species of plants would fail to be fertilized and would die out. It isn't only the flowering plants that depend on the services of the bee either. We think you'll agree that the world would be less pleasant without beautiful sweet-smelling flowers, although we could survive without them. But without the food crops the bees pollinate, mankind might well be in danger of extinction.

What is *Bee* Pollen?

Bee pollen is simply entomophile pollen, with the very important touch of magic added by the bee. Gathering pollen is not as easy as it may sound. Once a honeybee arrives at a flower, she settles on the stamen and nimbly scrapes off the powdery loose pollen with her jaws and front legs. She then moistens it with a dab of the honey she brought with her from the hive.

The enlarged and broadened tarsal segments of her legs are provided with a thick trimming of bristles, called pollen combs. She uses these combs to brush the gold powder from her coat and legs in mid-flight. With a skillful pressing movement of a rammer, called the auricle, she pushes it into her basket. The pollen baskets, surrounded by a fringe of long hairs, are a concave area located on the outside of the tibia. When her baskets are fully loaded, the microscopic golden dust has been tamped down into a single golden granule.

One of the most interesting facts about bee pollen is that it cannot be duplicated in a laboratory. Mother nature is keeping secrets from us. Although many thousands of chemical analyses of bee pollen have been made with the very latest diagnostic equipment, there are still some factors present in bee pollen which science cannot identify. The bees add some magic mysterious 'extra' of their own. These unidentifiable elements may very well be the reason why bee pollen works so spectacularly against so many different conditions of ill health.

Research From Around The World

In spite of all the solid documentation of the many, many benefits bee pollen offers mankind, U.S. scientists have shown scandulously little interest in the work of the bee. The following material comes primarily from the work of scientists and medical researchers around the world. In most instances, the work was published only in the language of origin, although a few papers do carry an English language abstract of a few sentences. For the most part, a full translation was necessary in order to fully comprehend the subject matter.

From the beginning, The C C Pollen Company shouldered the task of searching out the researchers working with beehive products, negotiated to secure copies of important published papers, and commissioned the necessary translations. The never-ending effort has been both time-consuming and costly. Of the world's bee pollen producers, only The C C Pollen Company exhibits such a high degree of professionalism. This is just one reason why The C C Pollen Company products are of superior quality.

Most of the papers we are reporting on in this chapter include scientific and medical terminology and are written in highly technical terms. When reasonably understandable, we quote extensively in the form of exact excerpts. This is where you discover the scientific basis for all those many, many testimonials. Settle back and relax. Space considerations make it impossible to give you a review of *all* the research on file, but this is still a very long, very interesting, chapter. We believe you will be surprised at the number of diverse conditions bee pollen successfully conquers.

Complete Nutrition

From *The Royal Science of the Naturalists of Mons* (Belgium) *and Borinage* (France) comes the almost poetically-titled work,

"The Secrets of the Life of Bees." Chemical analyses from research laboratories all over the world show that bee pollen provides all the nutrients mankind needs for complete life support. Because this particular paper is very nearly complete, we selected it to report on the various nutrients in bee pollen. In translation from the French, this twelve-page paper ably demonstrates the ability of bee pollen to completely sustain life and favorably influence the body. Although all the essential vitamins are present in bee pollen, the properties of the following specific vitamins are so important the author of this paper singled them out for special mention.

Chief Vitamins of Bee Pollen
Water-Soluble Vitamins

Thiamine (Vitamin B1) — Indicated for the treatment of the toxic effects of alcohol or certain medicines, industrial/occupational chemicals; the relief of sciatica, neuritis, neuralgia of the face and trigeminal nerve; the curing of edemas; the reduction of paralysis following poliomyelitis or diphtheria; phantom pains in stumps of amputees; the treatment of shingles; the heart conditions myocarditis and tachycardia; and in the regimen for diabetis mellitus.

Riboflavin (Vitamin B2) — In opthomology, necessary to cure conjunctivitis, disorders of retinal adaption; some skin diseases (non specific dermatitis and more); blepharospasms; labial moniliasis (an infectious disease); fissures of the breast and nipples of nursing mothers; chronic enteritis; migraine; abnormal redness of the lips and mucosa of the tongue; enters into the composition of numerous enzyme systems.

Pyridoxine (Vitamin B6) — Plays an important role in the exchanges and transformations of nitrogenous substances and lipids; required for the formation of hemoglobin; used to combat nervousness; neurasthenis; fatigue; stomach cramps; muscular weakness; Parkinson's disease; hemiplegias; brain tumors; arteriosclerosis of the brain; anemia; radiation sickness.

Nicotinic Acid (Nicotinamide) — Acts on the formation of blood; used in the treatment of dermatoses; in toxic overload; diabetes mellitus; gastrointestinal symptoms; urticaria; enteritis, chronic diarrhea; constipation; colitis; asthma; neuralgia. Possesses a vasodilating action on capillaries; also fights migraines and tinnutis (ringing) of the ears. Even more important, nicotinic acid lowers harmful cholesterol, while elevating the helpful high-density lipoproteins.

Pantothenic Acid (Part of B-Complex) — Effective action demonstrated on speeding the cure of wounds, especially those originating from electrical accidents. Cures gangrene; anal fistulas; varicose ulcers; herpes; inflammatory infections of the mouth; chronic ulcers; decubitus (bedsores); dermatoses; sunburns; colds; bronchitis; infectious hepatitis; fights dandruff; seborrhea.

Inositol (Part of B-Complex) — Indications for the need for inositol include disorders of hepatic metabolism; some inflammations of the conjunctival tissue. Has properties beneficial to heart and intestines.

Ascorbic Acid (Vitamin C) — Stimulating anti-toxic and anti-hermorrhagic effects; beneficial against colds, respiratory distress; required for the efficient use and metabolism of calcium (promotes the effect of calcium, eliminates toxic phenomena arising as a consequence of absorbing too strong a dose of calcium); reduces hypercalcification induced by excessive doses of Vitamin D.

Fat-Soluble Vitamins

Vitamin A (Retinol) — Vitamin A is known as the anti-infectious vitamin; the anti-xeropthalmic (excessively dry conjunctiva of the eye) vitamin; the night-blindness vitamin; the growth vitamin. Acts in a very important manner on human growth, assuring and regulating formation of epithelial (skin) tissue required for the external defense of the organism; protects against surface lesions; increases resistance to infections.

Vitamin E (Tocopherol) — Vitamin E is known as the vitamin of fertility, fights sterility; strong natural antioxidant (assists oxygenation at the cellular level); influences the assimiltion of lipids; acts on the reproductive organs; anticoagulant properties; improves blood circulation.

The Chemical Composition Chart (see chart below) is an important part of this landmark report on bee pollen.

CHEMICAL COMPOSTION OF BEE POLLEN
Quantitative Analysis of Valuable Components

Analysis of amino-acids
as percentage of total dry weight

Arginine	4.4 - 5.7
Histidine	2.0 - 3.5
Isoleucine	4.5 - 5.8
Leucine	6.7 - 7.5
Lysine	5.9 - 7.0
Methionine	1.7 - 2.4
Phenylalanine	3.7 - 4.4
Threonine	2.3 - 4.0
Tryptophan	1.2 - 1.6
Valine	5.5 - 6.0

Analysis of mineral substances and trace elements.
as percentage of ash

Potassium	20 - 45
Magnesium	1 - 12
Calcium	1 - 15
Copper	0.05 - 0.08
Iron	0.01 - 0.3
Silicon	2 - 10
Phosphorus	1 - 20
Sulfur	1
Chlorine	0.8
Manganese	1.4

Analysis of vitamins & hormones
in micrograms/gram

Thiamine	5.75 - 10.8
Riboflavin	16.3 - 19.2
Nicotinic acid	98 - 210
Pyridoxine	0 - 9
Pantothenic acid	3 - 51
Biotin	0.1 - 0.25
Folic acid	3.4 - 6.8
Lactoflavine	0.2 - 1.7
Vitamin A: Alpha/Beta Carotene	Avg. 1.53
Vitamin B2	16.3 - 19.2
Vitamine C	152 - 640
Vitamin D	0.2 - 0.6
Vitamin E	0.1 - 0.32
Inositol	30 - 40
Vitamin B12	Avg. .0002

Pigments
Some of the substances isolated:

Flavoxanthine; Xanthophyll epoxide; Carotene; epiphasic Carotenoids; Flavonols; Ethylic Ether; Quercitin; Zeaxanthine; Lycopene; Crocetin.

Percentage of water...	3 - 4%	
Reducing Sugars..	7.5 - 40%	(Av. 20%)
Non-reducing sugars..	0.1 - 19%	(Av. 5%)
Starches and other carbohydrates.......................	0 - 22%	
Etheric Extract (volatile fatty acids falsify the quantitative analysis of humidity beyond 70°C.) (Av. 4.5%)		0.9 - 14%
Proteins...	7 - 35%	(Av. 20%)
Free amino-acids (almost constant level).............	10%	
H.G.H. Human Growth Hormone Factor (not measured)		
Hormones (Gonadatropic estrogenic)		
Rutin (not measured		
Ash	1 - 7%	(Av. 3%)

Nutritional Tests

The nutritional test supervised by the station at Bures on hundreds of mice have demonstrated that pollen is a complete food and that it is possible to let several successive generations be born and live without the least sign of distress while nourishing them exclusively on pollen. The optimum of vigor and resistance to poor health and disease was obtained by adding a mixture of 20 percent bee pollen to their feed. Bee pollen is rich in rare and precious nutritive compounds; it works in a deep and lasting fashion.

We note the intestinal-balancing action of bee pollen obtained in stricken people, the favorable action of pollen on children who are anemic or lacking in appetite, as well as on adults in tropical climates who have had the surprise of seeing their red blood count normalized. Bee pollen stimulates the production of hemoglobin, the oxygen-carrying red blood cells. We have noted counts rising to 4 to 4.5 million. The large proportions of free amino acids, especially methionine, a specific medicine for the liver, explains the favorable action of bee pollen on that organ. The percentage of revivifying and rejuvenating elements in bee pollen is remarkable far exceeding those present in brewer's yeast and wheat germ.

Bee pollen contains all the essential components of life; it corrects the failings due to deficient or unbalanced nutrition, common in the customs of our present-day civilization of consuming in-complete foods, often with added chemical ingredients, which expose us to physiological problems as various as they are numerous. An organism weakened by a deficient dietary regimen becomes more subject to microbial infections and other disorders. Nutritional deficiencies and the breakdown of internal chemical balance generates diseased states for which the consumption of bee pollen works miracles.

A lecture by Gunther Vorwhol entitled *Pollen and Honey* was well received at a recent German Apiarist Convention held in Sontra, Germany. In translation from the original German, we are fortunate to be afforded an inside look at this workable and innovative approach to the problem of world hunger, excerpted as follows:

Because it contains all nutrients needed to sustain life, bee pollen is being used on an ever larger scale for human nourishment and health. In this connection, two considerations are of vital importance. As you all know, the human population on earth is continuously increasing. Standard food production cannot keep up with this population explosion. Much of humanity is threatened by hunger. Added to the inadequate general food production, there is the more pronounced insufficiency of foods rich in proteins. Large portions of the world are malnourished in this respect, in that their food does not contain suffcient protein.

Bee pollen is known to be a very protein-rich food for man. Besides all the essential amino acids present in bee pollen, many scientific studies confirm that the vitamin balance can be improved by eating this complete food from the bee hive. And there are other interesting active substances present in bee pollen as well. It offers rutin, for instance, which favorably influences the permeability of capillaries. Not to mention the important hormonal factors, the substances which act like the estrogenic or gonadatropic hormones which so greatly aid the human reproductive functions, both male and female. I should also point out the bacteria-inhibiting effects of the pollen collected by bees.

Science teaches that bee pollen contains numerous substances which make it healthy protein-rich nutritious food. Additionally, there are numerous reports from medical experience which show the benefits of bee pollen exceeds that of a simple food item. Repeated reports have been published about the positive influence of the ingestion of pollen in the case of prostate difficulties, the favorable influence bee pollen causes in cases of infertility, both male and female, and how it erases menopausal complaints. Because of the proven activity of the hormones in bee pollen, these cases are quite plausible.

More medical experience teaches that the ingestion of bee pollen is recommended in the case of digestion difficulties, arteriosclerosis, and liver dysfunctions. It also improves the hemogram (blood production). Lab animals sustaining purposely-inflicted wounds heal better if bee pollen is added to their food, and bone formation is also favorably influenced.

It's time to focus world attention on the utilization of bee pollen, the protein food of the bees. Bee pollen belongs with the protein-rich plant materials. Protein-rich pollen types are preferred by the bees. The protein content of blended bee pollen contains all the essential amino acids we must ingest every day, as the human body cannot produce them. The essential amino acids occur in pollen in free form, as well as bound to protein. Mixed bee pollens correspond favorably to other valuable protein foods, including eggs, cheese, and soybeans. And the bees do most of the work. As beekeepers, we must harvest more and more of this food from the hive and teach others to do the same, especially in the malnourished and starving areas of the world. Bee pollen can be the answer to worldwide hunger.

The following paper, entitled *Bee Products As Food & Medicine*, was written by Dr. Aleksander Jankovic. We have it in translation from the Yugoslav (Bratko Filipic, Ph.D., Institute of Microbiologia, Ljubljana, Yugoslavia). Dr. Jankovic opens this discussion with a look at bee pollen as a carrier of life and as the essential component in the production of royal jelly, as follows:

It has been determined that bee pollen represents the basis through which royal jelly is produced in the bee's body. The mechanism of such transformation remains mysterious. What is known is that, in order to change bee pollen into royal jelly, the bee needs water and honey also. This process is observed in young bees only.

In the case of older insects, bee pollen is consumed and metabolized as normal food with high biological value. Through analysis, it is found that bee pollen represents the most important source of proteins, essential fatty acids, sugars, and salts and is also the most important source of all vitamins, including thiamine, riboflavin, pyrodoxine, pantothenic acid, naicin, and ascorbic acid. The complete nutrient value and composition of bee pollen marks it as an important area for food scientists.

There are so many papers on the complete nutrition of bee pollen that we may be pardoned for excerpting only the concluding paragraph from a thirteen-page paper published by La Revue de Pathologie Generale et de Physiologie Clinique (Review of General Pathology & Clinical Physiology) entitled *The Physiological & Therapeutic Effects of Various Bee Pollen Extracts.* In translation from the French, this research is summed up as follows:

Conclusion: Bee-gathered pollens are rich in proteins, free amino acids, vitamins, including B-Complex, and folic acid. In addition, they contain variable quantities of an antibiotic potent against E.coli and Proteus, as well as a substance which significantly accelerates healthy growth of mice receiving a complete and balanced diet from other sources. The acceleration of growth is tied to a modification of the metabolism of carbohydrates. In human clinology, the effect of bee pollen acts favorably on the intestines, on the hemoglobin level of the blood, and in the renewal of strength in convalescents and in the aged.

All around the world, scientists and medical researchers praise the nutritive properties of bee pollen. Without going into the same depth of detail as we have given you above, still more documentation follows.

Institute of Apiculture, Taranov, USSR: "Honeybee pollen is the richest source of vitamins found in nature in a single food. Even if bee pollen had none of its other vital ingredients, its content of rutin alone would justify taking at least a teaspoon daily, if for no other reason than strengthening the capillaries. Pollen is extremely rich in rutin and may have the highest content of any source, plus a very high content of the nucleics, RNA and DNA."

Alain Callais, Ph.D., Academy of Agriculture, Paris, France: "Bee pollen is a complete food and contains many elements that products of animal origin do not possess. Bee pollen is more rich in proteins than any animal source. It contains more amino acids than beef, eggs, or cheese of equal weight. Bee pollen is particularly concentrated in all elements necessary for life."

Dr. G.J. Binding, MGE, FRHS, British scientist and world renowned expert on nutrition, sums up the subject of the nutritive value of bee pollen, as well as its health-restoring properties, admirably: "Pollen is the finest, most perfect food. It is a giant germ-killer in which bacteria simply cannot exist. The health restoring properties of honeybee pollen have been proven time and time again. Honeybee pollen not only builds up strength and energy in the body, but gives increased resistance to infection."

Medical Miracles

In translation from the French, this paper deals with several specific benefits of bee pollen as exhibited in on-going research with lab animals. This paper is entitled, *Techniques du Directorat des services Veterinaires.* We excerpt briefly as follows:

Products of the Hive - Pollen

In only the last tens of years have we seen beehive products return to the place of honor they held in past ages. Now, biologists, biochemists, doctors, researchers and scientists are carrying our precise researches into their use in human nutrition.

Pollen, a formative food, brings to the bees all they have need of beyond and above the sugars found in the nectar they transform into honey. Pollen is, then, a very rich food with a balanced composition. It suffices to maintain life and allows the colony to develop.

Without doubt, the most interesting point for the nutritionist is the presence of free amino acids at high levels, alongside those which are bound in the protein chains. The free amino acids in bee pollen are directly assimilable. Outside the work of biochemists on the composition of pollen, it is necessary to cite research carried out on the physiological action of this substance in laboratory animals.

It has been shown that mice can live on pollen and water

without showing the least signs of toxicity. Science shows bee pollen offers a very clear acceleration of growth which cannot be due to vitamin effects and which does not correspond with the nitrogenous supplement carried by bee pollen. There exists in bee pollen a principle which accelerates healthy growth.

Researchers have demonstrated that there is a substance in bee pollen which offers resistance to the development of numerous harmful bacteria. Experiments have shown that bee pollen contains an antibiotic factor effective on Salmonella and some strains of Colibacillus. On the clinical level, observations have shown precisely that a regulatory effect on intestinal functions may be attributed to bee pollen. The presence of a high proportion of cellulose and products allied to lignin in pollen, as well as the existence of antibiotic factors, all contribute to an explanation for this efficacious effect.

Working with lab animals has demonstrated that the ingestion of bee pollen has a salutary effect on the composition of blood. A considerable and simultaneous increase of both white and red corpuscles is observed. It is interesting to point out that clinical tests show bee pollen administered to anemic infants considerably increases their level of hemoglobin. In man, it has been observed that the ingestion of bee pollen entails a beneficial overall effect in convalescents and the aged. Strength returns rapidly and a characteristic euphoria is noted.

From Romania, a paper authored by G. Calcaianu and F. Cozma entitled, *Treatment with Bee Products of the Behavior Troubles in Young People in the Period of Puberty and Teenage,* offers special insight for the care of troubled youngsters, a subject often neglected in this country.

Opening Remarks: The important biological transformations which are produced during puberty and teenage are well known in medical pathology. There are periods of genuine biological crises which determine the healthy or unhealthy development of young organisms. Passage through these ages is often accompanied by clinical unrest, behavior troubles related to family, social, and school adaption, resulting in decreased performance in the education process.

Methodology: Our study concerns sixty-seven pupils, 15 to 18 years old. Clinical symptoms in this period of biological crisis were observed. We selected subjects exhibiting neuropsychic unrest, trophicity, with manifestations of paroxysmal, visceral, vasomotional and sensitivomotional problems. Our clinical and laboratory data were correlated with those obtained by school and familial inquiry referring to the behavior of these young people.

Conclusion: Given regularly, bee products (pollen, royal jelly, and honey) lead to favorable results. The results of our investigation determine us to believe that by adequate therapy we can prevent important behavioral troubles. In these periods of biological crisis, the young organism needs products with a rich content of bioenergetic substances.

In translation from the Spanish, a study of children comes from the Children's Hospital of Cordoba, Chair of Pediatrics, entitled, *Administration of Biological Pollen Products to the Undernourished.*

Opening Remarks: Swedish pediatrists observed the favorable action of the use of pollen in the treatment of children with influenza or with post-infection lack of appetite. Studies submitted to the Karolinska Institute of Stockholm confirmed the encouraging results achieved in pathological conditions of adults.

This experiment was carried out at the Children's Hospital exclusively with children hospitalized under the care of the Chair of Pediatrics, ensuring the accurate administration of medicines and guaranteeing a clinical control. Thirty children under two years of age with varying degrees of malnutrition were selected.

Results: The duration of the period of restoration varies in accordance with the degree of undernutrition reached. In our children, it varied generally between 20 and 40 days.

Biochemical Observations: Red blood cells and hemoglobin increased in 14 cases; calcium increased in 12 cases; urinalysis improved in 10 cases; proteins increased in 19 children. There was an 83.33 percent improvement in appetite.

A special reprint from the publication *Naturheilpraxis* offers an article entitled, *A Summary of Clinical Tests Concluded With Bee Pollen.* Along with all the other positive effects of bee pollen, it protects against atherosclerosis and heart disease in yet another important way. This article explores the rich composition of bee pollen, already well covered in this chapter. Here are the concluding remarks.

Conclusion: One can objectively observe a reduction of cholesterol and triglycerides and also of S-lipo-proteins and albumins, while K and S globulins increase. A normalization of cholesterol count was observed in 40 patients who suffered from cerebral sclerosis.

Bee pollen is a polyvalent vital substance which influences nutrient deficiencies favorably. A treatment with a combination of bee pollen, royal jelly, and honey has positive effects during the biological crises of puberty and adolescence, during behavioral disturbances, with problems of adjustment, learning disabilities, neurotic disturbances, and excessive neuromuscular sensitivity.

Bee pollen preparations increase mental work performance and favor blood circulation in the brain. In five out of eight children who were mentally lazy and doing poorly in school, mental performance and GPA improved significantly after taking pollen for 12 weeks. In ten patients, faulty memory and lack of concentration were improved after three months. In elderly patients, a significant change for the better is always observed.

One of the most important papers ever published on bee pollen came from our own Department of Agriculture. This paper, entitled, *Delay in the Appearance of Palpable Mammary Tumors in C3H Mice Following the Ingestion of Pollenized Food,* was the work of William Robinson, Bureau of Entomology, Agriculture Research Administration. It was published in the *Journal of the National Cancer Institute* way back in 1948, forty years ago. We are giving you pertinent excerpts.

Dr. Robinson started with a special strain of mice bred to succumb to tumors. He explains: "The age at which mice of this strain developed tumors ranged from 18 to 57 weeks, with an average of 33 weeks; and the *tumor incidence was 100 percent.*". The pollen used in this experiment was supplied by the Division of Bee Culture and "was the bee-gathered type." One group of mice was fed regular mice chow only; another group was fed mice chow with the addition of bee pollen at a ratio of one part bee pollen to ten thousands parts food.

The report states, "Particular attention was given to the weight of the treated animals, since underweight can in itself bring about a delay in tumor development. No decrease in weight occurred in the animals receiving pollenized food. Instead, a slight but fairly uniform increase was noted, possibly due to a nutritional factor in pollen. This increase is in agreement with the work of Vivino and Palmer who investigated the chemical composition and nutritional value of pollens collected by bees."

In his Summary, Dr. Robinson reveals: "In the untreated mice (not given bee pollen), mammary tumors appeared as expected at an average of 31.3 weeks and the tumor incidence was 100 percent. In the postponement series (given bee pollen with their food), the average (onset of tumors) was 41.1 weeks, a delay of 9.8 weeks being obtained. *Seven mice in this series were still tumor-free at 56 to 62 weeks of age,* when the tests were terminated." We emphasize that these mice were especially bred to die from cancerous tumors. Without the protection of bee pollen in their food, all mice developed tumors and died on schedule.

Dr. Robinson concludes: "It is suggested that the use of the extracted and standardized active principle from bee pollen might produce greater postponement. These experiments were based upon the postulation that *bee pollen contains an anticarcinogenic principle that can be added to food."*

Given the fact that cancer is the Number 2 killer in the U.S. (heart disease is Number 1), we all can certainly agree that this is an electrifying report. What happened? Nothing. Even the National Cancer Institute, which published it, failed to follow up this very promising line of research. It was dropped with no explanation.

But other medical detectives remain enthusiastic about the properties bee pollen displays against this dread killer.

L.J. Hayes, M.D., Apiculteur Haut-Chinois, Guebwiller in Mittelwigen: "Bees sterilize pollen by means of a glandular secretion which is antagonistic to tumors." This particular fact was also noted by the renowed Soviet science writer, Naum Ioyrish.

Sigmund Schmidt, M.D., the Natural Health Clinic, Bad Bothenfelds: "Bee pollen contains all the essential elements for healthy tissue and may well prove to be the natural cancer preventive all the world is seeking."

Ernesto Contreras, M.D., noted cancer specialist: "In the biologial treatment of cancer, proper nutrition is gaining more and more importance. To my knowledge, there is no better and more complete natural nutrient than honeybee pollen. Properly used, it should always give the expected results. A shift to natural non-aggressive agents in the management of cancer is mandatory for better results and happier patients."

More good news comes from the *University of Vienna* where Dr. Peter Hernuss conducted a study of 25 women suffering from inoperable uterine cancer. Because surgery was impossible, these women were being treated with chemotherapy. The lucky women given bee pollen with their food quickly exhibited a higher concentration of cancer-fighting immune system cells, their antibody production increased, and the level of their infection-fighting and oxygen-carrying red blood cells markedly improved. These women suffered less from the awful side-effects of chemotherapy as well. Bee pollen lessened the terrible nausea which commonly accompanies this treatment, they slept better at night, and hair loss was held to a minimum. The control group receiving a placebo did not experience relief.

In translation from the Yugoslav, a paper entitled *Therapeutic Effects of Melbrosin* in Irradiation Diseases* supports the results achieved at the University of Vienna. (*Swedish preparation of bee pollen, royal jelly, and honey.)

Opening Remarks: The undesired effect of irradiation on the organism is attributed, in addition to the direct effect of ionizing rays, to the toxic noxes induced by the emerging decomposition of the tissue proteins under the influence of X and gamma rays. The damage to the organism caused by irradiation can be interpreted as:

Disturbances in the metabolism
Vegetative troubles
Disturbances in hematopoiesis (blood constituents)
Endocrine disturbances

In order to make clinical studies, 84 female patients were separated from a group of tumor-dose irradiated patients who suffered from gynacological carcinoma and who showed clear signs of X-ray disease: fatigue, lack of dynamism, anorexia, nausea, vomiting, diarrhea, headache, unconsciousness, insomnia, heat and perspiration strokes, tachycardia, increased temperature, etc. The problems evolved from the fifth to seventh day of irradiation in doses of 1500 to 2000 rads. In some patients, the troubles were so severe we had to interrupt therapy temporarily. The patients for the clinical experiment were chosen at random, the youngest being 34 and the oldest 71, and were separated into two identical groups.

Results: After taking the preparation, 30.5 percent of the patients had no sign of fatigue; 66.7 percent felt light fatigue; only 2.8 percent still complained of severe fatigue; 38.9 percent no longer suffered from anorexia; 41.6 percent exhibited light anorexia; 8.3 percent moderate anorexia; 44.4 percent suffered no longer of nausea; in 50 percent, nausea was reduced to the mildest form; in only 5.6 percent did the intensity remain unchanged. Great improvement was also achieved in psycho and neurovegetative complaints.

Even in the most correctly applied method, technique, and dosage of irradiation, problems will develop in almost every patient because of the direct effect of the rays and of the toxic materials resulting from the decomposition of the irradiated tissue. As there is no specific medicine for irradiation disease, we have decided to apply this natural bioactive bee product substance, pollen and royal jelly. This preparation manifested a significantly positive effect in the morbid state caused by irradiation.

After we calculated the irradiation index, it was possible to conclude that improvement was obtained in 88.8 percent of the cases, which is indisputable proof of the positive effects achieved by the preparation.

From the *Argonomic Institute, Faculty of Zootechnics, Rumania,* we have a report showing the immune-strengthening effects of bee pollen. Given the state of the world today, this animal study should be of great interest to medical science, as well as the rest of us.

Results: The addition of pollen in the ration has instigated a diminution of dry material and an augmentation in the digestibility of mineral substances and in the coefficient of use of digestible nitrogen. The increase in lots given pollen can be explained by its biostimulating action, the best utilization of the ration, and the evaluation of its biologic value, especially with regard to proteins.

An increase has been recorded in the level of blood *lymphocytes, of **gamma-globulins, and of proteins in those lots given pollen in comparison with the control. The most significant difference occurred for lymphocytes. These results thus signify a strengthening in the resistance of the organic system.

(*Lymphocytes are white blood cells which are the 'soldiers' of the immune system. They are responsible for ridding the body of injurious and harmful substances, including infected and/or diseased cells (mutant and cancerous), viruses, metabolic trash and so on. **Gamma-globulin is a protein formed in the blood. Our ability to resist infection is closely related to concentration of such proteins.)

A paper read at the International Symposium on Apitherapy entitled *Pollen Preparations and Their Impact on Immunological Reactions of Test Mice* confirms the results reported above. We have only a brief English abstract of this lecture, which concluded as follows:

The fact that the immunological reaction is stronger (in mice given bee pollen) compared with the reaction of the animals given industrially prepared food may be attributed to pollen's nutritive effects. An addition of bee pollen to enriched food stimulated the immunological reaction, which might be due to the presence of specific stimulating factors in the bee pollen grains.

Reproductive & Sexual Function

There are many written reports on the powerfully potent action honeybee pollen exerts on a variety of sexual dysfunctions. This perfect food from the beehive has the seemingly miraculous ability to restore and rejuvenate tired and/or aging sex glands, both male and female.

Soma Health Magazine reports, "Bee pollen contains natural hormonal substances which stimulate and nourish the reproductive systems of both men and women. Sexual stamina and endurance are increased by the multitude of naturally nutritious components found in pollen. The bottom line is: Bee pollen does have a dramatic impact on sexual ability."

As an overview on this important subject, we turn to the writing of Dr. Morton Walker, long known as America's Number One Medical Journalist. Under the heading *Sexual Energy Using*

Bee Pollen, Dr. Walker says: "Honeybee pollen saves you the trouble of looking further for a food affording excellent energy potential. Along with its protein content, bee pollen contains natural hormonal substances which stimulate and nourish the reproductive systems of both men and women. It provides stamina for a muscular staying power of pelvic movement so you may attain the orgasmic sensation you crave. Bee pollen is a natural, organic and sensational food substance.

Honeybee pollen provides greater sexual vigor through the release of high-energy chemical bonds and the generation of adenoisine triphosphate (ATP). To satisfy sexual urgency, your body searches for required sexual vigor wherever it may be stored. If you have eaten wisely, sexual energy is found quickly in the stored energy from the bee pollen you have taken."

The natural hormonal substances in bee pollen that Dr. Walker talks about and which act so spectacularly on the sex glands have been isolated and identified. In clinical work, researchers have been able to document the glandular boost and therapeutic effects bee pollen provides.

In translation from the Yugoslav, this paper by Professor Dr. Izet Osmanagic of the University of Sarajevo documents the effects of bee pollen on *Reduced Sexual Potency.*

Opening Remarks: Sexual impotence in men is far more frequent than is generally thought, as many men are reluctant to consult a doctor. We established contact with the patients studied in this report through the person most concerned about a man's impotence, his wife. These women consulted the Gynacological Clinic at the University of Sarajevo about infertility. It was soon discovered that, in many cases, the man was to blame.

Materials & Methods: We studied 40 men between 20 and 52 years of age. In most cases the patients had lived in sterile marriages for two or more years. We examined economic situation, manner of life, conditions of marriage, and sexual habits. Patients were questioned about:

1. Sexual desire
2. Frequency of intercourse
3. Level of erection
4. Orgasm
5. Ejaculation

Seventy-five percent of the patients were found to be suffering from sperm deficiencies. Our patients took between 80 and 160 capsules of the bee pollen preparation, the daily dose being two capsules. During the 2 to 3 month periods of taking the preparation, the patients were interviewed and sperm count tested two or three times. The preparation was well supported by all. Undesirable side effects were not observed in any of the patients.

Results: After one month, the majority showed an improvement in their general and sexual condition, which had a significant effect on their performance during intercourse. The majority of patients showed improved sperm production. Two patients announced that their wives were pregnant, astounding proof of the effectiveness of this product. These fertilizations were made by men previously considered infertile.

We could reasonably conclude that a natural beehive product, the positive effect of which on general condition, physical health, psychological state and nervous stability has already been proved, would also lead to an improvement in sexual potency, which has proved correct.

Summary: Our tests were aimed at determining the effect of the prepartion on men with reduced sexual powers. Forty patients were examined. Eighty percent suffered from relative or absolute reproductive impotence and some from reduced capacity for intercourse.

On the basis of the recorded results, we were able to conclude that the preparation in the majority of our patients led to:
1. An improvement in the general state of health and subjective condition.
2. An increase in sexual activity
3. Improved sperm production

These results represent obvious proof of the positve effects of the prepartion in cases of reduced sexual and procreative potency.

The following paper reports on a joint Swedish/German study of 212 male patients in which twelve different urologists participated. As you will see, these men were suffering from chronic prostatitis, as well as a variety of sexual dysfunctions. The doctors who authored the paper are C.E. Alken, M.D., Professor of Urology, Hamburg, Germany, G. Johnson, Head of Urology, University Clinic, Lund, Sweden, and L. Rohl, M.D., Associate Professor of Urology, Heidelberg, Germany.

From the total of 212 patient case histories initially received, 40 had to be excluded because the patients had been treated with the bee pollen compound *in combination* with another antiprostatic agent, or because the observation period was less than three months.

Group I: Total 114 cases (none had exhibited previous urinary or focal infections), subdivided as follows:
75: Micturition trouble (difficulty passing urine)
66: Sexual dysfunction, broken down as follows:
25: Reduced libido (low sex drive)
22: Ejaculatio praecox (premature ejaculation)
21: Painful orgasm
20: Practiced coitus interruptus (a cause of sexual distress in 15, 5 without overt sexual distress)

18: Impotence (because of weak erection, or inability to sustain erection)

29: Initial pyuria (pus in urine; evidence of renal [kidney] disease)

47: More than 15 leukocytes (white blood cells) in exprimate

13: Positive bacteriological cultures of exprimate, including Staph. albus, Esch. coli, B. proteus.

14: Neurasthenic disorders (weakness or exhaustion of sinews)

Group II: Total 57 cases (all had exhibited previous urinary or focal infections), subdivided as follows:

26: Micturition trouble

14: Initial pyuria

12: More than 15 leukocytes (white blood cells) in exprimate

4: Positve bacteriological cultures of exprimate

4: Neurasthenic disorders

27: Sexual dysfunction, broken down as follows:

11: Ejaculatio praecox (premature ejaculation)

11: Painful orgasm

10: Practiced coitus interruptus (a cause of sexual distress in 6, 4 without overt sexual distress)

9: Reduced libido (low sex drive)

2: Impotence (because of weak erection, or inability to sustain erection)

Comments: The investigators thought it worthwhile to perform a trial of this drug (bee pollen compund) in representative material because the symptom complex known as chronic prostatitis is a definite reality in urological practice and many reports of the favorable influence of the compound on this condition have been published, especially by Scandinavian scientists.

It may be assumed that most cases of 'primary chronic prostatitis' were included in Group I, and most cases of 'secondary chronic prostatitis' in Group II. Concerning the 40 patients who were excluded from the investigation, 21 were found to have improved. Of these, 14 were treated with the bee pollen compound alone. Had these results been included in the final figures, the percentage of improvement achieved by the compound would further increase.

The number of sexual disturbances of any type occurring in the material was relatively high, 98 cases out of 176. Reduced libido, painful orgasm, premature ejaculation, and impotency occurred in about equal numbers. More than one of these symptoms of sexual dysfunction were present at the same time in many patients.

A tabulation of the results shows improvement in the total patient material evaluated averaged out at 44 percent (48 percent in Group I; 35 percent in Group II). This improvement percentage is surprisingly high. We also wish to mention that of the 60 cases in the entire material exhibiting a pathological exprimate, 24 improved. No appreciable adverse side-effects were observed.

Another study of the same compound on a common prostate complaint comes from Sweden alone. Dr. Gosta Leander of Stockholm authored a paper entitled, *A Menorandum Concerning a Statistical Evaluation of the Results of a Clinical Investigation of Cernilton.** (*Cernilton is a Swedish pollen prepartion.) The patients in this study were suffering from prostato-vesiculitis, an inflammation of the seminal vesicles and prostate gland. Dr. Leander reported truly spectacular results, as follows:

If the compound proved not to be superior to the placebo substance (given to the control group), the distribution of improved groups within the limits of chance would be the same. This was not the case. The probability that chance could result in the enormous difference between 92 percent improvement for the group given the compound and the 37 percent perceived improvement for the placebo is considerably less than 1:1000 (chi-square 31,254).

A group of 50 patients whose symptomatology may have been

more severe showed a 76 percent ascertained improvement in a test without blind controls. A comparison of therapy results obtained for the *same* patient following first placebo then the compound administration respectively, showed a statistically highly significant effect from the compound.

In summarizing, it can be confirmed that a statistically highly significant effect of the compound could be demonstrated in prostatovesiculitis, estimated on the basis of a double-blind control study of 93 patients, 50 of whom received the compound, and 43 of whom received the placebo. A 92 percent ascertained improvement was confirmed in the group given the compound. The effects of the compound found during the course of this study has been established as statistically highly significant.

A Japanese study originating from the University School of Medicine, Kyoto, Japan, provides yet more documentation regarding the beneficial effects of bee pollen on the prostate. This study is entitled, *Use of Cernilton in Patients with Prostatic Hypertrophy.* (*A medical term for an enlarged prostate.) As you will see from the opening remarks, this serious problem is on the rise in Japan.

Introduction: Today the only radical therapy for prostatic hypertrophy is a prostatectomy (surgical removal of the prostate gland) or transurethral prostatectomy (surgery performed through the urethra, which is the tube which carries urine). Prostatic hypertrophy is a kind of geriatric disease whose incidence in Japan has now increased as high as that in European countries. Frequently, this disease involves surgery not desired in aged patients.

This report concerns the authors' recent experience with a Swedish pollen product used originally as a prophylactic agent against infections in convalescent patients until its effectiveness in prostatitis was reported.

Materials & Methods: The subjects were 24 patients with prostatic hypertrophy seen at our Outpatient Clinic. The drug was given in doses of four tablets once daily in the morning over periods ranging from 25 to 150 days. In general, other drugs were not employed. The present report deals with 12 cases.

Discussion: From an absolute pathological point of view, formation of nodules in the urethral area of the prostate is an aging process seen in all males over the age of seventy. Some develop clinical symptoms and receive treatment for prostatic hypertrophy. Ten out of the twelve cases showed improvement in subjective symptoms; objective improvement in residual urine was obtained in six cases. No marked diminution in the size of the prostate on palpation was observed.

Of the ten cases which showed improvement, three were in the first degree of hypertrophy, four cases in the second degree, and three cases in the third degree. In two cases, symptoms recurred within one month after *withdrawal of the drug;* these patients eventually underwent prostatectomy. All patients in the third degree of hypertrophy subsequently underwent prostatectomy.

In other words, the drug is to be used in cases where surgical management is contraindicated, or to improve clinical symptoms when the disease is still in its early phase. Side-effects were observed in none of the cases treated.

Are you wondering why the 'drug was withdrawn' when improvement had been observed? So are we. Those patients who subsequently had their prostates removed are probably wondering too. The authors explain: "It (the drug) should not be employed indiscriminately for long-term administration for it may aggravate renal function and thus increase the risk in surgical operations." It may be that the combination of chemical ingredients in the Cernilton pollen compound pose a medical risk over time.

A later Japanese study of the same drug in a clinical evaluation of its efficacy in the treatment of chronic prostatitis achieved measureably higher percentages of effectiveness, as follows:

Discussion: Moore describes that chronic prostatitis is found
in more than 35 percent of adult males over the age of 35, while,
according to another report, it is found in 85 percent of adult males
over the age of 30. Participating factors include trauma, drinking,
and car-driving. In most cases, bacteria are either totally absent
or only sparsely detected, thus, positive use of antibiotics is not
justified. Long-term adminstration of anti-inflammatory drugs does
not always result in an improvement of symptoms. In this sense,
the pollen preparation points to a new approach. It may not be
effective in all cases of chronic prostatitis, but is certainly effective
in many such cases.

The cases of prostatitis selected for the present study were
mainly diagnosed on the basis of subjective symptoms and findings
on palpation. The fact that the rate of effectiveness was higher than
90 percent in the group griven the drug suggests there must have
been cases where the compound was indicated. This is supported
by the significant difference of effects registered in the cases where
both the drug and placebos were employed and further by the
fact that improvement of subjective symptoms was more difficult
to obtain in the placebo group.

Conclusion: Of a total of 15 cases in the Cernilton group, 10
cases were effective; 3 cases slightly effective.

Results obtained in the placebo group were much less
favorable; effective in 7 cases; ineffective in 9 cases.

Side-effects were observed in none of the 38 cases studied.

Bee pollen contains a gonadatropic hormone very similar
to the pituitary hormone, gonadatropin, which functions as a
sex-gland stimulant. Research conducted at the University of

Sarajevo, Yogoslavia with a group of impotent men shows that more than half of those treated with bee pollen exhibited a dramatic improvement in the production of sperm, gained a higher level of self-confidence, and were able to perform better sexually after taking bee pollen for just one month.

Noel Johnson (see Chapter 6), 89 year old author of *A Dud at 70 — A Stud at 80,* credits bee pollen with the full restoration of his manhood, as well as his return to health. Vigorous and virile today, Johnson, always the gentleman, doesn't 'kiss and tell.' He says simply, "I derive special nutrients from bee pollen. It give me the energy I need to engage in marathons... and other physical activities."

In their paper entitled, *The Gonad* Stimulating Potency of Date Palm Pollen Grains* (in translation from the French scientific journal *Experientia),* the Egyptian scientists F.A. Soliman and A. Soliman have this to say: "Several investigators have entracted estogenic materials from palm kernels and date pollen grains. Recently a gonad-stimulating principle was extracted from pollens. The gonadotrophic principles were extracted using the method of McShan and Meyer. The combined activity of the two hormones present in 1 gram of pollen is close to 10 I.U. When injected into immature male and female rats, it increased the weights of their gonads and activated them." (*Gonad is a generic medical term which refers to both the female sex glands, or ovaries, and the male sex glands, or testes.)

More work on the reproductive gland-stimulating properties of pollen comes from Rumania. The research report by

Gh. Salajan and Gh. Baltan is entitled, *Influence of Maize Pollen on Ovulation: Results of Incubation & Biological Value of Hen Eggs.* These scientists cited earlier work in their opening remarks, as follows:

Opening Remarks: Maize pollen is rich in proteins of great biological value and in mineral substances and stimulants which, if incorporated into food in quantities of 40 grams per day in calves and in proportions of 2 to 3 per 100 in the feeding of young pigs; in a proportion of 4 to 27 per 100 stimulates weight gain of chickens in growth.

It reduced the consumption of foods in a proportion of 6 to 22 per 100 and stimulated the functions of reproduction in young female hogs. Pollen protein can substitute for animal protein totally in the diet of young pigs and chickens. The mechanisms according to which this product stimulates growth, reduces appetite, and improves the nutrient value of food rations are well known. We present the results obtained in the *increase of ovulation*, in the *quality of incubation,* and in the *biological value* of eggs under the influence of maize pollen.

Of course, probably no one reading this book is planning to rush to Rumania and start a chicken farm. You probably think we are straying far afield in reporting this study. Nothing could be further from the truth.

The woman who wishes for a child, but is unable to conceive, may well be desperate to increase ovulation, thereby increasing her chances of being impregnated. The woman planning to bear a child may well be interested in the enhancement of incubation values bee pollen promises, even though she 'incubates' an infant in her womb, not in a mechanical device. And this same woman will certainly praise bee pollen to the heavens on finding that the biological value of an egg (or a baby) is improved when the diet of the mother (hen or human) includes the powerful natural hormones and complete nutrition of pollen.

This is a very long paper. We're not going to trouble you with all the scientific protocols necessary to set up the experiment, but the researchers took great care to insure that all factors were equal. For example, the hens were artificially inseminated using sperm from four brother roosters which had been tested for the quality of their sperm. The sperm from the four fathers-to-be was mixed together and fertilization of all hens, divided into six groups, was carried out immediately after the fresh sperm was collected. The results of this landmark study follow:

Ovulation — Ovulation increased in Groups 3 to 5, to which pollen had been added in proportion of 2 to 4 per 100 parts of the ration during the whole growth period of the chicks. Ovulation also increased in Group 6, to which pollen had been added in a proportion of 11, 57, and 6 per 100 only during the growth period. The intensity of ovulation increased in relation to the control group (not given pollenized feed) from 5, 57 to 16, 76 per 100 in Groups 3 to 5, and from 15, 28 per 100 in Group 6.

The maximum positive influence of the substances in pollen on the ovary is produced during the growth period of the chicks. From a practical viewpoint, it is necessary to administer the stimulant (pollen) during a period of one to 150 days. The qualitative and quantitative modifications that are produced in this period at the ovary level are those responsible for the production of eggs in hens.

Fertilization — The percentage of fertilized eggs and of eggs with a viable embryo increased in Groups 3 to 6, which reduced the percentage of eggs lost during incubation. Good results were also obtained in Group 5, where the percentage of eggs gained surpassed the control group in proportions of 9, 42 per 100.

These results confirm that pollen, added in a proportion of 4 per 100 to the ration, improves the quality of incubation. It should be administered to hens destined for reproduction during the growth period and also during the period of collection of eggs destined for incubation. The increase in the content of the eggs in dry matter and in the carotenoids of the yolk, as well as the more intense pigmentation, confirmed the best of the nutritive qualities and of the enhanced biological value of the eggs under the influence of pollen.

Conclusions — Pollen stimulated the development of ovarian function. The best results have been obtained with a pollen supplementation of 2 per 100 in the ration and with the substitution of animal proteins with pollen in a proportion of 5 per 100; the intensity of ovulation increased.

Parallel to the increase in ovulation, pollen also improves the ability of the eggs to withstand the incubation period. The best results have been obtained with a quantity of 4 per 100 of pollen added to the ration, a situation in which the percentage of eggs increase in a 9, 42 per 100 in respect to the control group. The application of pollen is recommended whenever the end result is obtaining eggs for reproduction.

Pollen also exercises a positive influence on the nutritive quality of eggs. It increases the consumable proportion of the egg, its content of dry matter, the biological value and the degree of pigmentation of the yolk. From this viewpoint, an optimum quantity of 2 per 100 of pollen is proposed. It is recommended to add pollen to rations during the growth period and also during laying, which will increase ovulation and also improve the nutritive qualities of eggs destined for consumption.

Other scientists are in agreement with the important findings reported above. In translation from the German, here's a concluding bit on the same subject from *Zeitschrift fur Tierphysiologie, Tiernahrung und Futtermittelkunde* (Periodical for Animal Physiology, Animal Nutrition, & Fodder Science).

Results: Maize pollen is a powerful biostimulant which has positive action on the organism, inducing a gain of weight and the development of impressive bodily dimensions, while also ensuring a better utilization of the feed among pullets. Maximum stimulation of growth is obtained by a dosage of 2 percent (by weight) of pollen. Further administration does not lead to an increase of weight, but does have positive effects on sexual activity, notably the production of eggs.

Because both these papers mention weight-*gain*, a subject of concern for many, it seems appropriate to add an explanatory note here. Because bee pollen synergistically boosts the *nutritive value* of food, cravings are eliminated, appetite is reduced, and you automatically eat less. By providing the body with all the natural elements it requires for the internal processing of each individual nutrient, the body finds it easier to extract and assimilate what it needs. Bee pollen will not add to a weight problem. Put that worry out of your mind for the moment. You'll find out why a little further along in this chapter.

Now back to the subject at hand, the wonders bee pollen works on the reproductive glands of women.

In translation from the Yugoslav, this next paper by L. Pokrajcic and I. Osmanagic is entitled, *The Treatment With Melbrosin* of Dysmenorrhea** in Adolescence.* (*Melbrosin is a bee pollen/royal jelly compound. **Dysmenorrhea is a medical term covering a wide range of menstrual problems.) The authors of this paper are physicians in a Yugoslav gynecology clinic. In this particular study, the doctors were treating young women with menstrual dysfunctions, as follows:

Remarks: The premenstrual syndrome and algomenorrhea are often encountered in the juvenile period of women. Despite numerous efforts by medical experts, the desired results were not achieved in treatment. Pain, affective emotional instability and psychic transformations not only hinder normal studies, they are an obstacle to any professional activity of girls, which makes dysmenorrhea not only a medical, but also a social, problem.

Analgesics, spasmolytics, sedatives, anabolic drugs, tonics and hormones have been used with the aim to eliminate problems connected with menses. In some cases, a therapy with radioactive, sulphuric and paraffin coatings, and similar, have been applied. Even surgical operations have not been avoided.

Methodology: One hundred twenty 15 to 20 year old girls with a normal or slightly weak body constitution and development of the genital area, all suffering from menstrual disturbances and who met the criteria of our experiments, were divided at random into two groups.

Neurovegetative, psychosomatic and particularly algomenorrheal disturbances were observed in all patients. The prevailing symptom was pain in the stomach before, at the beginning, or during the entire period of menstruation. In some patients the pain was manifested as a spasm with rising and falling intensity. In certain cases, the pain was so strong that the patients had to stay in bed for days. Localized hardships were often accompanied by general symptoms, including headache, neurosis swelling/bloating of the stomach, vomiting, unconsciousness, insomnia, and depression.

Our purpose was to examine the influence and action of the bee pollen compound, known in medicine for quite some time as a natural regenerating agent with beneficial effects on the entire somatic development of 14 to 20 year old girls, on the development of genitalia and breasts, on the regulation of the menstrual cycle whenever it is disturbed, on the alleviation or full elimination of menstrual pain, nervous and vegetative disturbances related to menstruation.

Studies had been previously made on the effects of the compound on the fertility of female mice. Female mice fed for 16 weeks on the compound with poor food were put into nests with male mice. The female mice were examined daily to see whether they had a vaginal plug as sign of accomplished copulation. Further, we followed the number of deliveries and health of the litters. Histological analyses of gonads, uterus, and tubes indicated the effectiveness of the preparation. These results were doubtless based on the effects of elements with a hormonal and fermentative orgin, present in the pollen and royal jelly compound.

Results: It has already been established that all our female patients had pain of varying intensity during menstruation. Following the application of the bee pollen compound during two full menstrual cycles, the situation improved in almost all patients. Symptoms persisted in only five cases out of the sixty given the compound. Such obvious results of the therapy were assessed as being very good. In the control group not given the compound, only two girls of the sixty reported any symptomatic changes.

Similar results were obtained with regard to the elimination of other problems with the menses. As the etiology of dysmenorrhea in adolescence is varied, it is necessary to undertake a detailed diagnostic procedure before initiating any therapy. Since the insufficient development of the uterus and of the parauterine tissue, as well as a weaker sensitivity of these organs to hormonal stimuli, are causes of the mentrual problems most often detected, they should be treated during adolescence when the most intensive somatic and psychic processes go on. Time when these processes can be influenced is limited.

The positive effects of this preparation, which may be applied for a long time, is easily tolerated and does not give rise to undesired side effects, are due to the anabolic and trophic effects of the herbal hormones phystosterol and auxin contained in the pollen and royal jelly.

For the first time in our country we attempted to influence painful menstruations and dysmenorrhea in the juvenile period by a natural preparation which contains pollen and royal jelly. Encouraged by the results of this experiment on patients with underdeveloped constitutions and irregular menstrual cycles, we have decided to initiate a thorough clinical testing of the compound in girls with difficult menses.

At the other end of the menstual cycle, Yugoslav researchers carried out a study of the effects of the same bee pollen/royal jelly compound on women suffering the effects of menopause. This one comes from the Endocrinological Department of the University Clinic for Women at the Medical Faculty in Sarajevo. It is entitled, *A Clinical Testing of the Effect of the Preparation Melbrosin on Women Suffering from Climacteric* Syndrome.* (*Climacteric is a medical term for the period that marks the end of a women's ability to reproduce, more commonly referred to as menopause.)

Methodology: Tests were carried out on women who expressly exhibited climacteric troubles in the cases of only partially preserved or totally extinct functions of the gonads (ovaries). The patients were in a condition of physiological pre-climax, climax, and menopause, with climacteric syndromes, also on patients on whom complete or partial castration (destruction of the ovaries) had been performed, either by surgery or by irradiation leading to climacteric troubles.

Cases were divided into two groups, according to the etiology of the complaint: The first group was formed of patients in which menopause had been induced artifically; the second group consisted of cases of normal cessation of the menses. Although the majority of patients were women in the 40 to 50 age group, ages ranged from 30 to 60 years.

Results: In our nomenclature, a good effect was achieved when symptoms had either completely disappeared after therapy, or had significantly decreased both in number and degree. In the majority of patients (90 percent), we were able to assess more or less excellent positive results of treatment.

Results were particularly favorable in the case of patients thrown into menopause by surgery or radiation treatment. The women of this category were aged between 30 and 60 years and were those on whom radical operations had been carried out for cancerous conditions of the female genital organs, leading to removal of their ovaries or the inactivation of their ovaries by large doses of ionized irradiation. The irradiated patients' complaints were especially serious. An additional factor contributing due to their hormones being depleted, was probably the damage caused to blood-forming processes and the liver as a result of irradiation.

We proved that the compound exerts a salutary effect throughout the whole system affected by irradiation. Thanks to the therapeutical action of the compound, these women have experienced a general improvement of their condition; they feel fresher, more dynamic, open to every activity, and mentally calmer. The compound is easily taken, very rarely causes side effects, and the beneficial effects of the preparation are noticeable after only 14 days of treatment.

Summing up, it may be said that in addition to causes of menopausal disturbances in general, this treatment offers justifiable indications that the preparation should be used in the treatment of all patients subjected to irradiation.

The Physically Active

If there's one thing that health authorities all over the world agree on, it's the basic need to provide our bodies with some form of regular exercise, as well as basic whole nutrients. In fact, science says that for every two hundred hours we spend in exercise, we gain an additional year of life. Therefore, the health and fitness lifestyle should encompass not only perfect nutrition, but an exercise regimen as well. It isn't only competing athletes who should be interested in this portion of the chapter, but all of us.

A two-year study conducted by former Russian Olympic coach, Remi Korchemny, now coaching the track team at Pratt Institute in New York, gives much insight into the part bee pollen plays in an active lifestyle.

This double-blind study fulfills all the criteria of scientific research. Korchemny's research has finally given us a solid foundation for the dynamic effects athletes taking bee pollen regularly have reported. What this study confirms is that bee pollen actually does improve the crucial recovery power of athletes after stressed performance. The runners Korchemny provided with bee pollen not only bettered their time in a second run around the track, their bodies quickly recovered normal heart-rate and blood pressure and they were ready to go again sooner. The team members taking a placebo couldn't keep up.

The British author and nutritionist, Dr. Maurice Hanssen, says, "I look on pollen as being part of the ideal athlete's diet. I define an ideal athlete's diet as that diet pattern which produces maximum performance when it is required, with no long-term harmful side effects. Your body is being continually renewed in the average half-life, which is the time taken for half to be replaced. Protein, for example, is in the body for 80 days, but the time differs with different tissues. Blood serum, heart and liver and kidneys are all 10 days, while bone, skin and muscle are 158 days.

"The extraordinary richness of pollen in micro-elements cannot be stressed too much. We just cannot be sure that a normal diet produces enough in available forms, but the absorption properties of pollen allow the trace elements to be incorporated into the body structure without excessive loss."

The British Sports Council has recorded increases in strength as high as 40 to 50 percent, and The British Royal Society has reported height increases in adults who take pollen.

In his book, *How Bee Pollen Slows Aging,* medical writer Harry McCarthy says, "Pollen contains mysterious ingredients which boost an athlete's performance further — and much more safely — than any 'pep pill' in existence. Sport super-stars in particular are using bee pollen."

Antii Lananaki, coach of the Finish track team that swept the Olympics in 1972 reveals, "Most of our athletes take pollen food supplements. Our studies show it significantly improves their performance. There have been no negative results since we have been supplying pollen to our athletes."

Alex Woodly, Executive Director of the prestigious Education Athletic Club in Philadelphia, says, "Bee pollen works and it works perfectly. Pollen allows super-stars to increase their strength and stamina up to 25 percent. This increase in strength and endurance may be the key to the secret regenerative power of bee pollen. Bee pollen causes a definite decrease in pulse rate.

The whole beauty of bee pollen is that it's as natural as you can get. No chemical, no steroids."

The German naturalist Francis Huber was a great proponent of this miraculous food from the hive. Huber said, "Bee pollen is the greatest body-builder on earth."

Weight Control

Bee pollen works wonders in a weight control or weight stabilization regimen by correcting a possible chemical imbalance in body metabolism which may be involved in either abnormal weight-gain or abnormal weight-loss. The normalizing and stabilizing effects of this perfect food from the beehive are phenomenal. In weight-loss programs, bee pollen stimulates the metabolic processes. It speeds caloric burn by lighting and stoking the metabolic fires. Honeybee pollen should be recognized as nature's true dietetic weight-loss food.

Bee pollen is a true low-calorie food. It contains only 90 calories per ounce, approximately two tablespoonsful. It offers 15 percent lecithin by volume; lecithin is a substance which dissolves and flushes fat from the body. This is one reason why bee pollen lowers cholesterol surer and faster than any other food.

By boosting the value of each nutrient present in the food you eat, bee pollen eliminates cravings. Its natural phenylalanine* content acts as an appetite suppressant. You just plain won't want to eat as much when you're taking bee pollen regularly. A study reported by *Aerospace Medicine & Life Sciences* proved that the average daily consumption of food falls by 15 to 20 percent when bee pollen is a regular item on the menu. This fact is confirmed by all the studies of laboratory animals reported on earlier in this chapter.

Phenylalanine is a natural amino acid the body requires. It acts on your appestat, the control center that signals hunger. Mother Nature knows what she's about. When you are over-weight, phenylalanine exerts a natural appetite-suppressant effect; when you need to gain weight, it works in the reverse.

The chemical drug in over-the-counter weight-loss tablets and pills is a manmade cousin called *phenylpropanolamine.* Phenylpropanolamine chemically depresses the appetite, whether you are fat or thin or just-right. It can also give you the jitters and leave you with a drug-induced 'hangover' and can be addictive. Phenylpropanolamine is also present in decon-gestants, explaining why one of the side-effects of these products is a loss of appetite. Products that include phenylpropanolamine as an ingredient must by law carry a warning that they should not be taken by persons with certain conditions, including thyroid problems and high blood pressure.

Health And Beauty

Basic beauty begins with the glow of good health that shines from within. A scrubbed and radiant complexion transforms any woman (or man) into a singularly attractive person. On the other hand, a dull muddy skin, often caused by poor nutrition, can detract from the most attractive. Studies have shown that unhealthy and/or aging skin will be dramatically improved by the consumption of honeybee pollen.

When it's included daily in the diet, honeybee pollen not only gives you the glow of health and aids in safe permanent weight loss, it can be blended into seemingly 'magic potions' to smooth, soothe, and rejuvenate every inch of the outside of your body, too. Several relatively inexpensive mixtures, used externally, will revitalize and rejuvenate the complexion.

In his book, *Bee Pollen & Your Health*, noted medical author Carlson Wade details several. Wade says that a pure, natural deep-cleanser can be made by simply mixing 1 tablespoon of honeybee pollen grains with the yolk of an egg, ½ cup milk, and half of a ripe avocado. To keep your complexion free of pollutants which can interfere with proper skin function, simply apply with cotton balls.

To slough off dead skin cells clear down to the shine, Carlson Wade recommends the following scrub. Mix 1 tablespoon honeybee pollen grains into half a ripe avocado (mashed) and blend in ½ cup fine cornmeal. After cleansing the face thoroughly, rub this mixture into any trouble spots. Remove with a damp washcloth and splash with cold water to close the pores.

For all-over satin smoothness, Wade suggests a blend of 2 tablespoons honeybee pollen granules mixed into half a ripe avocado (mashed) and ½ cup ordinary table salt. When thoroughly combined, rub all over your body with particular attention to any rough sports. Dead skin cells will slough away quickly. Shower off. Warning: This mixture is too strong for delicate facial skin.

For a fantastic skin rejuvenator, blend 2 teaspoons of honeybee pollen granules with ¼ ripe avocado (mashed), 2 tablespoons instant nonfat dry milk, and 2 tablespoons of water. Mix thoroughly until you have a pale green cream (a blender will help). Apply to clean skin and leave in place until your skin begins to tighten. Add another layer. When that dries (about ten minutes), remove with lukewarm water and a washcloth. Rinse well.

It was Dr. Lars-Erik Essen, M.D., a dermatologist of Halsinborg, Sweden, who pioneered the use of rejuvenating honeybee pollen. He has treated many of his patients successfully for acne by this method. Dr. Essen says, "Through transcutaneous nutrition, bee pollen exerts a profound biological effect. It seems to prevent premature aging of the cells and stimulates growth of new skin tissue. It offers effective protection against dehydration and injects new life into dry cells. It smooths away wrinkles and stimulates a life-giving blood supply to all skin cells.

"The skin becomes younger-looking, less vulnerable to wrinkles, smoother and healthier with the use of honeybee pollen. Taken internally or used externally, bee pollen exercises a suppressive effect on facial acne and is an important skin rejuvenator because it contains a high concentration of the nucleic acids, RNA and DNA, and a natural antibiotic."

Carlson Wade has developed a kitchen recipe for a bee pollen lotion which he says is a good thing to keep in your refrigerator at all times. Make this up in any quantity you wish, using the following proportions: For every cup of strained fresh lemon juice, add 1 teaspoon bee pollen grains and ½ cup water. Shake well. Use this astringent lotion as a quick facial, as a base for mixing with other ingredients, or as a splash to revive tired or aging skin. This will keep well in the refrigerator.

A nourishing all-purpose cream can be made easily by mashing a very ripe banana and half an avocado with 2 teaspoons of honeybee pollen grains. When thoroughly blended, Wade reports you will have a cream that can be easily applied with fingertips. This rich cream will help smooth out fine lines as it corrects dryness. Smooth on delicate facial skiin and leave in place for up to sixty minutes. Store any unused portion in the refrigerator, tightly covered, but plan to use the remainder within two days.

The French, long noted for their preoccupation with all things beautiful, have done a great deal of research on the use of bee pollen in cosmetic preparations. Dr. M. Esperrois, M.D., of the French Institute of Chemistry, explains that honeybee pollen contains potent antibiotics which act to reverse the effects age exerts on skin, correcting darkening, wrinkles, and blemishes.

Count Michael d'Ornand's research led to the conviction that aging of the skin, darkening, wrinkles, and blemishes can be treated with specialized preparations which employ bee pollen. The Count points with pride to the 'firsts' he created, some of which are still creating a stir in the cosmetic world. Count d'Ornand pioneered the use of chicken embryos as a skin renewing agent, and was first to introduce royal jelly. The wonderous effects of royal jelly on the skin led to his research with bee pollen, the stuff of which royal jelly is made.

In *Literature on Pollen Cosmetology*, R. Lunden, says, "Bee pollen contains all the known vitamin Bs, and also all the hydro-soluble vitamins, and it contains the three essential lipo-soluble vitamins: A, D, and E. Bees instinctively choose only the best kinds of pollen. Therefore, the mixed pollens gathered from their hives are not only richest in vitamins, but they are also richest in antibiotic substances."

Professors N. Mankovsky and D.G. Chebotarev, two Soviet scientists, confirm that honeybee pollen stimulates cell-renewal. The rejuvenation of skin and body cells can be encouraged by the adminsitration of the poly-vitamins, microelements, enzymes, hormones, and amino acids present in bee pollen, which are used by the body to form new tissue. They praise the properties of bee pollen as vital to a form of internal and external rejuvenation at the cellular level.

Mother was wrong. Beauty isn't only skin deep. Proper attention to good nutrition and health practices will do more than just keep the doctor away. Vibrant health imparts a glow no cosmetic preparation can manufacture. The 18th century poet William Shenstone said it best: "Health is beauty, and the most perfect health is the most perfect beauty."

Longevity & The Aging Process

Ponce de Leon didn't have to travel half-way around the world. He might have found what he was looking for in his own backyard, if he had been a beekeeper. Honey and pollen have been used as both beautifiers and food since the dawn of time — and just might be the legendary 'Fountain of Youth' fabled in song and story.

In Norse mythology, the secret of the eternal life of their many gods was reputed to be ambrosia. Ambrosia is simply an incredibly rich combination of raw honey and 'bee bread, another name for the bee pollen which bees store in the waxen cells of honeycomb. This same food was reserved for the original Olympic athletes of ancient Greece to increase their energy and performance. Ancient texts unearthed in Babylon, China, Persia, and Egypt agree this revered food contains the secret of eternal youth and health.

Honey is mentioned in the Bible sixty-eight times as specially blessed food. In pre-Biblical times and for many centuries, all honey was raw wild honey, was eaten with the comb, and was loaded with bee pollen. Since the discovery of centrifigal force, now used to extract liquid honey from the comb, honey is commonly strained and processed, removing all the pollen-rich particles. When the health benefits grandmother attributed to honey have been tested with the pollen-free modern version of this ages-old medicinal, science calls them greatly exaggerated and untrue.

Today, we know that it is the bee pollen suspended in raw honey that gives this sweet treat from the hive its health-promoting life-extending powers.

In translation from the German, *Bee Pollen: Valuable Good*

Nutriment & Remedy, a book written by G. Liebold, a Holistic Physician and Psychologist of Karlsruhe, Germany, explains how bee pollen works against the aging process.

Bee pollen should be used as prophylaxis and therapeutical treatment against all the disease of modern civilization. The people of today often consume too many calories, without getting a sufficient amount of the vital substances. First in the spotlight is the need to improve the general condition of the body affected by nutrient malnutrition, stress, and other negative influences.

Bee pollen is an excellent prophylaxis and therapeutical treatment against all the precocious symptoms of old age. It should be considered a universal geriatric treatment in the form of a natural remedy. Bee pollen causes an increase in physical and mental abilities, especially of concentration and memory ability, activates sluggish metabolic functions, and strengthens the cardiovascular and respiratory systems. This natural nutriment from the bees removes the causes of cardiovascular symptoms, such as arteriosclerosis, cerebral insufficiency, and toher sequelae. It prevents nutrient deficiency during old age, gravidity (pregnancy), and the lactation (nursing) period. Bee pollen accelerates convalescence after serious illness and/or an operation, increases the body's physical defensive powers of the immune system, stimulates mental and psychological resistance to stress, and creates a harmonizing of vegetative and hormonal disorders.

Bee pollen is very complex in composition. It contains nutrients and vital substances in such manifold content that this composition is unique in nature. Only the natural completeness of bee pollen explains its effectiveness.

Many small villages dot the landscape high up in the Caucausus mountains of Russia where the air is always clear and sweet. In summer, the breezes are perfumed with the scent of thousands of wild flowers. Here the villagers work their small farms and tend their kitchen gardens without the dubious 'benefits' of the space-age technologies employed by agribusiness conglomerates. This is one of the few areas left in the world where the old ways prevail.

The stalwart families who make their homes in the mountainous regions of the Soviet Union are some of the most long-lived people in the world. On examination, many exhibit signs of 'silent heart disease,' scars of 'silent' heart attacks which would have certainly been lethal to a modern man. The hard physical work they do every day well into what some of us in the so-called civilized world consider 'old age' plays a part in their remarkable healthy lifestyle.

This small paradise is where Dr. Nicolai Vasilievich Tsitsin, the USSR's Chief Biologist and Botanist and an acknowledged expert on geriatrics, came to investigate those hardy souls who had sailed effortlessly past the century mark. He was amazed to find more than two hundred individuals who were over 125 years of age, all still working every day and participating actively in village life. The hard facts of their daily existence partially explained the extended lifespan they had achieved, but Dr. Tsitsin remained puzzled. He knew there had to be some other factor entering into the equation. He set himself the task of finding the common denominator. Then he stumbled upon it.

These people kept bees. Beekeeping is a profession which in itself historically confers some sort of 'magical' life protection on its members, a fact confirmed by today's scientific research.

Still, only very well informed modern beekeepers are know-ledgeable about the many health-promoting benefits of bee pollen and regularly serve it at table. The villagers didn't fit the profile. Dr. Tsitsin dug deeper.

And found the answer. These beekeepers, happy and fulfilled though they might be with their almost idyllic pastoral existence, were very poor. Bartering among themselves with an exchange of homegrown and handmade products and services was the accepted way of life. They had little cash available to them, so they regularly harvested — and sold or bartered away — the pure clear honey from the combs of their hives. What they kept for themselves and ate regularly was the thick residue which accumulated on the bottom of the hives. When he was served some of the sweet sticky stuff in the home of one of the villagers, Dr. Tsitsin realized that this was the magic elixir that contributed to their remarkable longevity. The tasty but unattractive glob was rich with golden granules of bee pollen.

Dr. Tsitsin attributes the remarkable health and extended lifespans of these Soviets to the scientifically-documented action of bee pollen and says that, taken regularly and in sufficient amounts, bee pollen will prolong the lifespan of man for many years.

Another USSR scientist, Naum Petrovich Ioyrish, Chief of the Soviet Academy of Vladivostok agrees. In 1975, Dr. Ioyrish reported without any qualification, "Long lives are attained by bee pollen users. It is one of the original treasure-houses of nutrition and medicine. Each grain contains every important substance necessary to life."

The Best Gets Better

At this writing, High-Desert Honeybee PollenS, acknowledged around the globe as the best bee pollen in the world, is about to get even better. The C C Pollen Company is currently negotiating with Soviet authorities to purchase approximately 70 tons of Caucausus Mountain bee pollen every year. When the arrangements are concluded and the first shipment comes in, the bee pollen of the world's longest-lived peoples will be blended with the fresh clean sweet pollens of High Desert. It can't get any better than this!

CHAPTER 9

PROPOLIS

What It Is & Why We Want It

The name *propolis* comes from two Greek words, *pro*, which means before, and *polis*, which means city. This ancient term came into being centuries ago when some early Greek student of nature established the fact that honeybees use propolis to narrow the opening into their cities, or hives, to keep out unwelcome intruders. Many sources attribute the word to Aristotle (384 - 322 BC).

What is Propolis?

Propolis is the sticky resin which seeps from the buds of certain trees, the bees prefer poplar, and oozes from the bark of other trees, chiefly conifers. You might not notice propolis exuding from the new buds on the new shoots the poplar puts forth in séason every year, but we've all seen shiny dribbles of resinous sap on the trunks of trees.

The bees gather propolis, sometimes called 'bee glue,' and carry it home in their pollen baskets. It is blended with wax flakes secreted from special glands on the underside of the bee's abdomen. Besides reducing the size of the hive entrance, the bees use the propolis and wax mixture as a caulking compound to plaster up any unwanted holes or openings to the outside.

Propolis is used to slickly line the interior of brood cells in preparation for the Queen's laying of eggs, a most important procedure. With its antiseptic properties, the propolis insures a hospital-clean environment for the rearing of brood.

Propolis is also used to completely seal off any dead aliens who have somehow managed to penetrate the city's considerable defenses. A wasp or other foreigner who makes it inside the hive is immediately stung to death. If the intruder is too large to remove, the bees gather together and quickly cover the corpse with a thick layer of propolis, completely sealing it off and thus preserving the pristine cleanliness of their environment.

Unless they themselves harvest propolis for market, beekeepers find propolis a nuisance. Although it hardens in the cold, it remains soft and sticky during warm weather and gets all over the beekeeper's hands and clothes. Because the bees instinctively close up any extraneous spaces in the hive with propolis, they install a thick layer of the stuff around the edges of the comb. In order to harvest the full combs of honey, the beekeeper has to cut around the edges to free the comb before he can remove it from the hive.

On the other hand, migratory beekeepers who transport their hives long distances appreciate the industry of the bees. The propolis caulking helps hold all the parts of the hive steady as they are bounced around when being trucked to distant fields.

Propolis Through the Ages

The Frankincense & Myrrh Connection — Even theological scholars well-versed in the intricacies of Biblical language aren't sure of the exact constituents of frankincense and myrrh, mentioned in the holy writings of many civilizations.

In *Matthew 2:11*, we learn that frankincense and myrrh were considered so precious in ancient times that, along with gold, they were carried as gifts to the newborn Christ Child. In *Exodus 30:23-25*, the Lord God instructs Moses in the preparation of "An ointment compound after the art of the apothecary; it shall be a holy annointing oil." One of the principle components of this holy ointment is myrrh. In *Exodus 30:34-38*, the Lord God directs Moses "thou shaft make perfume, a confection after the art of the apothecary, tempered together, pure and holy." This holy perfume employs frankincense. There are other Biblical references to these two holy substances as well.

A modern dictionary tells us that frankincense is an aromatic gum resin from various trees used chiefly for burning as incense in ceremonial practices and in perfumery. Myrrh is defined as an aromatic resinous exudation from certain plants used chiefly in incense and perfume. What we don't know is how frankincense and myrrh were collected in Biblical times. Because both are resinous exudations, as is propolis, some authorities believe that the ancients gathered these holy substances directly from the hives of wild bees.

Many scientific writers of ancient times, including Celsus

and Dioscorides, mention propolis and detail its use in unguents, poultices, and, in powdered form, against mouth and lung diseases. Artistotle wrote of propolis and identified its presence in the hives of honeybees.

The refined Greeks developed an exquisite perfume named polyanthos, which had a propolis base. The formula included finely powdered propolis with olibanum, styrax, and banzoin, blended with aromatic herbals. When this perfume was burned on live coals, a very delicate aromatic incense wafted through the air of patrician mansions.

Pliny the Elder (23-79 BC), the great Roman naturalist, had much to say about this natural medicinal from the bees. Pliny's encyclopedic 37-volume *Historia Naturalis* talks extensively of propolis, separating it into three distinct categories: Commosis, which refers to the bees' habit of using propolis as a disinfectant 'paint' for brood cells and the interior of the hive: *Pissoceros*, the mixture of propolis and wax used to close holes and reinforce structurally weak areas; and *Propolis*, used to reduce the size of the entrance to the bees' 'polis,' or city. Pliny also identified the medicinal action of propolis, including the reduction of swellings, the soothing of pain, and the healing of the most hopeless sores.

The Koran mentions propolis and identifies it as being distinctly different from bee pollen. Before their destruction by the Spanish conquistadors, it is known that the Incas (circa 1600) used propolis topically against inflammations and swellings of all kinds. During the Boer War (1988-1902), propolis mixed with vaseline was used to disinfect wounds sustained in battle and to speed healing.

On the technical side, propolis has long been the raw material of choice for the production of an exceptionally fine and smooth varnish. It is a known fact that the famed Antonius Stradivarius (1644-1737) handmixed his own propolis varnish for the incomparable musical instruments he handcrafted so long ago at his shop in Cremona, Italy. In his lifetime, Stradivarius produced only 1,116 stringed instruments. Those which survive, chiefly mellow-toned violins, are priceless. It has been said by musicians fortunate enough to possess one that a Stradivarius 'plays itself.' Stradivarius' formula for varnish has been lost. This may be one reason why the workmanship of this acknowledged master has never been duplicated.

Electromicroscopic analysis of a Guardangnini violin dating back to 1750 reveals the presence of bee pollen, bee hairs, and pieces of propolis in the varnish. In 1961, German researchers Knopf and Ogait almost, but not quite, succeeded in producing a varnish identical in composition to the Italian varnish used by Stradivarius and Guardagnini. String instrument manufacturers in many countries still buy propolis regularly, presumably still hoping to duplicate the magic that Stradivarius instilled in his instruments.

In past centuries, propolis dissolved in alcohol was used to preserve the shining finish of the gold leaf which brightened statuary, moldings, and plaster ornamentation of walls and panels in fashion at many times throughout history. Propolis dissolved in turpentine or alcohol was often added to molten silver or tin to give the resulting leaves and bars a rich golden hue. Leather treated with propolis develops a superior luster, a process still used today in some areas of the world.

In Mongolia and Siberia, natives often diluted propolis with oil or turpentine and immersed their sleds in the mixture. It is written that wood so treated is able to withstand the worst snow and cold. Propolis has always been in demand in Russia and other areas of the world where the weather is intensely cold.

The Propolis Hunter

In spite of its importance to the colony, there are usually just a few propolis-gathering specialists in each hive. Bees of foraging age collect propolis only during warm days when the resinous exudate is soft and malleable. The propolis-gatherer flies to the source, bites into it with her sharp mandibles to free a bit, and finally tears off a tiny glob. If it is exceptionally sticky, she may take time to knead it into shape before transferring the bit to one of her pollen baskets. She then repeats the procedure, placing the next bit into the pollen basket on the opposite leg. She continues in this manner, placing the tiny globs in baskets on alternate legs to keep the load balanced. If the original source becomes exhausted and she has to search for more, it may take an hour before she has both baskets fully loaded with propolis.

Once she has her baskets chockful, she returns to the hive with her burden. There she is met by one or more worker bees whose task it is to help her unload. The helpers reverse the procedure, biting and pulling off one tiny piece of propolis at a time before pressing it firmly into the area of the hive selected for reinforcement. Because the helpers may be busily secreting wax flakes and blending the propolis into it as they work, this unloading procedure may take up to several hours before the propolis-gatherer's baskets are completely empty. After she is freed of her load, she flies off to forage for more.

It has been established that bees are impervious to any virus or bacteria. This innate ability to defend themselves against infectious diseases is very important. Any contagion could run rampant and rapidly destroy all 20,000 to 100,000 members of a colony living together in the very close quarters of the hive. Certainly the bee's good health can be attributed, at least in part, to a genetic immunity.

The bees are out and about in an increasingly polluted environment every day. They come in contact with many chemicals, some harmful, in a day's work, but they enjoy yet another form of natural protection. The experts point out that the bees are effectively 'decontaminated' as they pass over the propolis barrier guarding the entrance.

The Constituents of Bee Propolis

Chemically speaking, propolis is a very complex mixture that varies according to the source from which it comes. Colors range from brownish-green to reddish-brown to blackish-brown. A broad analysis reveals approximately 55 percent resinous compounds and balsams, 30 percent beeswax, 10 percent ethereal and aromatic oils, and 5 percent bee pollen. Many flavonols contribute to propolis. Other components include cinnamic acid, cinnamyl alcohol, vanillin, caffeic acid, tectochrysin, isalpinin, pinocembrin, chrysin, galangin, and ferulic acid.

The Properties of Propolis

Propolis is another wonder from the beehive. Research shows it offers antiseptic, antibiotic, antibacterial, antifungal, and even antiviral properties. Propolis is nature's premiere preventive. It is so powerful in action that it is often called 'Russian penicillin' in acknowledgement of the extensive research the Soviets have mounted on this natural medicinal from the beehive.

Propolis demonstrates strong antimicrobial properties against various bacteria and fungal infestations. Even streptococcus bacteria has been shown sensitive to propolis. The experts say that at least part of this documented bacteriostatic power can be attributed to the galangin, caffeic acid, and ferulic acid content of propolis.

For an overview of the many benefits of propolis, we turn to a paper entitled, *Propolis, Natural Substance, The Way to Health*, by the well-known naturalist and medical writer of Denmark, K Lund Aagaard. In this eight-page paper, Aagaard reports on extensive research conducted in Scandinavia, as follows:

During my long practice, I had the opportunity to examine certain affections and often experimented with propolis in its natural form. I obtained relevant results for the cases treated. Based on close cooperation, these experiments involved more than 50,000 persons all across Scandinavia.

The field of influence of propolis is extemely broad and includes: swelling of the large intestine, catarrh of the eyes, infection of the urinary tract, swelling of the throat, gout, open wounds, sinus swellings, colds, influenza, bronchitis, gastritis, cancer, diseases of the ears, periodontial disease, caephalea, intestinal infections, micoses, ulcers, eczema eruptions, pneumonia, arthritis, lung disease, stomach virus, headaches, Parkinson's disease, bile infections, sclerosis, circulation deficiencies, warts, conjunctivitis, and hoarseness.

Propolis has a refreshing effect both for regulating hormones and as an antibiotic substance which is in itself a stimulator of the natural resistance of the body. Propolis may be used by everybody, sick or healthy, as a means of protection against microorganisms. Propolis is also efficient in a series of affections caused by bacteria, viruses, or different fungi. Propolis cures almost all diseases because it is a special natural substance with strong effect.

The whole research program, with thousands of cases, had a single purpose, namely, to obtain a substance with the greatest efficiency against the greatest number of diseases mentioned. The numerous healings are relevant by themselves and the number of people who use propolis is ever increasing.

In Rumania, the medical researchers N. Popovici and N. Oita, zeroed in on one of the most important effects of propolis. Their paper is entitled, *Influence of Extracts of Propolis on Mitosis.*

Mitosis is a medical term for the process of cell division. In cancer, malignant cells divide and multiply out of control. Obviously, a substance which affects cell division is very important in the management of this lethal disease. Pertinent excerpts follow:

Opening Statement: Visible remissions in some cases of malignant tumors and leukemia reported by some authors as a result of the administration of propolis determined us to study the mechanism of the action of propolis on some vegetal meristems (embryonic actively-dividing cells) whose cells were genetically un-balanced, as is the case with cancerous cells.

Discussion: If we refer to the mitodepressive (repression of the proliferation of cancerous cells) principles of propolis on cells which are deranged by malignancy, the cases of remissions of cancerous tumors and leukemia mentioned at the beginning of this paper could be explained by a similar action.

A tissue never becomes entirely malignant; it will always con-tain some normal cells, but the activity of the normal cells will be affected or even repressed by malignant cells. By repressing malig-nant cells, propolis favors the activity of normal cells, helping the body to reestablish its normal condition.

Conclusion: Further experiments are necessary to determine the relation between remissions of cancerous tumors and leukemia as a result of the administration of propolis and the cytological ef-fects of this bee product.

One of the valuable properties of the natural products of the beehive is the fact that they exhibit true immunostimulating characteristics. Unlike many modern medical drugs, propolis (or bee pollen) does not depress the immune sytem. Instead, these beemade products boost the immune defense forces of the body.

The USSR has conducted considerable research on propolis. In a paper entitled, *Propolis Impact on the Immunogenesis in the Case of Immunization with Anatoxin,* Soviet scientists V.P. Kivalkina and E.L. Budarkova document the dramatic effects pro-polis exerts on the immune system, as follows:

Opening Statement: Propolis has drawn attention to itself more and more as being a nonspecific stimulator of the immunologic reaction. In the Department of Microbiology of the Kazan Institute, the favorable impact of propolis on immunogenesis has been established.

Discussion: Our present work studies the effects of propolis on the immunologic rates by simultaneous administration with anatoxin. Propolis was added to anatoxin in the form of alcohol extract. Two series of experiments were conducted.

Results: The antitoxin content from blood serum in rabbits immunized with propolis-anatoxin was higher than in those administered the same antigen levels without propolis. During the whole experiment, the titre (strength per volume) of the complement in the animals which received propolis-anatoxin was higher than in the control groups.

The data obtained demonstrate that the hyperimmunization of the animals with propolis-anatoxin stimulates specific and nonspecific factors. As the antitoxin accumulated in the animals' blood, the protective characteristics of the sera increased. The blood sera of the experimental animals protected them from death to a greater extent than the blood sera from the control group.

Research in the second series of experiments showed that as the antitoxin accumulated in the blood, the prophilaxis power of the sera increased. In all research periods, the blood sera of the propolis-anatoxin immunized animals protected them to a greater extent than in animals which received anatoxin without propolis.

Equally impressive results were obtained by V.P. Kivalkina, A.I. Balalykina, and V.I. Piontkovski, also of the USSR. This paper is entitled, *Plasmocitary Response in White Mice Immunized with an Antigen Associated with Propolis.* We excerpt from the opening statement and conclusion, as follows:

Opening Statement: The purpose of our present work is to study the impact of propolis administered together with an antigen on the plasmocitary (blood, bone marrow) response, which constitutes one of the main proofs of the immunologic altering of the organism which is present soon after immunization.

Conclusion: Cytologic (cell) analysis shows that the immunologic response is more intensely manifest in a very short time by an increase in the number of cells from the plasmocitary series in the regional lymphatic ganglions. (The lymphatic system is the base of operations for the immune system.) The aglutinynes titres in the blood serum of animals immunized with propolis-antigen were 3.7 to 4 times greater than those of animals inoculated with complete antigen combined with other adjuvants.

The conclusion is that propolis-antigens stimulate the plasmocitary response and the development of antibodies in the regional and peripheric lymphatic organs.

Chemical antibiotics destroy all bacteria in the body, both the friendly and necessary flora required for healthy functioning for the entire gastrointestinal tract, as well as the bad. And an individual who constantly takes prescribed antibiotics for one condition after another soon learns to his sorrow that drugs no longer work as well as they once did. As the bacteria gets 'smarter,' the drugs become less and less effective as time goes on.

It is a medical fact that some biologically harmful strains of bacteria develop a resistance to chemical antibiotics because they learn to defend against a drug. Some harmful microorganisms are able to subtly change their characteristics. Where once certain strains were easily detroyed by medical drugs, a bacteria can develop defenses that leave the body open to their destructive effects.

Propolis, the natural antibiotic, works against harmful bacteria without destroying the friendly bacteria the body needs. Propolis has also been proven effective against strains of bacteria that resist chemical antibiotics.

We excerpt next from an important paper published by Polish scientists S. Scheller, J. Tustanowski, and Z. Paradowski entitled, *Comparative Study on the Staphylococcus Sensitivity to Propolis and to Antibiotics*, as follows:

Opening Statement: Following recent prior research conducted in our laboratory, we have determined the range of sensitivity of bacteria to an alcohol-propolis solution, which proves the efficiency of this solution in the treatment of purulent dermatitis and gynacological affections.

During this test, we compare the sensitiveness of staphylococci isolated from pathogen sources with that of strains in our collection. Our second goal was to prove the possible correlation between the sensitiveness to propolis and antibiotics of the staphylococci isolated from pathogen sources.

Material: We tested 56 staphylococcus strains isolated from pathogen sources. The antibacterial effect of propolis, by inhibition of the development of standard strains, was determined for 3 mg/ml. The sensitivity of staphylococci to antibiotics was determined by the common method of discs. The antibiotics used were penicillin, ampicillin, meticillin, streptomycin, cloramphenicol, terramycin, erythrocyn, myacyn, and sulphathiazole.

Results: All strains whose sensitivity to propolis was certain were highly resistant to the tested antibiotics. Even strains with low sensitivity to propolis exhibited a wide range in degree of sensitivity to antibiotics, as did the resistant strains. For the last two groups, a general reduction of their sensitivity to antibiotics was recorded.

On the same subject, we proceed next with brief excerpts

from a paper from Czechoslovakia authored by L. Vechet. It is entitled, *Effect of Propolis on Some Species of Microorganisms and Molds.*

Opening Statement: A great deal of attention is being given at present to the study of propolis, not only in the domain of apiculture, but also in chemistry and medicine. I am interested in propolis not only as a beekeeper, which I am, but also as a chemist because I work in the industry of antibiotics. The purpose of this experiment is to draw some conclusions as regards to the antimicrobial effect of propolis on some microbes, molds, and yeasts.

Results: To establish the relative effect of propolis as compared to antibiotics, staphylococcus aureas was used as a microorganism for testing. Materials used: Propolis dissolved in ethyl alcohol (1:3); penicillin in units of 16, 8, 4. Propolis created inhibition zones, but penicillin did not.

For determining the propolis effect compared to the effect of a fungicidine, the yeast Saccharomyces cerevisiae was used as a microorganism for testing. Materials used: Propolis dissolved in ethyl alcohol (1:3); fungicidine in units of 100, 50, and 25. Propolis created a greater field of inhibition and its effects lasted longer than that of the fungicide.

The antibiotic effects of the propolis solution corresponds to the value of 16 units penicillin; the antifungal effects of the propolis solution to 25 units of fungicide.

Empirical Evidence

Empirical, or testimonial, evidence of the benefits of propolis are as many and varied as are those for bee pollen. Because propolis is not yet well known in the U.S., most of the following experiences have been culled from reports originating overseas. We bring them to you in translation from the language of origin, as written by various individuals.

The first is a modern account of the Yugoslav church painter, Rado Seifert, credited with the rediscovery of the benefits of propolis by Mitja Vosnjak, author of *The Miracle of Propolis*. According to legend, it was in the 1800s when Seifert earned two beehives as payment for restoring a shrine, which subsequently led to his first experience with propolis. Vosnjak tells how it happened.

"Seifert's health was threatened. Something strange began to happen to his left leg, his feet, and toes. The skin became increasingly dark purple, finally, almost black; his toes were ice-cold, completely without feeling, and on one, a large infected ulcer opened up and refused to heal. Every week he went to the doctor, who put ointment on the ulcer, jabbed his leg with needles, and established it really was without feeling. It was finally recommended, apparently as the only possibility, that half the leg be amputated straight away.

"Rado refused the operation and put on his boots. He would not give up so quickly. At home, he covered his leg with honey rich with propolis and bandaged it. After a few days, when he took off the bandages and cleaned his leg, he could not believe his eyes. The ulcer on his toe was gone, healed; his foot was warmer than before and no longer hurt him when he stood firmly on the floor.

"Once more he went to the doctor and there was no further talk of amputation. He could not resist saying, as he walked out, 'If ever someone else comes with the same problem, try propolis and honey first. Time enough for the scalpel later!'"

Rado collected pure propolis from his bees and kept it in the house. When his wife burned her fingers with boiling oil, he used some of the resinous stuff as an ointment. His wife's fingers stopped hurting. In just a few days, she was completely healed and no trace of a scar remained. After several more such experiences, Rado decided he had to share this great discovery with the village doctor, and proceeded to do so, saying:

" 'Look, Max, I've brought you this bee medicine to try. You have enough patients in hospital. You can easily find which ones it will help.' Quietly and patiently he waited for an answer. Doctor Max Kern shook his head 'no' firmly." Time passed. Then something happened which decided the doctor to try the bee medicine after all.

"The little girl, only four years old, was lying curled up almost asleep, but moving restlessly, sometimes trembling violently. In the morning, she had felt dizzy. Her mother and father decided she must stay home from kindergarten. Her throat hurt. Even when her mother boiled her an egg, she pushed the tray away. She took nothing but water, weak tea, or milk, for she was terribly thirsty and hot. By midday, she was no better, but she wanted more and still more to drink because she was so very thirsty.

"Then Uncle Max, her father's doctor-friend, came to visit. With a little persuasion and a few tears, little Barbara opened her mouth while Dr. Max pressed her tongue down with a spoon. 'Yes, yes,' he said, 'just as I thought. Bad tonsillitis again. That's the fourth time this year.' Barbara often had to stay in bed with tonsillitis, but this time the infection was supperating. Barbara always had to take tablets that were bitter and hard to swallow. Sometimes the doctor would come with a needle he put deep under her skin. 'She's quite hot,' the doctor said. 'Her temperature is 39.7 degrees (103⁰ F.). I'lll have to give her something.'

" 'What will you have Barbara, an injection or a sweet?' he asked. Little Barbara smiled and said she would rather have a sweet. Mother brought a lump of sugar from the kitchen. Dr. Max took a brown bottle from his pocket and put a few drops of the liquid on the sugar. Barbara put the propolis-drenched sugar cube in her mouth and smiled.

"Barbara slept. Two hours later, they awakened the peacefully sleeping child and gave her another of Dr. Max's special sugar cubes. Her father took her temperature and couldn't believe his eyes. In only two hours, her fever had dropped from 103⁰ to 99.7⁰. All night, the child slept quietly. When she awakened naturally in the morning, she asked her mother to take her to kindergarten.

" 'Wait a moment, sweetheart,' her father smiled, 'we must see if you have a temperature.' But she didn't! The thermometer showed normal. No high temperature; no infected throat; no more pain, only an enormous healthy appetite. Never before had she recovered so quickly. To put their minds at rest, the parents took her for a checkup with an ear, nose, and throat specialist.

" 'Why have you brought this child?' asked the surprised doctor. 'There's nothing the matter with her. The mucous membranes are nicely firm, no trace of infection in her tonsils. She's perfectly healthy.'

"That evening, the mother went to Dr. Max and asked if he would give her more of the 'miracle' medicine in case Barbara should have another attack of tonsillitis. Dr. Max gave her a medicine bottle and told her what it was, saying, 'It's nothing very special, just propolis dissolved in alcohol. It's something that comes from the beehive.'

"A decade passed by. Yet one thing did not change. Dr. Max still believed in the power of his propolis-drenched 'sweets,' and also in ointments, capsules, and various other medicines containing his precious natural healer, propolis, which he got from the beekeeper, Rado Seifert."

The remarkable power of propolis against throat infections has been discovered and rediscovered time and time again. Here is another account testifying to overnight healing.

"On June 3rd, 1967, I experienced an incident which led subsequently to unexpected consequences of great importance. I did not feel very well because of some throat trouble which I had for a couple of days, yet I was obliged to go on a business trip. At supper, the swelling in my throat became so annoying that I could not swallow anything and I found I had a temperature of over 40⁰C. (101.2⁰ F.) I decided to try some propolis.

"I crushed a bit of propolis in a mortar and dissolved the powder in a cup of warm water. I filtered it through a coffee filter and obtained a yellow infusion, like tea. I gargled with this 'tea' two or three times, then I drank the rest and went to bed. In the morning, I found myself in perfect good health. I had only a slight red spot left in my throat, which disappeared during the day.

"I drew the conclusion that propolis contains a very strong antibiotic if it could cure such a powerful infection and swelling in just five to six hours." *K.L.A. (Denmark)*

"In the summer I had a painful catarrh (painful inflammation of the mucous membranes) of the eye. The drops for the eye prescribed by the doctor did not cure me. When I saw that the sickness still persisted, I tried to treat it with propolis. I crushed a little dry propolis with the back of a spoon, then dissolved it in warm water. After I strained it, I dripped this solution in my eye with a dropper. The eye smarted a little, but I stood it. Next morning, the catarrh had disappeared." *Mrs. J.A. (Czechoslovakia)*

The following experience of a 42-year old man, F.W.S., was so remarkable that an account of his healing appeared in several European newspapers headlined "He Was Cured." Here is the story:

"I was diagnosed as having cancer and had a long operation. After my surgery wound was healed, they made me have 36 cobalt ray sittings (radiation therapy). Then I was sent home and could eat only liquids because I was nauseated and vomited solid food. My weight was only 54 kg (109 lbs) and I had two sores in my mouth, which the physicians tried to heal with medicines. Because my situation did not improve after eight months, the physicians decided that they would have to operate on me again, in a month's time."

The newspaper account explains: "This patient obtained propolis from a relative just six days before the operation. On being examined before the operation, the doctors noticed that the cancer ulcers previously operated on had completely dried and could be easily removed with tweezers. The operation was now considered unnecessary."

F.W.S. continues his story: "Thus discovering the effects of propolis, I went on taking it. I was able to resume my work and regained the 20 kg (45 lbs) I had lost. After six months, I stopped taking propolis, breaking the therapy for seven or eight months.

"Then the physicians found another malignant swelling on my pancreas, which they treated in hospital by normal methods and radiotherapy. I quickly resumed treatment with propolis. When the doctors asked me whether I had taken medications prescribed by them, I answered that I had taken only propolis. There was much surprise when the physicians found propolis was the only medicine I took. More surprise when today I can eat and drink anything, even a glass of beer or even plum brandy.

"For prophylaxis and maintenance, I continue to permanently take a half spoonful of propolis every day, together with food." F.W.S. (Madrid)

"I am a nurse and work in the free clinic in my city. I am constantly in contact with sick people, many of whom have some contagious disease. During the last viral influenza outbreak, I was just about the only worker in the clinic who did not get it. I am never ill and never catch anything. My associates marvel that I seem to have an inborn immunity. I have explained many times that I take propolis regularly as natural preventative medicine. I tell them that this miracle from the beehive is what gives me immunity. But they are too thoroughly indoctrinated in orthodox medicine. They laugh and will not listen. I am living proof of the power of propolis, but still they scoff. I know better. I will never give up my daily dose of propolis." *B.N. (Rumania)*

Because of its infection-fighting antiseptic and antibiotic properties, propolis works miracles against common skin afflictions, including stubborn cases of long-standing acne. One woman writes:

"Though I am in middle life, age 46, I have always had the worst complexion. Since I was in my teens, my face, chin especially, always has had ugly bumps of pimples that break open and weep pus. I want to hide my face so no one will see my shame. Doctors give me medicine for inside and outside, but nothing helps for very long. Still the pimples come again and again and stay a long time and more come after. I think my whole life will be like that. My daughters and son have the same thing and that makes me sorrow more.

"But then the sister of my neighbor came to our village to visit. She tells me that this need not be, that she knows what to do to clear up my face for always. I do not believe, but I listen and do what she say. This smart sister took some brown sticky stuff from the beehive that she say is propolis. She melted the propolis stuff in some honey and gave it to me in a little jar, telling me to smear it on my face at night and in the morning, promising it will work even though doctor's medicines do nothing. I do it.

"After two times, scabs come and weeping stops. I am happy and do the treatment on my daughters and my son also. Same thing happens with them. In two weeks, all our faces are clear and smooth. Even the scars from old pimples seem to go away. I am glad for this woman's great knowledge and kiss her hand many times for thanks. I make the propolis-honey myself now and will always to keep my family from the great embarrassment I have for many years before knowing this great secret."
M.E.S. (Hungary)

Down through the ages, beekeepers have developed many home remedies employing the products of their hives. One of the long established effects of propolis is its remarkable power against periodontal disease. Gum inflammations (gingivitis) and infected mucous membranes inside the mouth heal quickly. And, because propolis has documented anesthetic properties, it works fast to relieve the pain of toothache. A Georgian (USSR) farmer and beekeeper explains:

"I woke in the night with a throbbing pain all over the right side of my face. I knew it was the same infected tooth that bothered me so often, but the dentist of our village was away. I tried to sleep, but it was impossible. By dawn, the whole side of my face was swollen terrible and the pain was so bad I could hardly stand it.

"As soon as it was light enough to see, I prepared the smoker and hurried out to the hives. I knew the bees would be angry at being disturbed so early in the cool of the morning, they don't like to fly until the sun warms the fields, but I didn't care. I just knew I must get some propolis into my mouth as quickly as I could. I opened one hive and snicked off a big piece of propolis with my knife even though many bees were buzzing angrily around me.

"Then I hurried back to the warmth of the kitchen. The propolis was hard and brittle from the night cold. My good woman had the kettle boiling, so I speared the glob with my knife and held it in the steam coming from the kettle. As soon as it softened a little, I pulled off a chunk and put it in my mouth. I chewed it a bit on my good side and the bitter juice went down my throat. Soon I had it soft and was able to position it against my bad tooth. I molded it around the aching tooth with my finger. The gum was bad swollen up and almost covered the whole tooth. I wanted my tea, but was afraid even to sip it from the saucer for fear I would dislodge the propolis.

"Still, there was much work to be done and I went to tend the fields with my sons like always. Not so fast as I wanted, but soon enough the pain of my face eased and the throbbing in my tooth stopped. We worked until midday. By then, the swelling was down considerable and the propolis was almost entirely gone in juices down my throat. I was able to eat hearty. Before returning to the fields, I fixed another propolis wad and put it again around the tooth. When we came in at dusk to a big supper,

I felt good with no more swelling or pain. I had much vodka with much pleasure and laughed with my sons at giving the dentist no business that day." *G.V.M. (USSR)*

Old-Time Propolis Remedies

In the past, no household pharmacopeia was complete without a store of propolis, either in lump, tincture (alcohol solution), or tea (infusion made with boiling water) form. Now it's no longer necessary to brave the bees in order to put propolis in your medicine cabinet. This natural antibiotic is available in health food stores. However, we have it on good authority that these homely remedies from yesteryear are just as effective today as they were then. Here's a peek into the past.

Corns — To get rid of a corn, coat the area with a thick layer of propolis and cover. In ages past, country people wrapped soft clean cloth around the whole foot, but a bandaid will work just as well. Apply more propolis every night before going to bed. It is said that in just a few days the hard corn will soften and can soon be easily removed.

Sore Throat — For a sore throat, put a lump of propolis in your mouth and let it melt. The juice is bitter, but the results are remarkable. As you swallow the propolis-rich saliva, your entire throat is treated to a disinfecting antibiotic bath. Swelling is reduced and the infection usually clears up overnight.

Minor Burns — Treat minor burns with propolis-tea. Prepare an infusion of propolis by pouring boiling water over a lump and allowing it to steep. Pour the resulting propolis-tea in a sterile jar and keep it on hand. Should a burn occur, bathe the affected area with the propolis solution immediately. The area cools quickly and healing is speedy. (Note: Burns should not be treated with grease (including butter) or ointment. Greasy substances seal in the heat, instead of allowing it to dissipate. If you have no propolis solution ready, use cold water.)

Preventive Medicine — Steep a lump of propolis in pure food-grade alcoholic spirits (not rubbing alcohol). Vodka is excellent. The resulting brown liquid can be taken by the teaspoonful, on a sugar cube, or on a square of bread. Taken daily, this old-fashioned European folk remedy constitutes real preventive medicine.

Those country people of ages past knew what they were about. Modern scientific studies show that those who take propolis regularly escape winter colds and sore throats, never succumb to bronchitis, and actually develop a natural immunity to common viruses, including all the various strains of flu. It will work for you, too. Propolis really is strong preventive medicine.

CHAPTER 10

ROYAL JELLY

What It Is and Why We Want It

Royal jelly is the rich royal milk fed to the Queen bee for the whole of her life. Royal jelly plays an absolutely necessary role in the making of a Queen. Queen bees are made, not born. Although eggs to be reared as queens are laid in specially prepared super-size brood cells, the eggs deposited therein by the queen mother are identical to those eggs which are destined to become the sexless worker bees of the hive. They are not genetically superior in any way, as you will see.

The Rearing of Worker Bees

During the first three days of larval development, the baby worker bees are fed a diluted form of royal jelly liberally mixed with honey. This rich brood food is supplied so generously that the tiny young larvae actually lie in a pool of it within their individual brood comb cells. But this mass feeding period comes abruptly to an end after three days. The quality of the brood food changes and quantities are reduced sharply.

During the last three days of larval life, less rich food is supplied and is given only as it is needed. During the final stages, the development of the worker-larva's sex glands is suppressed. But the development of brood food glands, the glands which will secrete royal jelly to feed the Queen, mature and the wax glands develop fully. Should royal jelly, even in diluted form, continue to be supplied, a queen would be produced.

The Rearing of a Queen

Throughout her entire larval period, an egg reared to be Queen is supplied with highly-nutritive hormone-rich royal jelly. Without this rich royal milk, she would fail to develop properly and the result would be merely another worker for the hive. It is this royal diet which single-handedly transforms her into a Queen.

As she continues to feed on royal jelly past the three day cut-off for workers, the Queen grows a modified stinger. Unlike worker bees, the Queen's stinger is curved, not straight. The Queen's Guard takes care of hive defense, so she will never sting an intruder or give her life to protect the entrance to the hive. Because the Queen will use her stinger only to defend her royal right to rule, the Queen can retract her stinger after shooting out venom. Unlike a worker bee, the Queen does not die after stinging.

There are other major differences in the development process, too. As an adult, the Queen will have no wax glands. It is the worker bees who build comb. The Queen will have no pollen baskets on her back legs. It is the workers who forage for pollen and propolis. And the Queen will have no hypopharyngeal glands to secrete royal jelly. Nurse bees secrete royal jelly.

The Queen's sex organs progress to fully-ripe maturity as she passes through the larval and pupal stages of her development. When she emerges as a royal adult Queen, her body will be noticeably larger and clearly superior to those of her sisters, the sexless workers of the hive. An average queen bee measures 17mm. and weighs 200 mg, compared to 12 mm. and 125 mg for the worker bee. Royal jelly gives the royal beauty a 42 percent increase in size and a 60 percent superiority in weight over the workers of the court.

And nature builds in yet another advantage. Because the Queen is so necessary to the colony, her royal development to full adulthood is accomplished in just 16 days, thanks to her richly royal diet, compared to the 21 days it takes to rear a worker.

The Queen has another advantage, too. Her lifespan is measured in years, while a worker bee's lifespan is measured in weeks. A Queen will live *forty times* longer than the ladies of her court. (We emphasize that the figure is forty *times,* not a 'mere' 40 percent, although even that percentage would be impressive.) In the wild, a Queen will live productively for five to seven years. Worker bees are worn out and die at an average age of seven to eight weeks. Workers are expendable; the Queen is not.

During her remarkably extended lifespan, the Queen will lay around 2,000 eggs per day, and each batch of brood has a total weight greater than *two-and-one-half times her own body weight.*

The Queen feasts on royal jelly for her entire lifetime. It is this remarkable food alone which insures her superior development and incredible longevity. Remember, a Queen does not start off with an inborn genetic superiority at all. It is the direct feeding of each and every cell in her body with richly-nutritive royal jelly which first creates and then sustains the Queen for the whole of her extra-long life.

What Is Royal Jelly?

Because it is fed directly from the worker to the Queen, many beekeepers themselves have never really had a chance to examine royal jelly. Nurse bees between five to fifteen days of age secrete the rich royal milk. In the nursing phase, these workers practically force-feed themselves near to bursting on an incredibly rich diet of bee pollen and honey in order to be able to produce royal jelly. The queen drinks her fill directly from a nurse's hypopharyngeal glands.

This thick fluid is creamy in consistency and milky-white in appearance. Royal jelly is synthesized in nurse bees' bodies during the digestion of bee pollen, accounting for its remarkable quantities of hormonal substance and the strong proteins found in its highly nitrogenous composition. It has a slightly pungent odor. The Queen obviously thinks royal jelly is delicious, but we find it very bitter on the tongue.

Royal jelly is chemically very complex. A broad chemical

analysis reveals a moisture content of 66.05 percent; proteins 12.34 percent; lipids 5.46 percent; reducing substance 12.49 percent; minerals .82 percent; with unidentifiable elements totalling 2.84 percent. And here we are again with the 'magic' of the bee. Like bee pollen, science still hasn't been able to completely identify and isolate all the important constituents of royal jelly, let alone synthesize a satisfactory 'substitute' in a laboratory.

It is known that royal jelly is exceptionally rich in natural hormones, offers an abundance of B vitamins (including thiamine, riboflavin, pyridoxine, niacin, pantothenic acid, biotin, inositol, and folic acid), plus vitamins A, C, and E. With twenty amino acids, royal jelly is a highly concentrated source of rich proteins, including cystine, lysine, and arginine. It possess important fatty acids, sugars, sterols, phosphorus compounds, as well as acetylcholine. Acetylcholine is important in the transmission of nerve messages and assists in the production of glandular secretions. Royal jelly is rich in nucleic acids. The nucleic acids in royal jelly include DNA (deoxyribonucleic acid) and RNA (ribonucleic acid), the very stuff of which life is made. Gelatin, one of the precursors of collagen, is another component of royal jelly. Collagen is a powerful anti-aging element that keeps us youthful.

The presence of gamma globulin, an infection-fighting and immuno-stimulating factor has been documented in royal jelly. And, not surprisingly, royal jelly also contains decanoic acid, which exhibits strong antibiotic activity against many bacteria and fungal infestations. Without this built-in antibiotic factor, science points out that the richness of royal jelly would offer an excellent growing medium for all kinds of harmful microbes. Mother Nature takes care of her own.

Harvesting Royal Jelly

To collect bee pollen, a beekeeper merely puts a pollen trap on his hives. To collect propolis, a beekeeper merely cuts away chunks with a knife. It's messy, but not difficult. However, it's not easy to harvest royal jelly. Imagine trying to 'milk' a nurse bee and you'll have some idea of the problems, and some idea of why royal jelly is so expensive. Still, as demand for this rejuvenating cell-food continues to escalate, beekeepers have come up with workable methods.

To produce royal jelly on a small scale, a beekeeper can simply take the Queen out of the hive. The entire colony will then frantically rear queens the queen-mother previously deposited in the large emergency queen cells scattered around on ordinary brood comb. After cutting away these cells, the beekeeper can harvest the royal jelly deposited there for the tiny larvae. But this method isn't really very efficient. The hive can't stay queenless for very long. Without a queen to lay eggs, the population will decline quickly, honey and bee pollen production will suffer, and gradually the colony will die out.

For the large production of royal jelly, we turn to the mass production of queens. Because most commercial beekeepers now routinely requeen their hives every year by purchasing young healthy commercially-reared queens, the commercial production of queens is something we already know about. This queen-rearing process can be modified to insure a continuing harvest of royal jelly. Here's how it is accomplished.

Young worker larvae, 8 to 24 hours old, are plucked out of their tiny brood cells and quickly transferred into artificial queen cells, which can be made of either plastic or beeswax. These queen brood chambers are fitted into a special frame, making removal easy. Each queen cell is primed with a drop of royal jelly. Young nurse bees eagerly take up the task of feeding and caring for up to 45 occupied queen chambers, but some colonies will accept fewer cells than others.

By the end of the third day of intensive feeding by the nurse bees, each queen cell will contain the maximum amount of royal jelly. The frames are then removed and the queen cells are cut down to about the level of the pool of royal jelly with a sharp, hot, thin-bladed knife. The unlucky larvae are quickly removed with tweezers and discarded. The tiny puddle of royal jelly in the bottom of the cells can be removed with a tiny spoon, or sucked out with a thin-nosed vacuum apparatus. Each queen chamber will contain between 148 to 281 mg of royal jelly. To produce a pound of royal jelly, an average of 1,000 three-day old cells must be harvested in this painstaking manner.

The royal milk is immediately strained to eliminate any bits of debris. The quality of royal jelly deteriorates by the hour. Twenty-four hours after removal from the hive, studies show that the nutrient content of royal jelly is sharply reduced. Lypholizing (freeze-drying) *on site* immediately upon harvest is the only way to insure that all beneficial properties will be available in the finished product. Only if the royal jelly is to be used within a day, is refrigerator storage at 35⁰ F. considered sufficient. Don't be fooled. The liquid royal jelly some companies offer in small vials cannot be as biologically-active and has most likely been 'stabilized' with chemical processing.

The Properties of Royal Jelly

Royal jelly has long been credited with miraculous rejuvenating and regenerating properties. Legends tell of oriental potentates who regained renewed sexual powers and attained remarkably long lives with a diet of royal jelly. The basis for the long-held belief that royal jelly possesses some mysterious magical elements that extend life are based on the scientific fact of the Queen Bee's existence.

But what about studies on the royal substance itself? From The C C Pollen Company files, we report on the ongoing hard scientific research with royal jelly.

For an excellent overview on the oral ingestion of royal jelly, we excerpt from a paper entitled, *Biology, Biochemistry & The Therapeutic Effects of Royal Jelly in Human Pathology.* This paper was written by Dr. A. Saenz, who held the important position of Head of the Laboratory of the Anti-Rabies Institute of Montevideo, Uraguay before joining the staff of the Pasteur Institute in Paris. Note particularly that Dr. Saenz cites the work of many other scientists in his very comprehensive 12-page paper. We excerpt extensively, as follows:

Opening Statement: Each day man enlarges the therapeutic arsenal which he uses to battle against senescence (aging), the term of his life cycle (longevity), and against diseases which disturb his biological equilibrium for as long as he exists. The numerous physiocochemical and pharmacodynamic constituents of royal jelly, as well as rigorous bacteriological analysis, assure the integrity of the different elements in its composition. The use of royal jelly has spread widely and continues to be of interest more and more to the scientist, the biologist, and the physician.

Discussion: Numerous studies undertaken during the last ten years have demonstrated the existence of fractions in royal jelly which correspond to 97 percent of the substance, plus an unmeasurable and undetermined fraction whose presence could explain the remarkable and mysterious properties of royal jelly.

All the hydrosoluble vitamins of the B group are found together in royal jelly. Speaking generally, all physicians and biologists realize the prime role of the B vitamins in most phenomena associated with cellular respiration and in the metabolism of carbohydrates, lipids (fats), and proteins. The vitamins in this group are those advocated by Dr. A. Lariviere in his gerontological practice precisely because a properly conducted treatment with royal jelly allows us to obtain most conclusive results. A detailed analysis of the function of each vitamin shows that:

Thiamin (B1) — Works in cases of neuritis, in the neuro-anemic syndrome. Possesses a tonic action on the central nervous system.

Riboflavin (B2) — Returns life to the skin, has an anti-wrinkling effect, corrects glossitis and fissured tongues, keeps body free from muscular cramps.

Pyridoxine (B6) — Combats cerebral sclerosis and muscular asthenia of the aged. Used successfully both orally and by injection.

Nicotinic Acid (niacin) — Abundant in royal jelly, acts essentially as a vasodilator, indicated in disorders of the peripheral circulation and in vascular spasms so frequent in the brains of the aged. Its rapid action avoids anoxemia of the comprised region.

Psychiatrists have observed its auspicious effect in senile psychoses and have even administered it as a preventive measure.

Biotin — This important B plays an absolutely essential role in the fertilization of the ovum, in cell mitosis (cell division) and in the metabolism of lipids and carbohydrates.

Inositol — Studied intensively by Canadian biochemists. Inositol is a growth factor, is anti-baldness, a remarkable hepatic (liver) protector, fights fatty degeneration of the liver, protects against cirrhosis. Considered a specific anti-arteriosclerotic agent as it favors the synthesis of phospholipids and reduces cholesterol, inhibiting the infiltration of the walls of the blood vessels, as demonstrated by Morrison and Wolfson. With inositol, blood vessels remain supple as in youth and without atheromatous plaque. According to studies instituted by Auguste, Paris, Claynes, and Helleu, inositol augments the esterificated fraction of blood cholesterol at the expense of the free fraction, thus reducing the tendency of cholesterol to be precipitated on the endothelium.

Pantothenic Acid (B5) — Considered by some investigators as the 'longevity factor,' pantothenic acid is of prime importance in biology. Acts as a catalytic factor in the utilization of nutrients, has a direct effect on the skin, hair, and mucosa; increases resistance to infection. During his experimental studies, Gartner observed a significant increase in the life span of white mice beyond the norm when a sufficient amount of pantothenic acid is added to their feed.

Therapeutic Effects: Royal jelly, a biogenetic product, has been in use since 1952 in human clinical practice. Its field of action is becoming progressively extended, thanks to the research of that great French biologist, Boyer de Belvefer. Royal jelly has rendered valuable aid to a great number of sick people.

The most tolerance to and the harmlessness of royal jelly are outstanding. Most research scientists and clinicians advocate taking it via the buccal pathway (by mouth), the dose being generally one ampule per day. In cases of serious organic deficiency, two ampules per day are generally indicated.

Arteriosclerosis — The action of royal jelly in arteriosclerosis is extremely interesting and rests on experimental verification. Russ, Eder and Ban note the relationship existing between arteriosclerosis and an increase of lipoproteins and cholesterol. Arteriosclerosis is the consequence of a disturbed lipid metabolism; lipoproteins increase considerably with age. Blood electrophoresis of atherosclerotic victims in a state of hypercoagulability show an abnormal reading. When those who are suffering from arteriosclerosis are subjected to royal jelly treatment, the readings correct themselves. This correction of the plasma protein dispersion thus reestablishes normal activities of the metabolic process where lipoproteins originate.

Varicose Veins — Royal jelly offers excellent results from the clinical viewpoint, plus very significant improvements in another arterial disorder, thromboangeitis obliterans (Buerger's disease).

Deficiency States — States of malnutrition and, in general, in all states of convalescence, royal jelly benefits the organism. Simple stress, physical or mental exhaustion, so frequent in modern life, is rapidly corrected by treatment with royal jelly.

Sexual Deficiencies — In manifestations of sexual involution, as well as in endocrine asthenias, royal jelly in association with classic therapies accelerates the normal re-establishment of disturbed functions by means of its action on the adrenal cortex.

Pediatrics — Sarrouy, Raffi and Leuteneger have treated cases of serious hypertrophy in nursing infants; the effect of royal jelly on weight is made clearly evident and the authors show a general tonic effect on the child. Antibiotics and blood transfusions given in similar cases do not offer such rapid recovery.

Further, during the meeting of the Congress of Medicine at Bologna, Italy, Professor Malassi and Dr. Grandi announced their observations on the effect of royal jelly in the feeding of premature infants, concluding that royal jelly ought absolutely to be part of the biological therapy given such children.

Various clinical trials have established the effectiveness of royal jelly in serious dystrophies of childhood by rapidly promoting necessary weight gain and by promoting the nutrition of the sick child, as well as in the cases of convalescent adults.

Psychiatry — Professor Decourt praises the stimulating action of royal jelly, which mimics that of amphetamines without the harmful side effects. Binet demonstrated its effectiveness with psychic asthenias of the aged and in cases of senility in general.

Truly spectacular results were obtained by Gautrelet in several cases of anorexia nervosa. One published case involved a 16-year old girl considered medically incurable who was hospitalized and kept alive only with blood transfusions and transfusions of hydrolyzed proteins. When given royal jelly, the girl regained 5 kg (almost 10 pounds) in one month and was able to eat normally once again.

Cases of anxiety, depression, shock, and senility all benefit by royal jelly treatment. Several cases of long-standing insomnia have been corrected as well.

Gastroenterology — Professor Izar stresses the importance of royal jelly in the treatment of gastroduodenal ulcer. Its specific action is due especially to the presence of pantothenic acid, known to be necessary in the protection of the mucosa and the healing of ulcerations.

Arthritis — In rheumatology, clinical testing of royal jelly is currently taking place. Dr. Livaditis of Greece has published several studies of patients suffering from arthritis and chronic evolutive arthritis who were helped by royal jelly.

Neurology — A satisfactory remission of Parkinson's disease has been obtained by royal jelly, including a marked reduction of the trembling caused by this affliction. These early clinical trials suggest further study is indicated to understand the beneficial action royal jelly offers victims of neurological disorders,

Dermatology — Royal jelly acts as a bactericide and antibiotic while revitalizing the skin. Several specialists have employed royal jelly treatment with success in eczema, in neurodermatitis, and in impetigo. Its use is indicated in skin ailments with a very alkaline pH. Royal jelly has an acid pH which re-establishes the acid mantle of the skin.

Conclusion: We are not yet fully acquainted with all the mysteries of royal jelly, but many therapies of royal jelly have been crowned with success. Physicians ought to use royal jelly above all else in diseases where a disorder of the lipoprotein metabolism exists since it activates the basal metabolism and increases cellular oxygenation up to 38 percent.

What is astonishing from the biological viewpoint is royal jelly's extreme concentration as compared to human blood plasma. The beneficial action of royal jelly is due to the presence of, and the synergy between, various substances harmoniously bound to one another and mutually reinforcing their effect.

Royal jelly allows man to re-establish his biological balance and to confront aging with optimism and serenity. Nature has created here in the extremely complex biological product which is royal jelly a genuine 'panacea' for the aged and even, to put it simply, for the adult who aspires to push back the limits of his natural aging.

Researchers in Argentina have been working with royal jelly for a considerable length of time. The following paper, authored by J.R. Lamberti and L.G. Cornejo, is entitled, *Presence of Gamma Globulin in Injectable Royal Jelly and Its Use in Revitalizing Processes.* Gamma globulin is medically defined as a protein formed in the blood. The ability of the body to resist infection is closely related to a concentration of this important element. This work was confirmed by Professor Dr. E.L. Mandrile of the National University at La Plata and shows the protective effects of royal jelly.

Even more exciting, these scientists have documented important elements in royal jelly which slow down the aging process. It just might be that we are close to discovering a factual basis for all those stories of rejuvenation and longevity.

Opening Statement: After many chemical, analytical, and clinical-therapeutical investigations of royal jelly, we can state that we have determined in its composition the presence of the globulinic amino-acid frequently called gamma globulin. We discovered this element in the composition of royal jelly by direct observation of a series of persons who were administered royal jelly and who subsequently showed an increased resistance to bacteria and viruses.

We determined the dosage of gamma globulin in injectable royal jelly solution reached a value equal to 10 UT/centrilitre. Our discovery was confirmed by electrophoretic analysis of globulin solution identified in the royal jelly solution.

Discussion: Gamma globulin is of incalcuable value to the living body. Gamma globulin is the most important component of proteins which participate in the fight against bacteria, viruses, and toxins.

The proteic group of royal jelly also includes a gelatinous amino acid, which is a basic component of collagen. This sustains the mesenchyme of reticulo-endothelial system, whose deterioration is obvious in and specific to the aging process. Once it was said that human beings had the age of their arteries, but at the present time one can say more precisely that human beings have the age of their collagen.

The old organism should maintain and remake its collagen, an element of first importance for the body. In addition to polyvitamins, pluriminerals, and pluriamino acids, royal jelly also includes gamma globulin, which becomes an element of particular importance for the treatment of aging. It is known during the aging process that the psycho-physical functions of the body diminish progressively. For this reason, it is necessary to apply an early prophylaxy for controlling these decaying organical stages.

We have to resort immediately to elements having a visible revitalizing action. The most important of these is royal jelly, a substance which benefits mankind and which reduces the destructive effects of time. At present, we can state that royal jelly makes a matchless contribution in this direction and is a first-rate therapeutic. Its gamma globulin and gelatinous collagen content is of high value, particularly when injected because direct assimilation assists blood chemical composition dramatically.

Clinical Results: Before commencing the experiments, patients were analyzed for gamma globulin levels in their blood; a dermic (skin) exploration of the reticuloendothelial system was conducted by a dinitrofluorobenzene solution. Patients were then administered subcutaneous injections with royal jelly solution daily.

After treatment, new analyses were made regularly to establish the therapeutical effects of the substance. Analysis revealed a visible increase in the activity of the protective mechanisms of the body, with a marked revitalization of the trophysm of cells.

Conclusion: The results we obtained with injectable royal jelly administered to the human body particularly in pathologic stages were promising and encouraging. With the documentation of gamma globulin and the precursor of collagen among the components of royal jelly, these results become of paramount importance for medicine.

The injectable royal jelly solution is a medicine which justifies thorough studies toward offering mankind a complete therapeutic, particularly to the aged which are too often neglected.

From the University of Sarajevo in Yugoslavia, we excerpt from a paper entitled, *Clinical Value of Royal Jelly & Propolis Against Viral Infections.* Many studies exist showing the documented antiviral effects of propolis. The authors of this paper, B. Filipic and M. Likvar, wanted to know if the addition of royal jelly, another powerful beehive product, would improve antiviral action. Here's what they found:

Opening Statement: Lately a number of laboratories have been trying to find effective antiviral drugs for a number of different viruses. Generally, antiviral substances can be divided into two groups: chemically synthesized and natural antiviral compounds. Opinions about the value of these two groups differ, but natural antiviral substances are the more valuable as they are not toxic to living cells and organisms. Should they prove ineffective, they still cannot harm.

From the natural antiviral substances, we must mention natural bee products, including royal jelly and propolis, which have a clinically pronounced antibacterial effect. From natural substances, the best known antiviral substance is interferon. It is very effective against herpes viruses, influenza viruses, VSV virus, and vaccinia virus.

Discussion: In our preliminary clinical experiments, a total of 220 perons were treated. From these, 63 were treated with royal jelly-propolis compounds of varying strengths; 157 were nontreated controls.

Results: In high concentration, royal jelly and propolis alone have an antiviral effect. A proper combination of royal jell, propolis, and honey had a very obvious antiviral effect, especially against influenza, even diluted 1:10. The combination with 2 percent royal jelly was very effective against vaccinia virus. Against visicular stomatitis virus, the most effective mixtures included 10 percent royal jelly (without interferon) and 2 percent royal jelly (with interferon added).

Among those persons treated with royal jelly-propolis compounds, only 6 percent suffered viral infections. In the unprotected control group, close to 40 percent became ill.

If you have been paying attention, it probably won't come as a surprise to learn that royal jelly, like bee pollen, exhibits strong properties against cancer, witness the following paper.

This work is a joint effort of three prestigious Canadian

facilities, Ontario Agricultural College, Guelph, Department of National Health & Welfare, Ottawa, and the University of Toronto, Toronto. It is entitled *Activity of 10-Hydroxydecenoic Acid From Royal Jelly Against Experimental Leukemia & Ascitic Tumors.* We excerpt as follows:

Opening Statement: As part of a long-term study on the chemistry and biological activity of royal jelly, we have recently investigated its possible anti-tumor properties. We report that the admixture of royal jelly with tumor cells before inoculation completely suppresses the development of transplantable mouse leukemia and the formation of ascitic tumors in mice. Fractionation studies have established that this anti-tumor activity resides in the main fatty acid of royal jelly, 10-hydroxydecenoic acid.

Discussion: The criterion used in these experiments was survival; the mice either developed leukemia or tumors or were protected; control mice died from ascitic tumors in less than 14 days, while mice receiving appropriate mixtures of cells and royal jelly all failed to develop tumors. Protected mice were kept under observation for 90 days after death of the control mice. They were then sacrificed and autopsied to confirm the absence of tumors.

Conclusion: Results indicate that 30 mgm. of fresh whole royal jelly, or 1.5 mgm of 10-hydroxydecenoic acid, per ml of cell suspension completely inhibited the development of transplantable leukemia in mice. This effect was obtained only when the active material was mixed with the cancer cells prior to administration. Attempts to demonstrate protection after tumor implantation or by separate administration of royal jelly and leukemia cells have as yet been unsuccessful. Further studies are in progress to determine whether the active material in royal jelly causes death of the tumor cells before inoculation.

These results have been confirmed repeatedly on nearly 1,000 mice during a two-year period and show a striking effect: either all the mice die quickly, or all survive. Two groups of mice which received tumor cells plus royal jelly remained alive and healthy more than 12 months after inoculation, while sister mice which received the same number of tumor cells without royal jelly died within 12 days.

You already know the products of the beehive are truly remarkable. But here's a real surprise. Ch. Kalman of Israel has written a paper entitled, *Royal Jelly Effects on Faded Eyesight.* In this paper, Kalman merely relates two stories. Because there is nothing really scientific about this paper, these stories have to be considered as testimonials. Still, they can act as guideposts for further research.

Opening Statement: The mechanism of the human body is very complicated. A deficiency of one part in a million percent of some nutrient, even a lack of a tiny milligram of some component, can cause body discomfort or serious illness.

Discussion: A man came to me asking for royal jelly, as fresh as possible. He asked me how much he should take. I told him a tenth of a gram per day for at least three weeks. I did not ask him why he needed it. A week later, he came to me and shouted excitedly, "I can really see!" When I questioned him, he told me he was under the strict observation of an opthalmologist because he could not see clearly. The doctor had not found any inflammation or deterioration or any detectable fault, but had told the patient, "Take royal jelly. Try it. I read in a medical journal that it can improve eyesight."

Another man came to me sometime later following a lecture I had given on the on the dietetic and medical of bee products. He was the director of a big technical enterprise. He told me, "I can't see clearly, everything is almost blurred and I have double vision. I am a very careful dirver, still the reason why I don't kill people in the streets is because I've been lucky." He asked for royal jelly, which I supplied. Two weeks later, he came to see me and offered me a big sum, which I did not take, saying, "Now I am another man. I see clearly and I'm no longer afraid I will kill someone when I'm driving. I am much calmer and feel very well."

Conclusion: Neither of these two men are elderly. One was 35 years, the other 45 years. I believe both lacked certain vital microelements which are present in royal jelly. It is surprising that such a small amount of royal jelly restored their deficiencies and corrected their vision in such a short period of time. But man is such a complicated mechanism that a few milligrams of required material restores us to a normal condition.

For the benefit of mankind, it is my belief that it is worth while scientifically investigating the effects of royal jelly on problems of eyesight under clinically controlled circumstances.

In conclusion, we turn to a paper by the German physician Hans Weitgasser, M.D., entitled *Gelee Royale Medizinische Kosmetik* (Royal Jelly in Dermatological Cosmetics), which includes material subtitled *Experiences with Royal Jelly in the Medicinal-Cosmetic Practice.*

Unlike most of the papers in the CCPC files, this particular translation from the original German is very sketchy, at best, and there is no indication that the controlled double-blind studies science requires were employed. However, it's very much worth reading between the lines. Dr. Weitgasser has compiled some amazing results obtained by his countrymen with the use of royal jelly. In spite of the title of this paper, not all involve the effects of royal jelly on the skin, as follows:

Through local application, as an ingredient in face masks, creams, and lotion, royal jelly has tremendous effects at the cellular level. In regular use, the skin becomes soft and wrinkles disappear. When royal jelly is used topically as a salve on skin damaged by the effects of radium treatment, the skin heals rapidly and symptoms disappear.

According to Dr. Elfriede Kerschbaumer, royal jelly promotes the growth of tissue in the case of underdeveloped breasts; stimulates the circulatory system in the case of circulation problems; works against cases of depression, vegetative dystosis and exhaustion. In the treatment of patients with alopecia (abnormal hair loss or baldness), royal jelly trials produced increased hair growth.

Ninety percent of Kerschbaumer's patients with seborrhea, dry skin, red spots, abnormally colored skin on the insides of extremities, excessive sweating, hair loss, fatigue, sagging of skin (tissue, muscles, breasts), swollen legs, digestive problems, obesity (three obese patients averaged a loss of a pound per week without diet or exercise), failing memory, lack of concentration, and insomnia reacted favorably to royal jelly therapy.

Royal jelly reduced nervousness and depression, increased the size of breast tissue (an 18-year old woman gained 1 kg (2 pounds) growth of breast tissue in three months), re-established hair growth (in six weeks with no side effects), promoted healthier circulation, and all patients experienced a feeling of increased well being.

Neurovegetative disorders in a 48-year old man, including impotence, depression, lack of concentration, blood pressure 115 over 100, no involved organs. Treatment: Three drops of royal jelly in water three times daily. In three weeks, symptoms gone.

Royal jelly normalizes and increases sexual activity in both males and females; royal jelly increases androgen hormones in men, estrogen levels in women.

Diffuse hair loss in a 21-year old man, also suffering severe headaches. Treatment: Fifteen drops of royal jelly three times daily, ten 2-15 minute treatments with high-frequency heat lamp. In fourteen days, headaches better; in three months, stronger hair growth.

Seborrhea on face and head of 26-year old woman, plus under-development of breasts, sleeplessness, inability to concentrate, sweating spells, large inferiority complex leading to depression. Treatment: five ampules of royal jelly daily; at same time, ten face and breast treatments with royal jelly cream. After one treatment, sleep came easier; after four, concentration improved, sweats and depression disappeared; in four weeks, a 4 cm increase in bust tissue was observed; after eight weeks, all complaints were gone; larger breasts remained.

The Euphoric Effects of Royal Jelly

It's easy to understand why a young man suffering from impotence and losing his hair into the bargain might feel euphoric on discovering that royal jelly has alleviated both symptoms. It's also easy to understand why a young woman self-conscious and depressed because she was flat-chested and suffered from disfiguring acne into the bargain might feel euphoric on finding that royal jelly has eliminated both conditions. And it's easy to understand why anyone suffering from any condition of ill health might feel euphoric at being restored to perfect health. But that's not what we're talking about here.

The term *euphoria* comes from the Greek and identifies 'a state of well-being.' In the jargon of the psychologist, euphoria has come to mean an *exaggerated* feeling of well-being, one which has no basis in truth or reality.

In the case of royal jelly, its euphoric effect has been well established. It is very real. But physicians call it a 'false euphoria' and warn against the feelings this incredibly powerful and potent substance from the beehive provides. Here's why: The natural high that royal jelly brings travels through the body like a jolt of electricity. Even someone taking royal jelly for the first time will usually feel a dynamic energy and well-being pulsing through his entire body.

The entire organism responds dramatically to an influx of the concentrated nutrients present in royal jelly. Energy levels peak and a feeling of invincibility pervades the body. Even those who are ill suddenly feel almost miraculously better after taking royal jelly. And therein lies the danger. It is important to understand that the euphoric effects of royal jelly are sometimes so strong that they can actually mask symptoms which require the close attention of a doctor.

On the other hand, the scientifically documented benefits of the ingestion of royal jelly are many and varied, as discussed in this chapter. And who can deny that it's wonderful to feel full to bursting with youthful energy and well-being? Just be sure that the wonderful feeling of euphoria that royal jelly brings doesn't stop you from seeking necessary medical treatment, should a condition arise that calls for a visit to your physician.

In Conclusion

We conclude this chapter with the closing statement from a lecture given before the German Medical Association. The topic is *Royal Jelly in Diet, Prophylaxis, and Therapy;* the speaker is H.W. Schmidt, M.D. Dr. Schmidt says:

"The action of the active substances and nutrients contained in royal jelly takes place throughout the entire body and acts to regulate all the functions of the body. From all the investigations and observations regarding royal jelly, it is apparent this is a powerful agent composed of hormones, nutrients, enzymes and biocatalysts which starts up and revives the functions of cells, the secretions of glands, the metabolism, and blood circulation. To summarize, it is the interplay of all the complex factors present in royal jelly which works to preserve life and strength in the organism, which delays the aging process, and which retains for as long as possible the youthful physical freshness of the body, elasticity of the mind, and psychic buoyancy."

CHAPTER 11

BEE POLLEN
FOR ANIMALS
The Not-So-Surprising Benefits

You've read all those studies where animals ranging from the usual laboratory mice to sheep to hens to rabbits and even cows were used in researching the benefits of bee pollen. (Chapter 8). These closely monitored double or triple-blind clinical animal studies document the effects of dietary bee pollen very scientifically. So it surely won't come as a surprise to find that this perfect food from the beehive is just as right for *domestic animals* as it is for people and lab animals.

The C C Pollen Company has any number of stories in their files from families who started sharing their High Desert pollen with a family pet who was ailing, with dramatic results.

My favorite has to do with an aging Irish Setter named King. King came to the Antol family as a wobbly-legged youngster of eight weeks. Although this pedigreed pup had a very fine bloodline and was descended from a long line of champion show dogs, he was purchased as a family companion. As large as King was, the big baby slept curled at the bottom of the bed of either of the two young sons in the family.

In the mornings, King was first up. His usual routine included making a tour of the house, checking out every room, and padding up and down the steps. If he was lucky, he found the family cat, a little black named Sukey, and tried to coax her to play. Sukey was sometimes agreeable, but sometimes let King know with a snarl and a swipe of her paw that she didn't care to chase or be chased. When the cat definitely didn't care to be disturbed, she lept from the breakfast bar to the top of the refrigerator and preened herself well out of King's reach.

Once King had finished his rounds, he nosed open the door of the master bedroom and came bounding in. If he wasn't greeted immediately, he danced around impatiently, nosed the sleeping Papa Antol, and 'talked' in a curious soft sharp bark until the master of the house gave up, got up, and took him out for his morning run.

King quickly learned his manners and, for the most part, followed the rules. For example, he knew he was allowed to nap on top of a (washable) bedspread, but wasn't allowed to scramble up on an unmade bed. Dear as he was, Mama Antol didn't care for silky red hairs (or dirty paw marks) on the sheets. After his morning outing, he waited patiently until the boys had pulled their covers into place and half-heartedly straightened their spreads before he jumped up and settled down in his place at the end of the bed with a sigh of satisfaction.

King demanded his share of attention while the boys were

dressing. They took turns tussling with him, often tossing a knotted old sock across the room for him to fetch. Tug-of-war was a favorite game. King took a firm grip on the knot with this teeth, set his legs, and shook his head back and forth while one of the boys held onto the other end. King growled deep in his throat with delight and the boys laughed as their small arms were flung around. When they were very young, it took both of them to hold the sock while King tried to wrestle it from them.

Time passed and King grew into a very handsome and happy animal with a sleek and shining red coat. As he matured, he discovered the female of the species. Whenever King sniffed the air, barked frantically and scaled the fence to escape his backyard run, the family knew he was off and running to locate a mate. Once over the top, true to his hunting dog instincts, King quartered the field with his nose until he located the female's scent and took off.

It was a good thing that this big friendly clown was a favorite in the neighborhood. He was impossible to catch when he was on the trail. No amount of hollering or coaxing or chasing worked. When King was in joyous single-minded pursuit of a female in heat, there was only one way to track him down and get him back home. You may not believe this next bit, but the family swears to the truth of it. When the boys and Papa Antol came home exhausted from their fruitless chase, Mama Antol sent Sukey out to bring King home. Within an hour, the little black cat and the big red dog came trotting home side by side.

Papa Antol's hobby was cooking and he was a wizard in

the kitchen. The family feasted on good whole freshly prepared foods, no fast-food junk-food was permitted. King loved to eat and was treated to healthy wholesome bites from time to time. He sat alertly and waited patiently beside the table when the family was at dinner. Because he was so large, his head was level with the top of the table. Mama Antol objected and wanted to send King from the room, but when Papa Antol taught him to daintly take a morsel from a fork, she gave in. King would pull back his lips, bare his teeth, gently clamp down on the fork, and slide off his bite. Soon a fork was placed on the table for King and it became a family ritual to spear a bit of meat and present it to the dog. King, always the gentleman, was never demanding.

As the years ticked by, King's muzzle became gray and grizzled, but his happy disposition and devotion to the family never wavered. With the help of the vet, he was nursed through hip dysplasia, a condition common to the breed. But, in spite of the love and care lavished on him, the day came when the old gentleman was no longer able to make it up on the bed. He was content to sleep in his big wicker dog bed made cozy and soft with blankets.

And there were still more trials awaiting this dog and his family who loved him. The time came when King was off his feed. Even tidbits from the table no longer tempted him. It was all too apparent that King was getting very old and the family was worried. Although he didn't seem to be in any pain, he had a great deal of difficulty getting around and often had to literally be helped to his feet. An appointment was made to take him to the vet.

Although King had always enjoyed a bath and brush, he was no longer eager for a grooming. Mama Antol discovered why as she was combing out his long silky hair before taking him to the doctor. Running her hand down the side, she felt a series of hard lumps deep under the skin. The vet confirmed that King was suffering from wide-spread deep-seated cancer and recommended he be put to sleep. An agonizing decision faced the family, but they were not ready to give up and put down their old friend without making an all-out effort to save him.

This family had all taken *High Desert Honeybee Pollen* granules for a very long time and were big bee pollen fans themselves. Mama Antol began sprinkling a liberal handful of bee pollen on top of the special canned dog food prescibed by the vet. At first, King sniffed at the pollen-laced food and merely licked the granules off the top. Then he slurped some water and sank heavily to the floor. But after just a few days, he ate some bites of food along with the bee pollen. Within a month, the stiffness in his hindquarters seemed less and he was eating a full dish of food. After two months, although he wasn't frisking around like a puppy, he was more like his old self than he had been in the past year and his appetite had come back full force. It was hard to tell, but it certainly looked as if his cancerous lumps were getting smaller as well.

Then the day came when they found King up on a bed. The family cheered and fussed over him and petted him and called him 'good dog.' They were certain the worst had passed, and they were right. Once again, King enjoyed his walks. He never sniffed the air and took off like a shot at a female's scent again, but he padded alongside a family member in contentment when taken outside, and he still stopped to investigate an interesting tree or two along the way.

For a full two years after the crisis that almost took King from them, the Antol family cared for and loved the aging animal. That love was returned in full. Still, as it must to all living things, the time did come when King just couldn't make it outside without help. The old gentleman looked embarrassed and whined an apology when he wet his bed. His back legs had finally given out completely and he could no longer support himself or drag himself to his feet.

Because King had always hated taking a trip to the doctor, and he always knew when that was where he was going, Mama Antol phoned the vet and arranged a house call for a time when everyone was out of the house. With much love, she hoisted the now-fragile animal to the bed, wrapped him carefully in his own blankets, and kissed him goodbye. She stroked his head and hugged him close while the vet administered the lethal injection. With a gentle sigh, the great dog closed his eyes and slept the good sleep forever.

King was 15 years old, the equivalent of 105 human years, and had lived an extraordinary long and very full life for his breed. There is no doubt that bee pollen inhibited and controlled the cancer which had invaded his body, allowed him to overcome the stiffness of arthritis which made it so difficult for him to move, and restored him to a measure of health. Thanks to the nourishing and medicinal properties of bee pollen, King had lived a happy and contented two full years beyond the time allotted him by his doctor.

All the many Antol family pets which followed King, and at one time the family had six dogs and three cats, are given *High Desert Bee Pollen* from the time they join the household. It is stories like this one that led The C C Pollen Company to develop *Pet Power*, the bee pollen tableted formula especially blended for cats and dogs.

Love Isn't Enough

There is a growing body of evidence which shows that a lifetime of eating commercial pet foods can shorten your pet's life, make him fatter than he should be, and can contribute to the development of such common disorders as cystitis and stones (in cats), glaucoma and heart disease (in dogs), diabetes, lead poisoning, rickets, sodium poisoning and serious vitamin and mineral deficiencies.

Dr. R. G. Broderick, Director of the Animal Clinic at Southdown, located in Huntington, New York says, "We spend approximately $8 billion dollars every year on pet products. And, still, with all our care and concern, we often don't do the right thing for these special members of the family. Remember, your pets are unable to communicate their nutritional needs. They are totally dependent on you."

Consumers Digest (November/December 1979) published this warning: "Almost all commercial pet foods fail to nourish a pet with special needs where vitamins are concerned. Many vitamins are killed during processing. Remember that brands with less sodium, sugar and additives are preferable. If you feed your pets commercial diets, they will do better if you give them vitamin and mineral supplements."

The C C Pollen Company's *Pet Power* contains 53 mg High Desert Bee Pollen, plus barley, dandelion root, garlic, honey, hops and kelp. The box carries suggested use instructions tabulated according to the weight of the animal. These tablets are all-natural and qualify as the best vitamin and mineral supplement around for the domestic animals who brighten your life. *Pet Power* contains no sodium, no sugar, no chemical additives, and no artificial flavors or colors. To really appreciate the fact that this product contains none of that disgusting red dye that colors so many dry cat and dogs foods (and Kool Aid), just try getting a stain made by that dye out of your carpet.

Just as High Desert is 'health insurance' for people, *Pet Power* is 'health insurance' for your beloved pets. Chances are you make sure the rest of your family takes vitamin and mineral supplements and 'eats right.' Doesn't your pet deserve the same care and consideration?

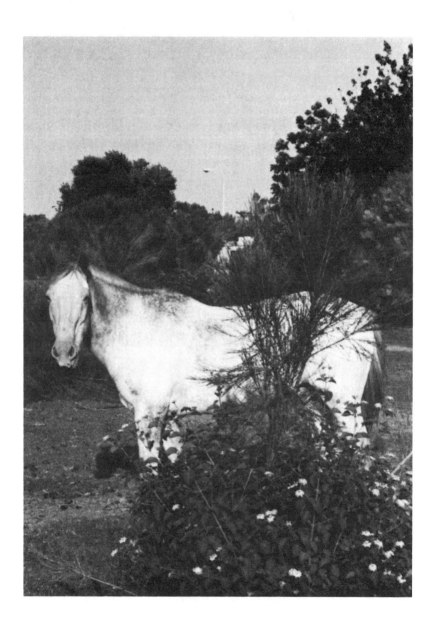

CHAPTER 12

THIS OLD GRAY MARE
IS *BETTER* THAN
SHE USED TO BE

The Birth of Winners Bee Pollen

In 1986, *Winners Bee Pollen,* The Equine Division of The C C Pollen Company, was born. The story which follows is told by Buzz Kennedy, the founder and President of Winners Bee Pollen. Here's the progression of events which led to all the excitement in racing circles. Buzz tells how it happened:

When I was in the market for a stable pony five years ago, I ended up coming home with a little gray filly. Mind you, she wasn't really what I was looking for. In point of fact, I guess you could say that she chose me. I was talking to a buddy when she stretched her neck over the door of her stall and nipped me on the behind. I clutched the spot, hollered, "ouch," and turned around to see the gray laughing at me. I swear that little gal had a twinkle in her eye. She shook her head and whuffed at me and got her nicely combed 'please buy me' mane in a tangle. I glared at her and walked on.

243

What I needed, of course, was a *stable* stable pony, a work horse, not a prima donna. I looked over the rest of the stock, but I kept coming back to that little gray filly. There was just something about her. Anyway, I ended up forking over $700 and took her home to the ranch.

Soon after that, a neighboring rancher dubbed her Mary Poppins, because she was such a good 'nanny.' When she was working, she tended to business and worked hard. And, believe me, my bloods got a real workout keeping up with that high-stepping little gal. But when Poppy (for short) was 'off duty,' she still frisked around like a colt even as she got older. She gave herself airs and pranced like the thoroughbred she wasn't when she took one of the high-bred bloods out to the paddock. With her friendly nature, Poppy became one of the family and a favorite with the hands. Like a mischievous child, Poppy exasperated me sometimes, but I've never been sorry I bought her.

As the years went by, Poppy got tired. She'd come back from the first run of the morning blowing and short of breath. She began jerking her head up and down and her sides would heave as she tried to get enough air. We gave her longer and longer breaks between workouts. But eventually, we had reached the point where the pedigreed bloods weren't getting enough exercise anymore. I tell you, folks, I felt bad. Poppy had been a good and faithful employee for five years. Even more than that, she was a friend, and I was reluctant to replace her.

Then Poppy lost interest in eating. Even oats didn't tempt her anymore. Oh, sure, I tried a little extra molasses and some special vitamins, even liquid food supplements, but those old standbys didn't work. She was off her feed for sure. Then I remembered reading about the spectacular results Charles Whittingham had been racking up ever since he started feeding his horses bee pollen back in 1981. I knew that The C C Pollen Company, the oldest and largest harvesters of bee pollen in the world, was located in my home state of Arizona. When I was looking over the stock at the horse show in Scottsdale Horse Park in February of 1986, I gave those friendly folks a call and got some bee pollen for Poppy. At first, she didn't seem to like it, but she did nibble a few grains from the palm of my hand. I guess the fresh, sweet taste won her over. Soon, she was watching for me and nuzzling around and sniffing my pockets looking for her morning bee pollen treat.

Then I started sprinkling some bee pollen on her mash, and her appetite came back full force. It wasn't long before she was chomping hay again and prancing out in the morning eager for a hard run. Instead of needing a break between exercise sessions, she snorted just like she used to and signaled her readiness to go again. The dullness disappeared from her coat and it became glossy and thick. Even her *attitude* improved. She got that old mischief back in her eyes.

When I saw what these golden granules had done for Poppy, you'd better believe I became a believer. Whittingham was onto something. We started giving all the stock a ration of bee pollen, and that's when we saw some very interesting side effects. Even after a hard workout, there was less puffing and blowing. Not only Poppy, but the thoroughbreds seemed ready to go again immediately. That in itself was terrific, but we had another surprise coming as well. All the horses seemed to be traveling better when we hauled them from track to track around the country. Even the bloods with their delicate digestive systems adjusted quickly to the differences in hay and water wherever we went. We didn't have to factor a time lag into the schedule for adjustment any longer when we went on the road. I decided to look into this phenomenon and, knowing they had research from the laboratories of the world on bee pollen, I went back to The C C Pollen Company for some answers. And got 'em.

Bee Pollen As A Superior Supplement

It turns out that bee pollen is a complete food. It contains all the nutrients needed to sustain life. In other words, bee pollen is so richly endowed that the only other requirements for life and health are air and water. Another thing that I really liked was that this golden powder is perfectly balanced by nature — unlike manufactured supplements, which are sometimes top heavy in one nutrient or another and deficient in others. What this told me was that I didn't have to buy a variety of different vitamin and mineral supplements any longer trying to piece together a complete complement of nutrients for the stock.

In addition, bee pollen is completely organic. All these live vital nutrients are totally assimilable and available to the animal's system. The ingredient panel of some supplements may look good, but if some of the elements are inorganic (and they don't tell you that), the body can't absorb, assimilate, or make use of them. Here's a few highlights:

Enzymes: Bee pollen provides the live digestive enzymes and coenzymes all animals need for efficient metabolism. Expensive feed (or just plain old hay) gives up more food value when enzymes are supplied. Enzymes are also vital for fast recovery after worming.

Vitamins & Minerals: Bee pollen offers them all, including every vitamin known to science, plus all 27 mineral salts (and all the trace elements) necessary for good tissue, muscle, and bone development.

Rutin: A known strengthener of capillary walls, rutin protects blood vessels against bursting during the extreme exertion of a race. Research shows it can also restore equine bleeders in regular use.

Proteins: Bee pollen provides more essential amino acids than any other plant food — and, surprisingly, more than meat, cheese, fish, or eggs of equal weight.

Hormones: Unlike steroids, the natural hormones present in bee pollen build muscle and muscle tone. Assists in building fertility and readiness to mate. Hormones stimulate tissue and bone growth as well.

Carbohydrates: With both simple and complex carbos, bee pollen provides short-term energizers for a fast start, and long-term fuel to sustain high levels of energy for the distance.

The Benefits of Bee Pollen

As 'manufactured' by mother nature, bee pollen is a complete *food*. It contains no drugs, legal or illegal. There's some very real benefits connected with supplying bee pollen to horses (or any other living thing). Remember, all of these effects are backed up by hard scientific data. Here's a sample of what you can expect:

Recovery: In a two-year double-blind study, it was shown that subjects eating bee pollen recover quickly after stressed performance and require less time to re-establish normal body rhythms (blood pressure, respiratory system, etc.) than the controls. Even more dramatic, some subjects actually bettered their time on a second go around the track immediately after completing a hard run.

Swelling: Clinical tests show that the swelling of limbs and joints common after a hard race can be markedly relieved by the regular feeding of bee pollen. Up to a half-inch reduction in swelling just twenty minutes after going the distance has been documented.

Red Blood: Maybe your stock are all 'bluebloods,' but they run on red just the same. Studies show that bee pollen can increase the red blood cell (hemoglobin) count by up to 30 percent.

Oxygenation: As the production of healthy hemoglobin is stepped up, richly oxygenated blood courses swiftly through the body, resulting in a measurable increase in strength, stamina, speed, and endurance. This important advantage enables an animal to stay the course and finish tougher.

The Birth of Winners Bee Pollen

To say I was impressed with the mountains of scientific data on 'the world's only perfect food' is an understatement. I was even more impressed with Poppy's near-miraculous turn-around, and extremely pleased with the increase in stamina and endurance our thoroughbreds showed when we added bee pollen to their feed. My mama taught me to share the good things of life, and bee pollen certainly qualifies.

Since I established *Winners Bee Pollen,* the Equine Division of The C C Pollen Company, in 1986, I'm proud to tell you that we're putting out some mighty powerful bee pollen products, especially for horses: The pure powdered *Winners Bee Pollen,* and the same high quality *Winners* powdered bee pollen with dried honey, and a number of specialty products (detailed later in this chapter), too. Mind you, these products are composed of *blended* American bee pollens from a variety of clean and unpolluted areas — and that's important. We all know that man-made contaminates seem to be just about everywhere. And, in many areas of the country (and the world), the soil is lacking certain vital elements. Only a blend of quality bee pollens from a variety of uncontaminated sources can offer all the nutrients — and all the benefits — and that's what *Winners Bee Pollen* delivers.

Here's What They Tell Us

We're getting a lot of feedback from owners, trainers, and

breeders about the great effects of *Winners* products. We know *Winners Bee Pollen* is the best, but we've had a few surprises all the same. If we'd thought about it, we might have predicted that regular *Winners* feedings would stop a stable full of horses who insisted on gnawing on the sides of their stalls. After all, wood-chewing is a sure sign something's missing in the feed. In their own words, here's how Dick and Boo Hooker solved the problem:

"Winners Bee Pollen is terrific. Here at West-End Stables (Rupert, Idaho), we see a lot of horses. Although in good health and not too bored, they'll chew on wood, any kind of wood. We pride ourselves on our horse care ability. We feed good quality third-cutting alfalfa hay. These horses receive calcium, protein, and many other important nutrients, but the soil is phosphorus poor. We knew we had to give them a phosphorus-rich supplement and have tried many products. For one reason or another, we found them below par.

"Winners Bee Pollen is easy to feed and the horses eat it nicely. It's easy to store, comes in a reuseable bucket, *AND* the horses have stopped eating the corrals. In addition, our winters can be rather nasty at times. Thanks to your wonderful product, the horses don't seem to feel the cold. Their coats are full and thick and feel 'bouncy' to the touch. The hair is holding in more air for added warmth. And they still have that nice summer shine.

"We at West-End Stables say thank-you for your fine product. We hope others will try it, so they too can enjoy its benefits."

A lot of nationally known trainers and breeders are feeding

their famous winners *Winners Bee Pollen,* too. The leader of the pollen pack is Charlie Whittingham, of course, with so many winners to his credit that it's hard to name them all. Whittingham is on the board of El Rancho Murrieta. And there's more famous names you'll recognize. The giants in the racing world, greats like Mel Studi, D. Wayne Lukas, Jack VanBerg, and Jim Maple, are all feeding bee pollen. Even Jack Klugman is getting into the act. As a newly licensed trainer and long time consumer of bee pollen himself, it's a good bet that Klugman is serving his big stallion, Jackie Klugman, a heaping helping.

You'll also be hearing about some up-and-comers, like the Willards down in Panama City, Florida who specialize in running quarter-horses. Virginia Willard says they hauled two colts to a Florida track last spring and found they were matched against two really good fillies trained by the top trainers of the state. She says, "Their horses looked magnificent. Needless to say, we were a little taken aback by them, and by the trainers as well. But one of our little colts broke straight and ran his heart out — and won. The other came in third. So far, we've had two more winners, and we've got stud colts on the bee pollen, too. We've had some great results. We've very happy and really excited about the benefits of this feeding program."

Common Market

An owner runs a horse he wants to get rid of in a claiming race. A prospective horse buyer can pick up a 'good bargain' horse (or a 'dog') for the entry price of the race. You pay your money and take your chances. On June 20th, 1987, Common Market ran last in a claiming race. Even worse, he was a bleeder. Nevertheless, this unhealthy bony gelding was claimed by W. Landolf of Mokena, Illinois for the sum of $6,500.00. Landolf took the horse home and his optimism faded as his worst fears were confirmed.

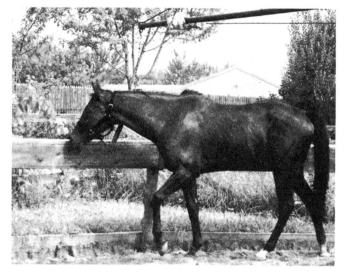

Common Market on July 15, 1987

Common Market was apathetic and disinterested and stood around the exercise yard (see above). When led, he barely lifted his feet from the ground and merely plodded along, head down. In spite of the good care and good feed he was given during the short month after Landolf bought him, the horse refused to eat right and steadily lost weight. His hair came out in the curry comb and he looked terrible. Landolf called the vet in and had Common Market wormed. He also asked for and got some medication for hair loss. But orthodox medical treatment didn't work. This was all to no avail.

The day after the above picture was taken, Landolf started Common Market on Winners Bee Pollen Powder in pure desperation. The horse refused to eat the bee pollen at first. Certain that what he was doing was right, Landolf mixed three to four ounces of Winners powdered pollen with water and used a syringe to get it down the horse's throat. He continued this force-feeding procedure for a week.

After ten days, Common Market was no longer losing weight and had begun to gain. He ate Winners Bee Pollen Powder mixed in with his feed readily and his appetite returned full force.

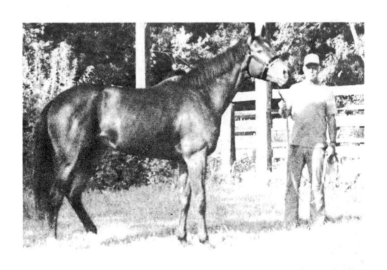

After 30 days on Winners Bee Pollen Powder,
this is Common Market on August 20, 1987.

The difference between Common Market's appearance in July and as pictured above is almost unbelievable, but pictures don't lie. Even his coat looks healthier and his ribs are barely visible under the thicker fuller coat of hair he exhibited here.

By September 13, 1987, the horse was no longer stressed, but relaxed and alert. In just forty-five days of supplemental feeding with Winners Bee Pollen Powder, Common Market gained 200 pounds of much needed weight. He was eating very well and was up to 12 quarts of grain per day, plus his Winners Bee Pollen. No longer a bleeder, his coat was sleek and shining and he no longer lost hair in a comb. His ears perked up when he heard something and he took an interest in his surroundings and stepped out smartly when ridden.

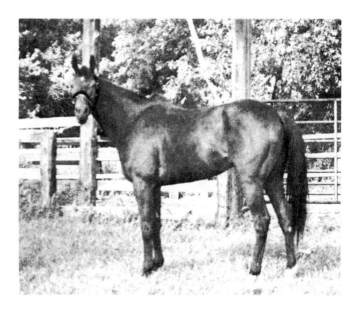

Common Market on September 13, 1987.

Soon Common Market was feeling frisky and chomping at the bit to get going. On December 12, 1987, Landolf entered him in a race and was pleased when he took second place. He ran him again on December 22nd, and again he finished second.

But it was the spring of 1988 that told the tale. On March 15, 1988 at Sportsman's Park in New Jersey, Common Market ran the six and a half furlongs and came home a winner. The following month on April 28, 1988, he repeated his win on a mile romp. With barely a breather in between races, he went a mile and 16th to win by a very impressive seven lengths. Common Market had come a long way back.

There is no doubt in Landolf's mind but that it was Winners Bee Pollen alone that caused the dramatic turn-around for Common Market. He says, "Winners Bee Pollen Powder sure makes all the difference!" Just one look at the *before-during*-and-*after* pictures of this great horse proves it. Thanks to Landolf's persistence in feeding Winners, he was well repaid for his hunch. Common Market's 1988 winnings alone totaled $14,000.00! That $6,500 gamble that Landolf took paid off — big.

Ronas Ryon

They call Ronas Ryon the millionaire quarter-horse. In 1986, this gallant horse streaked to victory and laid claim to the $2 million All American Futurity.

Trained by Arnold Simmons, Ronas Ryon was awarded an invitation to the prestigious Champion of Champions, resulting in his Derby win at Los Alamitos Race Course in California.

Simmons says, "I fed Ronas Ryon *Winners Bee-Bleeders Free* for two and one half weeks before the All American Derby trials. Ronas Ryon did not bleed! I ran him back in the finals and the rest is history. I'm satisfied it is a good product."

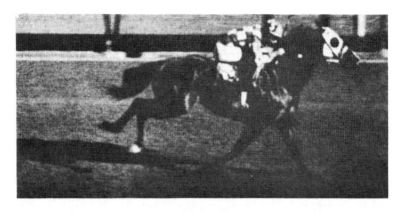

Well ahead of the pack and all alone at the finish, Ronas Ryon takes the All American Futurity in 1986.

Ridden by veteran jocky Jerry Nicodemus in the Derby, Ronas Ryon took a half-length lead as the gates opened. During the entire 440 yards he was never seriously challenged and he rocketed effortlessly past the finish line. He set a new stakes record of :21.32 and his All American Derby win made him the second horse in the history of the All American to come home a winner in both the Futurity and the Derby.

The Derby victory earned his owners a $361,000 check, taking Ronas Ryon's lifetime earnings to an impressive $1.73 million dollars. Ronas Ryon is now the fourth richest quarter horse in the history of track.

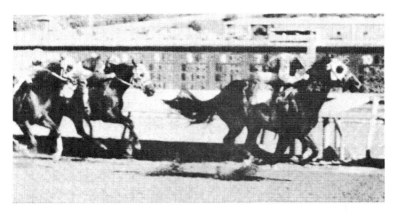

Making history: Alone again, Ronas Ryon crosses the wire to win the 1987 All American Derby, setting a new stakes record.

Zany Tactics Wins It With Winners Bee Pollen

That's the headline of a news release that went out from Winner Bee Pollen back in 1987 when this great horse set a record that still stands. Running at Turf Paradise in Phoenix, Arizona, Zany Tactics made a lot of people in-the-know some money. Keep reading. Here's the whole story:

They say Zany Tactics, who now holds the American track record on turf and the world's record on dirt, runs holes in the wind. This legendary six-year old brown gelding is by Zanthe out of Escort Lady. Just two and one-half months ago, Zany Tactics set an American turf course record at 6 furlongs. Then on March 8th, this dynamic and powerful horse exhibited a lot more than incredible stamina and staying power as he pulled away from Faro at the one-eighth pole and went on to win the Coors Phoenix Gold Cup. With lightning speed, Zany Tactics streaked to a world record on the dirt course at Turf Paradise with a time of 1:06-4/5, thereby erasing Grey Papa's 1972 time of 1:07-1/5 from the record books.

The winner's trainer, Blake Heap, told jockey Jack Kaenel to forget about strategy, explaining: "I just told Jack to let the horse run his own race. That horse knows how to win." Heap was laughing when he said, "Funny thing. Nobody wanted this horse. The Brunettes got him because the breeders didn't want him. He ended up in Utah for awhile, but no one seemed to get anything out of him."

Heap has been feeding the horses in the Vera and Don Brunette barn Winners Bee Pollen since October of 1986 — and gives no other supplements at all. He was heard enthusiastically telling friends in the stands just before the Gold Cup field went off about the dramatic improvement in speed and willingness Zany Tactics in particular had been showing. Heap says, "This is such a kind horse now. You can do anything with him. It's like a dream come true." Does Heap think Winners Bee Pollen turned Zany Tactics into a Winner? After the impressive finishes Zany Tactics has made his last two times out, it's not surprising to learn that Blake Heap personally endorses Winners Bee Pollen. He says the owners are high on it, too. Watch for the new Brunette silks, as golden yellow as Winners Bee Pollen and sporting two honeybees on the back.

Since the Equine Division of The C C Pollen Company opened for business, the division has been producing superior quality Winners Bee Pollen products for horses. The parent company, C C Pollen, is the oldest and largest harvester of bee pollen in the United States. Whether producing bee pollen products for horses or humans, they have the experience and expertise to do it right.

Unlike foreign pollen products, Winners Bee Pollen is harvested under strict supervision right here at home, an important factor in assuring quality. Because they are not stored in a deep freeze, foreign pollens are old and nutrient-impaired by the time they reach our shores, most are tainted with chemicals, and too many pollens (both foreign *and* domestic) are heat treated to retard mold, resulting in the total destruction of all enzymatic action. Winners Bee Pollen products are never heated. They are guaranteed to contain all the enzymes and essential nutrients all horses need for perfect conditioning.

Winners Bee Pollen is a multiblend of pollens harvested far from the environmental pollutants that drift through our skies, and the agribusiness chemicals that are tilled into the earth or dusted on food crops to improve yield. It is a sad commentary on the times to find that there are no agricultural areas left anywhere that still offer a perfect growing medium. Every state in the union registers substandard soil, documented by data collected by the U.S. Department of Agriculture. California, one of our most prolific producers of fresh fruits and vegetables, is a good example of this phenomenon. Citrus grown in California contains only half as much Vitamin C as fruits harvested elsewhere, and the soil of California is mineral-deficient and calcium-poor. California soil tests out lower in calcium than any other U.S. state.

Winners bee pollen is born in the cold, rocky, rugged mountainous areas of the country and is mated with pollens gathered in the oppressively hot desert states. It takes very hardy superior quality natural growth to survive in these rugged climatic areas. The pollens the bees gather in areas like these are fairly bursting with lifepower. What this means to you is that this fresh, clean blend of powerful superior quality bee pollens offers a full complement of each and every nutrient needed to sustain life abundantly. The only other elements your horses must have for sleek, strong, vigorous, and supremely healthy bodies are water and air.

As far as we know, Winner Bee Pollen is the only natural horse food supplement on the market that comes with a money-back guarantee. Horses taking Winners Bee Pollen improve rapidly. Look for improvements in strength, stamina, endurance, staying-power, and coat-conditioning. These are just a few of the improvements your horses will exhibit. Winners Bee Pollen helps build and repair blood cells, vitally important for a perfectly functioning system. When your horse is protected by a daily measure of Winners Bee Pollen, the animal will be less susceptible to fractures and many other problems.

Winners Bee Pollen has been well received by the racing industry in all parts of the United States. Winners products have been endorsed by California trainers running small, medium, and large barns. Blake Heap, Jack VanBurg, D. Wayne Lucas, Jude Feld, Bill Heaton, Alex Moffit, and Walter Greenman all feed Winners, to name just a few.

Chuck Badone

It wasn't just the dramatic performance of Zany Tactics at Turf Paradise that taught Chuck Badone the value of bee pollen. Badone has been a professional handicapper for thirteen years, functioning as the official track handicapper at both Turf Paradise in Phoenix, Arizona and Monmouth Park in Oceanport, New Jersey. Badone's track selections are featured in the Arizona Republic and the Ashbury Park Press in season.

It goes without saying that Chuck Badone is well acquainted with the horse trainers wherever he goes. It was a broken leg that convinced Gene Johnson, a top trainer at Turf Paradise, that bee pollen is a super perfect 'people' food, as well as 'the world's only perfect food for horses.' In an article Badone recently wrote for the Turf Paradise newsletter, Johnson is quoted as follows:

"I'd been taking bee pollen myself for about a year when I broke my leg. Two weeks after the accident, you couldn't see the fracture. I was supposed to be on a walker, but after a short period of time I kept forgetting to use it because my leg felt so good. I get up before dawn and was accustomed to getting in a nap in the afternoon. But I have so much more energy since taking bee pollen that I work right on through."

Johnson feeds all nine of his horses bee pollen, as well as himself. He says, "I've been feeding Winners since March of 1987 and I'm convinced my stock has shown a gradual but steady improvement. Many trainers who try it don't stay on it long enough," he explains. "It's not like a drug that floods the horse's system immediately with chemicals and gives it a hard jolt. You have to keep on feeding bee pollen and you really will see an improvement. I especially like the attitude the horses have after feeding Winners. It seems to satisfy something in their systems. My horses are less stressed now, relaxed, and they are able to go farther than before."

Another trainer, Bob Garvey, a top Turf Paradise conditioner for the past two decades, feeds his entire stable bee pollen. "They eat it up," Garvey says, "I've been using it for about a year now and I've never had a horse who wouldn't eat it. It's easy to administer, which is very helpful if you have a large stable. The horses don't back off their feed." Garvey says he especially likes the source of quick energy it provides his horses. Although he regularly feeds bee pollen, Garvey reveals, "I give them an extra portion two days prior to racing. They show a definite improvement since I've been feeding it." This trainer, too, eats bee pollen himself and says he really appreciates his renewed energy levels.

Orson Lanca started using bee pollen last spring and is more than pleased with the results. He has nine head in training at this writing and remarked he is especially impressed with the improvement in the healing process bee pollen provides. "When one of my horses got a hard bump on the knee joint, the injury healed very rapidly. I'm also impressed with the way my horses eat it up."

"I've been feeding Winners since August of 1987 and I expect to continue to feed it to all my horses that are running," says Lanny Sharp. Sharp won four of his last eight starts, including a stakes event with Dance Director. He then ran Dance Director in Santa Anita. The horse was a winner in an allowance race. "I also really like the way bee pollen makes their coats shine right away," says this veteran trainer.

Chuck Badone has compiled a list of trainers using bee pollen. He says, "Of the horses fed bee pollen, twenty percent have won races. But, more importantly, an astounding fifty-five percent have finished in the money. Considering that some real 'losers' have been turned around with bee pollen, these figures are even more surprising.

"In the relatively short time that bee pollen has been used as a food supplement for race horses, it has rapidly gained in popularity and the results have been remarkable. As the track handicapper at Turf Paradise, I have been able to recognize the sharpness of horses given bee pollen. Knowing which trainers have their horses on bee pollen has become an important bit of knowledge I apply when making my selections.

"When I see a horse well spotted in a race, I give extra consideration to him when I see he is trained by someone I know feeds bee pollen. If this trend continues and the results are as significant as they are now, I figure I will have to place more and more emphasis on bee pollen as a factor when handicapping. With the obvious success rate enjoyed by trainers using bee pollen, it seems likely that more and more horse conditioners will start using it. It may eventually reach the point where it will be difficult for a trainer to remain competitive without it.

"Testimony for the use of bee pollen goes on and on. There's a lot of printed studies that document its benefits. The bottom line is, if you aren't already feeding Winners Bee Pollen, you'd better start."

Badone holds a B.S. degree from St. Lawrence University and masters degree from Westfield State College and Arizona State University. He has earned the respect of racing professionals and fans alike across the nation. His book, *Secrets of a Professional Handicapper*, is considered a classic on handicapping. If you're interested in racing, don't miss this important book.

Winners Bee Pollen Products

The two basic products produced by the company include pure, unadulterated Winners Bee Pollen, a nutrient-rich golden powder, and the same sunshine gold powder enriched with dried raw honey. Both products are sold in reusable buckets in quantities as small as 6 pounds.

Buzz Kennedy, President of the Equine Division of The C C Pollen Company says his Equine Division has a number of specialty Winners Bee Pollen products for horses on the market. Kennedy revealed in confidence that many of these products are in direct response to needs expressed by some of the top breeders and trainers across the country. Here's what to look for:

Bee-Pain Free: Unlike almost all standard pain killers, *Bee-Pain Free is totally natural*, and can even be given freely on the day of a race. This product has no toxic side effects and no upper limits of ingestion, yet it affords the horse better and faster relief from pain than the conventional chemical drug products currently on the market.

Bee-Bleeders Free: Studies show that 80 to 90 percent of all horses which put forth maximum effort are bleeders. This product strengthens arteries, veins, and capillaries to offer the maximum protection against bursting, and even assists in restoring damage that has already occurred. Both of these products were released in April, 1987.

Bee-Fertile: Research coming out of the University of California estimates, on average, that a mare will foal only five times in ten years. Failure to foal is expensive and frustrating to the horse owner. Now, thanks to this newly formulated product, a horse owner can improve the odds. This product is especially designed to assist mares (and stallions) to produce foals between eight and ten times in ten years.

Bee-Worm Free: When a horse is wormed with chemical drugs, toxins accumulate in the tissues and all intestinal bacteria are destroyed, including the necessary friendly bacteria. Without the digestive bacteria needed to process nutrients, the horse gradually loses energy and vigor, and ages before his time. When Bee-Worm Free is fed routinely, the horse will not require chemical de-worming several times per year. Bee-Worm Free is a superior health maintenance product, and a very efficient *natural* preventive.

Bee-Joint Right: This new product has been especially formulated to assist those horses which have joint problems, knee problems, arthritis, bursitis, and so on. We have seen some dramatic effects occur in the short-term, but look for benefits over the long term and you won't be disappointed. These three products were introduced in May, 1987.

Bee-Jet Lag Free: Especially formulated to overcome the stress suffered by horses when flown (or hauled) from one locale to another for an important race. *Bee-Jet Lag Free* is designed to eliminate the typical "after moves" and "after flight" tiredness and lethargy. When Bee-Jet Lag Free is used as directed, it will no longer be necessary to factor recovery time in the schedule when moving horses.

Bee-Trot Free: Digestive upsets abound after a move into an area where horses are fed different hay and different water from the norm. Diarrhea can drain the animal of strength, endurance, and stamina just when they are most needed. This worry can be a thing of the past when Bee-Trot Free is used according to instructions. Bee-Trot Free is especially effective when given in combination with Bee-Jet Lag Free. Both products were released in June, 1987.

Bee-Electrolye Right: An *all-natural* electrolyte-rich additive available in powdered form designed to be given in a measued program over a period of days (instructions included) when maximum effort is expected, such as an important race. The chemical analysis alone on the label is guaranteed to create a lot of excitement. Look for it. Bee-Electrolye Right became available in July, 1987.

Bee-Hoof Right: To maintain a healthy, trouble-free hoof, this high nutrient product is synergistically potentiated with Winners Bee Pollen to give maximum results in the shortest period of time. Bee-Hoof Right gives horses a secondary benefit as well:

the shiniest most beautiful coat you've ever seen. Ask for it by name.

Bee-Heel Right: Far too many horses suffer from cracked and splintering heels. A horse's heels are especially sensitive to damage in sandy or rocky or hard clay soils, as found on so many race tracks. This unique product incorporates both Winners Bee Pollen and Winners Balsam of Peru paste. Heels have been restored in as few as two days with this product.

Bee-Fly Free: Early laboratory tests show that Bee-Fly Free can drive even embedded ticks out of the hides of horses (and dogs) and will keep the flies away, even hard to control stable flies and mosquitoes. Anyone who keeps animals in barn or stable will appreciate this one.

As you can see, the Equine Division of The C C Pollen Company has formulated a complete line of Winners Bee Pollen products for horses. We emphasize that all Winners products are legal in every state, including *Bee-Pain Free*. When a product from the Winners line is given, rest easy. Your horse will pass any spit box or test barn. These trademarked, patented, and copyrighted products contain no drugs, herbicides, pesticides, poisons, or toxic substances of any kind. When you select a Winners Bee Pollen product, you can be sure that product will have no toxic side-effects. Because these products are composed of *natural food substances* only, they are non-addictive and carry no contraindications of any kind. They may be fed at will without risk to the life and health of a horse or animal.

Winners Bee Pollen derives its marvelous health-maintaining

and health-restoring properties from the fact that it contains every essential nutrient needed by every animal for the life processes, plus all the trace elements required for perfect conditioning and perfect health. No other product is so richly endowed... naturally!

Winners Bee Pollen products are now available worldwide. Anyone wishing more information on this natural product, *"created by the Maker,"* may call 1-800-950-0096. Dealer inquiries are also welcome.

A Closing Word from Buzz Kennedy

BEEWARE! Speaking of a dynamite breeding program, I've had my best stallion and a really spectacular brood mare on bee pollen for quite some time. They're both getting all charged up and really feisty, quite probably from all those live hormones in the pollen. When the time is right, I'm going to mate these two. The colt of this union will be getting the benefits of *Winners Bee Pollen* from his mother as a fetus, from birth in the milk of his dam, and forever after.

If you ever have an animal running against this 'miracle baby,' it won't be a fair race — unless your entry has also enjoyed the advantages that *Winners Bee Pollen* provides. I guess it's only sporting of me to wish you luck.

CHAPTER 13

SHOPPING FOR THE PRODUCTS OF THE BEE

Beeware. Not All Beehive Products Are Created Equal

M y personal fascination with the bee and her products had its origin in England in the 1940s. It was before America's entry into World War II that I joined the Royal Canadian Air Force as a fighter pilot. I was based in London and flying with the British Royal Air Force when I was introduced to bee pollen by a fellow pilot I was lunching with in the officer's mess. His description of the benefits of these gold grains was over-enthusiastic, to say the least.

When I laughed at him, he gave me an article to read which had appeared in the London Times. This article extolled the properties of bee pollen and explained why bee pollen was a miracle food substance which would, in time, cure everything. I was skeptical. I just couldn't believe such a simple little bee-food could possibly be the miraculous substance the article claimed it to be. I promptly forgot all about it.

By the 1950s, I was back in the states, married, the father of two, and was associated with the Brighton State Bank in Brighton, Colorado. I ran across some articles on bee pollen relating some interesting studies conducted abroad which seemed to bear out the truth of the statements my friend had made fifteen years before. I still wasn't convinced, mind you, and I promptly forgot about bee pollen again.

Sometime in the 1960s, I read about bee pollen for the third time and decided I really should investigate this 'miracle from the beehive' that so many people were calling 'the only perfect food on earth.' These articles piqued my curiousity again. I decided I'd find out for myself about the true nutritional value of bee pollen.

By now, we had relocated to Arizona. I started first at the Phoenix Public Library, but there wasn't much on bee pollen back then. I ended up at the Arizona State University libraries. This great teaching institution proved to be a gold mine. I proceeded to read every article, every book, and every bit of information I could find about bee pollen. I reached the inescapable conclusion that those three articles I had read over the years were not only true, but may have actually understated the facts.

I decided to try bee pollen for myself. I purchased a packet of bee pollen tablets in a local health food store. They were hard and dry and not very tasty, but I insisted the whole family partake. I didn't know it at the time, but these tablets were made with imported Spanish bee pollen. We all took them regularly and it did seem we all stayed pretty healthy. But we were following a generally healthy lifestyle, so this little personal experiment with bee pollen was hardly conclusive.

As I continued on with my health research, I learned the bee pollen tablets we were taking were made from a single pollen source, the Jara flora. They were old and stale. My research dictated that I find a bee pollen product that was kept beehive-fresh by deep freezing, and one which was composed of pollen from many floral sources. My patriotism demanded I buy American.

I began searching for fresh bee pollen. Local beekeepers weren't much interested in harvesting bee pollen for me. I finally found a California beekeeper who agreed to sell me a multicolored pollen, proving his bees had gathered it from many pollen sources. He froze his pollen as soon as he took it from the beehive, too. This was the beehive-fresh pollen I was looking for. He packaged it for me in 30-pound buckets and I probably purchased about 210 pounds per year for many years. What a difference! Those fresh granules actually tasted good!

By the early 1970's, it became apparent that *something* was making a difference in our household. Year after year, both of my children received awards for perfect attendance at school. Not one of us was ever sick, not even a sniffle or a bout with the flu. We didn't even have a family doctor. We had no need for one.

I was convinced. It simply had to be the bee pollen that was keeping us well. It was then that I determined to do some serious in-depth research on these golden granules from the beehive.

At that time, I was in a partnership involved with the stock market, providing a highly successful and financially-rewarding investment advisory service. But once I started ferreting out and reading the research and double-blind studies on the incredible potency of those little golden grains from the bees, I was hooked. I lost interest in the stock market, sold the investment advisory service, dissolved the partnership and devoted myself full-time to the study of bee pollen.

It wasn't easy accumulating this material either. Much of the research on the products of the beehive was (and still is) conducted in the Soviet bloc countries. It took time, money, perseverance, and determination to persuade them to provide us with copies of their research reports. And, once received, we still had to have them translated.

Yet, the more I found out, the more I wanted to know. I was aware back then that I still didn't have the whole story. According to published scientific reports, researchers in the laboratories of the world were making incredible discoveries on the nutrient value of bee pollen. Still others were documenting the medicinal qualities of bee pollen. There seemed to be worldwide agreement that bee pollen possessed remarkable near-miraculous health-promoting properties.

Knowing what I know now about the miraculous benefits of the natural products of the bee, I'm very thankful that I persisted. I was more determined than ever to search out and chase down everything there was to know about bee pollen. I put my staff to work on the problem with a statement that seemed to cover everything: "I want the best bee pollen in the world. Yessir. I want the best bee pollen the whole world can provide."

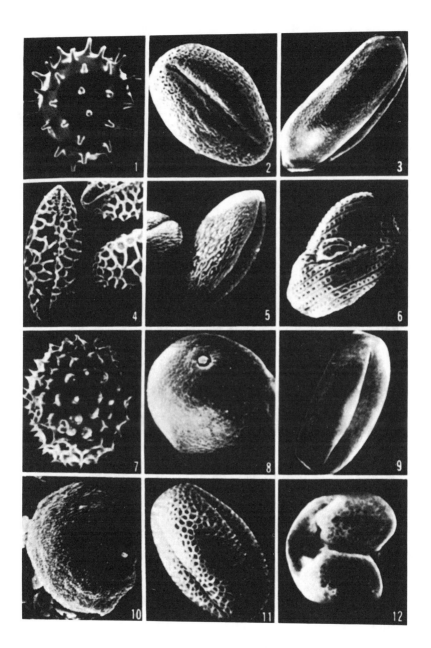

Bee Pollen

Tracking the Facts: Published studies from authorities around the world confirmed that heat-treated pollen was robbed of many vital nutrients. Excessive heat destroyed vital enzymatic action as well. This information led me to make two trips abroad to investigate foreign beekeeping methods. I was disturbed to find that most foreign pollens were, of necessity, heat-treated because the granules were harvested in humid climates and deep flash-freeze storage facilities were just not readily available to those beekeepers.

Further research revealed that pollen loses up to 76 percent of its nutritive value during a year when it is stored at ambient temperatures without freezing. And there was still another factor. Because foreign pollens cannot reach the American consumer much before they are four to six months old, I concluded that this combination of heat-processed dried pollen and age was devastating to the quality of the finished product. These were not the bee pollens I was seeking.

The decision to harvest naturally-dry high-desert Arizona mountain pollen was prompted by the research done by Dr. Nicolai Vasilievich Tsitsin, the gerontology expert of the U.S.S.R. (For Tsitsin's complete findings, see chapter 8). Dr. Tsitsin discovered the centenarians of the Soviet Union, people documented to be over 125 years of age, used bee pollen and honey collected in the high, dry, desert-like climate of the Caucasus Mountains in upper Russia as their main source of nourishment. Dr. Tsitsin attributed their longevity to the dramatic benefits of the naturally-dry pollen these beekeepers harvested from high desert plants. His published report concluded with the hypothesis that bee pollen taken regularly in sufficient amounts will extend the natural lifespan.

When I discovered that equally well-accredited scientists around the world confirmed Tsitsin's basic premise, I was elated! The climate of my own state of Arizona met Tsitsin's requirements for high quality bee pollen perfectly.

I promptly searched out and began working with a Master Beekeeper. We fitted his beehives with pollen traps, The C C Pollen Company was formed, and High Desert Honeybee Pollen was born. We harvested bee pollen that was sweet, fresh, and delicious. I began to believe I had fulfilled my vow of finding the "best bee pollen in the world."

Another Problem to Overcome

But we couldn't rest on our laurels just yet. When I was in San Antonio, Texas lecturing to The Texas Beekeepers Association about trapping pollen, Dr. Norman Gary, of the University of California at Davis, stated bee pollen is encased in two outer husks which protect the inner nutrients. He explained that these coatings preserve and protect pollen granules, quite literally for eons. Then he pointed out that the age of an object can be established by dating pollen granules clinging to it, pollen millions and millions of years old, preserved by those two husks. Dr. Gary said these nearly impenetrable exine jackets are not totally digestible in the human gut.

To say I was upset and disappointed was the understatement of the year!

As soon as I returned home, we started intensive research to discover how to burst the two husks on the granules without the use of heat, chemicals, radiation, or alcohol. Almost by accident, the process was discovered and The C C Pollen Company's *High Desert Honeybee PolllenS* have had the benefit of this proprietary 'Dual Fracture' process for many years.

The CCPC 'Dual Fracture' process double-cracks both exine coatings to permit the High Desert granules to burst when the grains come in contact with the digestive juices, thereby releasing all the vital life-giving nutrients for nearly instantaneous digestion and assimilation.

No other brand of bee pollen claims to have mastered this secret process.

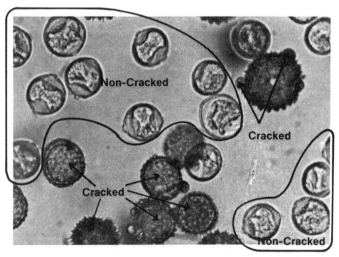

Demonstrating extrusion of contents of pollen grains subjected to the secret The C C Pollen Company process.
Photo magnified by use of an electron-microscope.

Yet Another Problem

After successfully solving that situation, I was just about ready to sigh with satisfaction and proclaim "we do it right." But the fates weren't finished with me yet.

When continuing research showed even my High Desert pollens harvested in the virgin mountain areas of Arizona were deficient in potassium, and other important soil nutrients, I did a quick study of the Phoenix Yellow Pages. I was surprised when I found pages and pages of listings for chemical fertilizer and pesticide dealers. I sent a member of my staff to the Public Library to check out the Yellow Pages of all U.S. states. Not surprisingly, the report was that the phone books of all states carried pages and pages of chemical fertilizer and pesticide dealers. It made no difference where we checked, California, Montana, Iowa, Wyoming, Idaho, Texas. Everywhere the results were the same, pages and pages of chemical fertilizer and pesticide dealers. And you can bet they were all making money.

If the nutrients aren't in the soil, they can't be in the bee pollen harvested from plants grown in such substandard soil. And I wasn't at all pleased to be able to correctly surmise that chemical fertilizers and pesticides were being used at an alarming rate to try to correct the soil deficiences man had caused in the first place.

I was devastated. What to do? I was searching for the best bee pollen possible. I still felt our Arizona High Desert bee pollen was the best bee pollen currently available on the world market. But I also realized even High Desert could be improved.

Three and a half years of intensive research on soil nutrients lay ahead. Every Federal government source, every U.S. Agricultural Department source, every County Extension agent, and every other source we could find was contacted. One very knowledgeable authority is Professor Albert Albrecht of the University of Missouri. Professor Albrecht has spent a lifetime studying the nutrient balance of the soils of the world. His studies show that when the annual rainfall equals 25 inches per year, the soils start to lose nutrients at a rapid rate. When the annual rainfall reaches 35 inches annually, the soils suffer a marked loss of all water soluble nutrients, as well as many very important trace elements.

Painstakingly, we gathered together reports on the nutrient deficiencies and excesses of the soils of all 50 states. We then laboriously consolidated and extensively analyzed this mountain of information. What we found was frightening. Thanks to man's tinkering with the environment, there is not one state in the union, indeed, not one place in the entire world, excepting the Caucausus Mountains of Russia and Hunza Land, which still has all the nutrients present in the earth that nature intended. Sad, but all too true. Environmental soil studies conducted by the U.S. Department of Agriculture all across the nation lay bare the facts.

We now have the general soil nutrient profile of each of the U.S. states. For example, North and South Dakota, some parts of Colorado, New Mexico and Arizona have high concentrations of selenium in their soils. But the entire northern areas of the

U.S., which were once covered by glaciers, the East Coast, most of California, all of Oregon and the entire state of Washington have soils deficient in important minerals, including selenium, zinc, and iodine, and all water-soluble nutrients.

States on the East coast and in the midwest are universally deficient in many trace elements, including selenium, one of the important minerals science says protects the heart. The soil in these states also tests very low in the water-soluble nutrients, including selenium, iodine, all the B-Complex vitamins and ascorbic acid (vitamin C).

The soils of California test lowest of all fifty states in calcium. Here's another surprise. Citrus fruits grown in the golden state contain 50 percent *less* vitamin C than the citrus grown in Texas and Florida. So it's important to include some Texas and Florida citrus bee pollen in blending bee pollen. However, the California climate offers something no other state can match. California has Eucalyptus trees that live a thousand years, making it important to include California Eucalyptus pollen in the High Desert blend.

It was certainly apparent to me that the only way to deliver as near-perfect bee pollen as possible was to blend pollens from many areas. We really didn't want to go to the trouble and expense of mixing pollens harvested in many different areas. Why? This is a very costly procedure. We realized that the blending process would inevitably result in excessive powdering of the fragile granules and we would lose a high percentage.

However, I reluctantly concluded we could only hope to

achieve "the best bee pollen in the world" by mixing and blending pollens harvested in many different areas of this country. Yes, we should even blend in bee pollen from the Caucausus Mountains of the Soviet Union, from the mountains and desert regions of China, from the Rocky Mountains and deserts of Central and South America, with the best of the U.S. to create the ultimate in bee pollen, the perfect bee pollen blend. To end up with the best finished product, the perfect blend, *the best bee pollen possible,* it was absolutely vital we mix bee pollens from areas having a high concentration of certain soil nutrients and a low concentration of other elements with pollens from areas having the opposite percentages.

We were forced to start harvesting bee pollen from the Dakotas, all of the Rocky Mountain states, and most of the Western states in order to achieve the mixture most desirable to provide "the best bee pollen in the world." Today, we blend pollens from as many as twenty different states to create the High Desert Honeybee PollenS blend.

Our expanded and extended range of bee pollen harvesting leads us to believe that *only* The C C Pollen Company goes to the bother and expense of mixing pollens. We believe this unique blending procedure of many, many pollens from widely diverse areas is the only way to insure highest potency and complete nutrient content.

As things stand now, we believe The C C Pollen Company is the *only* food producer in the entire world both aware of these documented soil deficiences *and* doing something about it. High

Desert just might be the only nutritionally complete natural food available anywhere on this planet.

As a case in point, in translation from the German, a study entitled *Bee Pollen: A Valuable Part of Holistic Therapy,* has this to say in part: "Being concerned about the widespread development of disease and the detrimental effects of modern civilization, often caused by our refined, beautified, and mostly denatured foods, termed *mesothropy* (semi-nutrition), it becomes clear we must seek the solution where nature still functions. Fortunately, the world of the bee is such a bastion of nature."

When soil samples from around the world are taken wherever foods are grown, the results always show a great depletion of essential nutrients, as the U.S. studies prove.

In my extensive travels, I have made a point of investigating methods of beekeeping around the world. Here's a brief review of bee pollen harvesting as practiced in other countries.

Australia: Nearly all Australian pollen comes from the Jarrah tree and the Marri tree. These trees produce pollens at different times of the year and, by my definition, are inferior because any single source pollen is inferior to blended bee pollens. Most of the pollen harvest 'down under' carries a high moisture content and must be heated, baked, or hot-air dried to remove the moisture and prevent mold growth. Virtually no Australian honeybee pollen is refrigerated. Worse, some is chemically fumigated. Due to shipping, handling, and storage problems, Australian pollen is from four to six months old (or older) before reaching the U.S.

Canada: Most Canadian bee pollen is gathered in the North Peace area of northern British Columbia. Virtually all Canadian pollen is from a semi multi-floral source in a humid area, meaning it must be sun-dried, hot-air dried, or heated. Consequently, Canadian pollen is usually heat-dried, not stored under refrigeration or frozen.

English & French: Almost all English and French honeybee pollen carries a high moisture content at time of harvest and must be heat-treated to remove harmful moisture. Although these pollens usually come from multi-floral sources, refrigeration is seldom used for storage. Pollens imported from England and France are at least four to six months old before they are displayed on health-food store shelves.

Spanish: Spanish bee pollen is commonly harvested at an intermediate altitude, from 2000 to 4000 feet above sea level. Due to the habits of Spanish beekeepers, usually pollen is not shipped abroad until long after harvest. Before it can be consumed by the American public, Spanish pollen reaches the ripe old age of six months or more. Much of the Spanish bee pollen is chemically fumigated; most is heat-dried, baked, or sun-dried to remove excess moisture and slow down the development of mold. Refrigeration is seldom used.

Traditionally, Spanish bee pollen is priced lower in U.S. stores than most other sources. It's easy to see why. Unfortunately, producers of bee pollen tablets or capsules often buy Spanish pollen because it costs so little. They fail to state the source of the pollen on their labels.

You Be The Judge

When selecting a bee pollen tablet or capsule formula, it's very important that you purchase from a reliable producer of beehive products. If the label does not state the origin of the bee pollen, it is most likely cheap Spanish or Chinese bee pollen. You won't be able to tell if the bee pollen in the finished product is good, bad, or indifferent once it's been ground up and mixed in with tableting or capsulizing ingredients.

But you don't have to be an expert to judge fresh honeybee pollen. You can *see* the difference; you can *feel* the difference; and, best of all, you can *taste* the difference. Trust your senses.

See: Pour out a bit of fresh pollen from the package and take a good look at it. Although most honeybee pollen granules are varying shades of gold, a good multisource bee pollen will exhibit a mixture of colors. These colors can range from a very pale straw shade all the way across the spectrum through oranges, browns, and purples to almost black. Occasionally, some pure reds and beautiful blues show up. Treasure these rarities.

Feel: Roll a granule around between your thumb and middle finger. It should be soft and springy. Rock hard pollen grains have been over-cooked. If your bee pollen crunches in your mouth and refuses to dissolve on your tongue, you can be sure that most of the live nutrients and all vital enzymes have been destroyed in the processing.

Taste: The proof of the pudding is in the eating. Although some high-heat treated pollen tastes rather good, though very hard and crunchy, you might as well eat potato chips for all the nutrient value it offers. Worse, a lot of imported pollens, even some harvested here at home, are chewy and gummy and musty-tasting. Stale pollen granules are unpalatable. They just plain taste 'nasty.' Even some nitrogen-canned bee pollens have this telltale taste. If they go into the can old and stale, all the nitrogen flushing in the world won't make them taste good.

But, ahh. . . Fresh raw bee pollen kernels taste like flowers smell, faintly sweet and as field-fresh as a sunny meadow filled with spring flowers gently dancing in a warm breeze. Think of chewing on a tender blade of grass or nibbling on a flower petal when you were ten and you'll come close. This is the taste of the High Desert Honeybee PollenS. And, because they go in the can fresh, the nitrogen-flushed pollens we offer have this same delightful taste.

The Challenger

Although we had fought the good fight and were well satisfied we were delivering the best bee pollen in the world, The C C Pollen Company faced yet another challenge. Another source of pollen hit the American market in 1984, pollen collected directly from planets without the benefit of the bee's benevolence. They called it 'Flower Pollen' and bombarded the consumer with literature that attempted to support their claims of the superiority of flower pollen over bee pollen.

These claims were ridiculously easy to refute. We excerpt from an article published in *Health Freedom News*, The Journal of the National Health Federation, in April 1984, as follows:

There is a wealth of documentation on the general efficacy of bee-gathered pollen versus the 'flower pollens,' which are now being marketed to U.S. consumers. We have analyzed the various claims of the 'flower pollen' people and the bee pollen producers. We present the following facts for your review.

For example, in a paper entitled *Bees Sterilize Pollen by Means of a Glandular Secretion Antagonistic to Tumors,* Guebwiller of L'Ariculteur haut-rhinois states, "Bees produce a very fast-acting substance in their bodies which sterilizes the pollen they gather."

Remy Chauvin, M.D., of the Institute of Bee Culture in Paris reports that bee pollen possesses bacteriostatic and antibiotic qualities pollens collected directly from plants do not. Dr. Chauvin points out that salmonella and E.coli cannot live in bee pollen, but live abundantly in the so-called 'flower pollens.'

Dr. William Robinson of the USDA published results of a 1948 study entitled *Delay in the Appearance of Mammary Tumors in C3H Mice Following Ingestion of Pollenized Food.* This paper concludes with the following statement: "Results indicate the development of mammary tumors can be influenced by the ingestion of pollenized food. These experiments were based on the postulation that bee pollen contains an anticarcinogenic principle which can be added to food."

Dr. Naum Petrovitsch Yoirisch, publishing in the USSR in 1976, says, ". . .none of this pollen, the male element of the plant, becomes a complete natural food until the bee gathers, annoints, and enriches it with its own nectar."

The Journal of Economic Entomology reports pollens hand-collected directly from plants "acquired a decidedly rancid odor within a few days." Interestingly, the *Journal* article concludes: "There was no noticeable change in any of the bee-collected pollens."

In *Literature on Pollen Chemistry,* the respected Grana Palynologica of Stockholm states, "The mode of collecting pollen must be considered when judging analytical results. Bee-collected pollen always contains large amounts of reducing sugars. Mechanically-collected pollen is heavy in non-reducing sugars. Another remarkable observation is that pollen carried by bees contains carotenes, whereas no carotenoids were detected in anemophile (wind-carried flower) pollens."

The old master, Dr. Alin Caillas, in a 1933 paper entitled, *L-Abeille de France,* writes: "It can be said that inactive pollens are almost exclusively the pollens of anemophilous plants. Conifers, in particular, always supply pollens having the least biological value and whose effect on longevity is rather negative."

Dr. Caillas notes that 'flower pollens' are harvested from maize, rye, pine, spring grass, orchard grass and alder and says, "All are overlooked by the honeybees because of their very low biological value."

Why do dispensers of mechanically-collected 'flower pollens' rely on the pollens the bees don't want, instead of those of great biological value which the bees bring back to the hive?

Dr. Caillas says it is because a pharmaceutical product must contain a constant and regular composition in order to be approved by the government, and the composition of bee pollens varies widely.

The consumer is well advised to question claims made for mechanically-collected 'flower pollens' bereft of the mysterious and well-documented 'magic' of the bee.

And that was just about the end of the 'Flower Pollen' challenge. The American health-food consumer is no dummy.

Natural Health Insurance

When you rely on food crops grown in soils which have been depleted of important nutrients and/or polluted with agribusiness chemicals (or the meat-animals fed on feed grown you are just not receiving the full and complete balance of nutrients our bodies must have to live in perfect health. If the giant food producers would switch from manmade chemical fertilizers and use instead natural decomposed organic matter to enrich the soil, we would be on the right track. But, except for small farmers who specialize in producing organically-grown foodstuffs, this is not a realistic hope for the future.

You can, of course, try buying foods grown in different areas of the country, but that has to be a real exercise in frustration. When you shop in a supermarket, you'd have to buttonhole the produce manager and question him to find out exactly where the broccoli, or anything else, was grown. Bagged potatoes usually carry a label identifying the state or origin, but trying to make sure you get a full complement of nutrients by attempting to shop for foods grown in different states is all but impossible.

The solution is obvious. Whenever possible, shop those markets which feature organically-grown fruits and vegetables. And here's another tip. Kosher butchers really do answer to a higher authority. Kosher meats are clean-processed and uncontaminated with chemicals. Yes, these especially produced foods cost more. And, yes, it's worth spending the extra dollars to safeguard your health.

The same problems apply when you rely on single-source bee pollen, especially when that pollen is harvested in areas where the soils are chemicalized with manmade fertilizers, and/or the surrounding environment where the hives are located is polluted with the detritus of man's passing.

There's an easier way to make sure you're providing a balance of all the natural nutrients every hungry cell in your body needs. Bee pollen is the only natural food that can be scientifically mixed and blended to deliver the proper and correct array of all the essential nutrients. And by now you understand why that's very, very important.

Incidentally, the belief that *local* bee pollen is somehow 'better' than bee pollens produced by giant pollen harvesters seems to have its basis in 'old wive's tales.' In the not too distant past, raw honey was administered by great grandmother as treatment for many minor ills, including seasonal allergies, with great success. Today we know that the effective substance in raw honey fresh from the farm beehive was actually the microscopic pollen spores suspended in unprocessed honey.

Using quality blended bee pollen to desensitize someone suffering from seasonal hay fever and other pollen allergies works even better than supplying raw honey. (See chapter 8). As we have discovered, a single-source pollen is always deficient in one or more elements. A blend of bee pollens is always more effective than a single-source pollen from a localized area.

The C C Pollen Company delivers the best bee pollen in the world. I believe I have achieved my goal. We now harvest and market High Desert Honeybee Pollen*S*, the capitol '*S*' signifying the all-important blend, beautifully trademarked as '*The Pollen of 10,000 Flowers.*' This single innovation alone makes High Desert preeminent in the field and puts all The C C Pollen

Company bee pollen products clearly in a superior class by themselves, far ahead of any other pollen products currently available anywhere in the world.

Of course, all High Desert bee pollen products are preserved with cold, not excessive heat. The fresh granules are frozen at harvest by the beekeeper and held frozen until shipment to us. Once they are packaged or formulated into finished products, all are held in deep-cold storage at minus 5 degrees F. until shipment to the purchaser, as extensive research dictates.

Today, I can honestly say I have actually achieved the goal I set for myself so many long years ago. I'm proud of the chemical analysis of High Desert Honeybee PollenS, reproduced for your review on page 290.

HIGH DESERT® HONEYBEE POLLENS™ CHEMICAL ANALYSIS

PROTEIN
7.1 GRAMS PER OZ. (RDA 12 GRAMS)

Standard chemical analysis identifies only 18 or the 22 amino acids present in pollen.

AMINO ACIDS	MGs PER OZ.
Cystine	36.8555
Lysine	366.360
Histidine	138.590
Arginine	292.520
Aspartic	542.440
Threonine	236.856
Serine	289.680
Glutamic	585.040
Proline	505.520
Glycine	585.040
Alanine	309.560
Valine	280.592
Methionine	94.004
Isoleucine	230.040
Leucine	377.720
Tyrosine	139.440
Phenylalanine	236.850
Tryptophan	49.700

Note: "Realities of Nutrition" states a person using the RDA to choose protein foods might not get enough of all essential amino acids. Bee pollen contains all essential amino acids.

MINERALS	MGs PER OZ.
Calcium	42.383
Iron	2.118
Potassium	158.675
Phosphorus	121.706
Sodium	2.693
Iodine &In MCGs)	6.237
Magnesium	27.675
Zinc	1.460
Copper	.221
Boron	.604
Barium	.136
Chromium (less than)	.010
Mangenese	1.395
Strontium	.094

MISCELLANEOUS	GRAM PER OZ
Carbohydrates	5.15
Fiber	1.02
Reducing Sugars	8.25
Ash	.65
CALORIES PER OUNCE	.90

VITAMINS	MGs PER OZ
A- 232,470 I.U.*	
Alpha Carotene	.031
Beta Carotene	.122
B1 (Thiamine)	.198
B2 (Riboflavin)	.459
B3 (Niacine)	2.551
B6 (Pyridoxine)	.119
B12 (Cyanocobalamin)	.00002
Biotine	.002
Folic Acid	.201
Pantothenic Acid	.198
C - (Ascorbic Acid)	1.304
D - 9 I.U.*	
E - 2.194 I.U.*	
* International Units	

RUTIN - Abundant. (Not measured in analysis) Of great importance for capillary strength.

ENZYMES. Active enzymes are needed to digest and assimilate nutrients. Chemical analysis measures only three of the many present in bee pollen.

ENZYME	UNITS PER GRAM
Amylase (USP Unite)	2.550
(Needed to break down starch)	
Protease (USP Units)	64.400
(Needed to spilt proteins)	
Lipase (mm Units)	.085
(Needed to emulsity fats)	

FATTY ACIDS 2.807 GRAM/OZ
Essential fatty acids, with carbohydrates and sugars, supply our energy requirements.

— CHOLESTEROL — 0 PERCENT —
Bee pollen contains a higher content (11) of the healthful unsaturated fatty acids as opposed to saturated (9).

NOTE: Bee pollen also contains elements science is not yet able to isolate and identify. Some authorities believe it is precisely these elements, often called the "magic" of the bee, which make bee pollen so effective.

NOTE: This important chemical analysis was conducted by an independent testing laboratory on the justly famous enzyme-active High Desert® PollenS™ blend. It does not apply to any other brand of bee pollen in the world. If you see this analysis, or any portion thereof, reprinted elsewhere you may be certain propriety material is being used both incorrectly and illegally to persuade you another product has the same documented high nutrient count as blended High Desert®.

You'll discover your favorites among these High Desert Honeybee PollenS products in your local health-food store:

Fresh High Desert Granules: This is the justly famous High Desert multifloral blend in bags of one pound and five pounds. Take a peek through the clear bag and notice the many colors. You'll find this one in the refrigeration case.

Nitrogen-Flushed High Desert Granules: The same multifloral blend, of course, but packaged in a can with a special food-safe lining. Once these granules are measured out and the can filled, the can is topped off with nitrogen (an inert gas) to force out all oxygen. Thus vacuum packed, the granules stay fresh and flavorful on the shelf.

Pollenergy: In handy tablets or easy-to-take capsules, these 520 mg and 1500 mg tabs and caps offer a convenient pre-measured *unadulterated* (nothing added, nothing taken away) form of High Desert with all nutrients and important properties live and intact.

Honey/Vanilla Tablets: A gentle 130 mg of High Desert lightly sweetened with honey and vanilla makes these chewable tabs pleasant to take. One tablet per day is the recommended amount for females; two tablets per day for males. The rationale for this suggested use is that the average female will ingest three pounds (or less) of food daily; the average male will ingest six pounds (or less) of food daily. These proportions equate to one-part bee pollen in 10,000 parts of food.

In 1:10,000, the studies conducted by William Robinson, M.D. (see Chapter 8) showed that these properties provided amazing protection against cancer.

Bee-Thin Tablet Formula: Contrary to commercial over-the-counter weight-loss preparations, Bee-Thin is not dangerous to your health and won't leave you jittery or with a drug-induced 'hangover.' Offers the natural appetite-suppressant action and satisfying nutrition of bee pollen. Average weight loss is a healthy one pound per week.

The C C Pollen Company also produces a number of bee-pollen based specialty products, including *Aller-Gone*, the basis for a program of natural desensitization that works against seasonal allergies; *Bee-Sleepy*, a natural aid for overcoming insomnia; several specially-formulated nutritive supplements for retarding the natural aging process, such as *Bee-Young* and *Forever Young* (with nicotinic acid), *Bee Young II* (with niacinamide); and *Bee-Stress Free*, which provides much-needed nutrient support in this stress-inducing modern age we live in.

You also should know about *Elixir*, the *High Desert Bee Pollen* liquid extract which is probably the most powerful and concentrated food product in the world; *Bee Jet-Lag Free*, which prevents jet lag on flights lasting up to 27 hours, *Bee Pain Free*, highly successful against the worst arthritic pain, even of the spine; *Bee Stronger*, especially developed to promote strength and guaranteed to work; *Bee Faster*, called amazingly successful by top athletes; *Diarrhea Bee Gone*, which can prevent and/or correct the most common problem arising during travel (often called 'Montezuma's Revenge' and known as 'the trots'); and *Wrinkles Bee Gone*, especially formulated to penetrate the skin surface; helps boost collagen levels of the connective tissue, thereby strengthening the facial muscles to pull the skin back in place and eliminate the wrinkles.

These specialty products can be found in major health food stores, or inquire directly of the company.

And then there's those very popular High Desert Bee Pollen Energy Bars. I tell you, folks, we have a hard time keeping these highly nutritive bars in stock. They come in a counter-top display of 24 bars. They're so good you often find them in the 'candy' department.

For a quick energy pickup, an easy way to take a daily measure of High Desert Bee Pollen, or as a satisfying substitute for a high calorie meal in a diet regimen, they're both winners.

The President's Lunch: This is a chewy delicious combination of healthy good-for-you natural ingredients, including 260 mg of High Desert Bee Pollen, oats, peanut butter, sunflower seeds, raisins, honey, kelp, and more. Calories total just 150.

The First Lady's Lunch: This is another delicious confection of just 150 calories featuring 260 mg of High Desert Bee Pollen, plus sunflower seeds, oats, kelp and honey, but with almonds and dates (instead of raisins and peanut butter).

Royal Jelly

For many years, I personally ate my way through a pound of liquid royal jelly every two months, at the rate of one teaspoonful of the bitter-tasting acid royal milk per day. During this period of time. The C C Pollen Company handled only liquid royal jelly. Knowing my determination to have only the best bee product of its kind, of course, I believed back then this was the best royal jelly obtainable.

It was not until 1981 that I discovered I was mistaken. Here's how it happened. For many years, I had been acquainted with Betty Lee Morales, of The Eden Ranch, Topanga, California. I not only subscribed to her very informative newsletter on natural self-care health-care, we had developed a friendship and often communicated on a personal level. When she was killed in 1987 in an automobile accident, the world lost a very knowledgeable and influential natural healer and I lost my good friend. I believe Betty Lee Morales was the greatest female authority on natural health-care who ever lived.

It was Betty Lee Morales who brought royal jelly to the attention of Hollywood stars right after World War II. In the late 1950s and early 1960s, the royal jelly craze was at its height. Betty Lee's royal jelly formulae were based on strong scientific documentation, as were all her nutritive products. She held to a very high standard and offered only the best, most purely-formulated products. And she knew exactly was she was doing.

As the word got out, it seemed as if everyone wanted royal jelly. Betty Lee's success led to imitators galore. Unfortunately, some unscrupulous manufacturers jumped on this particular bandwagon. The claims for royal jelly got wildly improbable, and many of the products that came into the marketplace were less than pure. The Federal Drug Administration moved in and stopped the importation of all royal jelly, including Betty Lee's shipments.

Nonetheless, her research was solid. When Betty Lee explained the facts to me, it was very apparent that she knew more about royal jelly than anyone else, except the bees themselves. She convinced me that the liquid royal jelly I was eating with such confidence was not the royal jelly served to the Queen bee. She explained that it is impossible for a consumer to get liquid royal jelly that's fresh enough to have all potent nutrients intact. In liquid form, royal jelly begins to deteriorate immediately on harvest.

The royal jelly the Queen bee feasts on is never more than 24-hours old. When Betty Lee Morales tested the biological activity of 24-hour royal jelly and compared it to the activity of royal jelly that was 48-hours old, she documented the results. What she discovered was that 24-hour royal jelly is close to four times more biologically-active than royal jelly just 48-hours old.

Betty Lee assured me that the 24-hour royal jelly manufactured in the pharyngeal glands of the nurse bees on a rich diet of bee pollen accomplishes many miracles. When the hive is without a queen, the bees feed ordinary larvae royal jelly and rear another queen. It is her royal jelly that develops the strong pheromones (scent) of a Queen bee. This scent, individual to the Queen, permeates the hive. Her pheromones are such a powerful stimulant that the worker bees literally work themselves to death for the benefit of the colony.

The fresh 24-hour royal jelly the Queen feasts on causes

her physical development to be greatly superior to her sister-workers. The Queen bee is from 150 to 200 percent larger than the female workers of the colony.

And it is 24-hour royal jelly alone which insures the fertility of the Queen Mother. The Queen is impregnated just once in her lifetime. The act occurs during the mating flight of a young queen. The sperm of the strongest drone, the only one to reach her as she flies higher and higher, is deposited in a reservoir. After this one impregnation, in nature, the Queen will remain fertile for 5, 6, 7, and even 8 years. On her exclusive diet of 24-hour royal jelly, the Queen Mother will lay more than her body weight in eggs every day. She will deposit more than 2000 eggs in the brood chambers each day, each one fertile.

The worker bees of the hive, who are forbidden the royal milk, have an average life expectancy of little more than a month, six weeks at the outside. The Queen bee's diet of 24-hour royal jelly extends her working lifespan from five to eight years.

Betty Lee pointed out that the Queen dines on freshly manufactured 24-hour royal jelly, not aged liquid royal jelly preparations sold on the open market similar to the one I was taking. Although Betty Lee wasn't telling me anything I didn't know about the inner workings of the beehive, I just hadn't put all the facts in the proper perspective. She was right, of course.

The conclusions were obvious. It is 24-hour royal jelly that gives the Queen Bee her powers, not ordinary liquid royal jelly. 24-hour royal jelly is the greatest rejuvenating food in the world. 24-hour royal jelly is the most powerful sex-gland stimulant for both male and female ever known.

The purveyors of liquid royal jelly don't want you to know when their product was harvested, she explained. Due to the time required to harvest, process, package and ship, most of the liquid forms of royal jelly are at least 30 to 90 days old. Betty Lee concluded that 24-hour royal jelly is perhaps *50 times* more biologically active than royal jelly that is a month old.

I learned from Betty Lee that the only way to call a halt to the rapid deterioration of royal jelly is *lypholizing* (freeze-drying) it on-site directly after harvest. Lypholizing is simply a super-quick way of removing all moisture in a substance. What's left behind is a freeze-dried powder that contains every bit of the substance, except the water. And that's how the best, most biologically-active royal jelly is handled. Once a quantity of royal jelly is 'vacuumed' out of the artificial queen cells where the bees deposit it (see Chapter 10), it is hustled to special lypholizing chambers and freeze-dried so quickly that none of its amazing properties is lost.

Betty Lee Morales had my full attention. She made me see that the liquid royal jelly I had been relying on was a great deal less than the best obtainable. Then she carried my education a giant step further.

The royal jelly formula Betty Lee favored contains 24-hour royal jelly, plus bee pollen and bee propolis. This mating of all three of the most active products of the beehive is a natural. She explained that her research showed that 24-hour royal jelly is immensely potentiated by the addition of pollen and propolis.

Then she revealed another fact. She had experimented with the formula by adding other natural substances in her search for absolute perfection. Her tests showed that the natural form of vitamin E (D-Alpha Tocopherol Succinate) also greatly potentiates 24-hour royal jelly.

Although I expressed my gratitude to her very fully, I still owe a great deal of thanks to Betty Lee Morales for her generous sharing of all the research she had done over the years. I promptly converted all that knowledge into the development of what I believe to be the best royal jelly formula in the world.

As a daily supplement, suggested use is one tablet daily for those forty years of age or younger. Those over forty may wish to take two tablets daily. Beginning ingestors are reminded that royal jelly may cause such a strong feeling of euphoria and well-being that they will be tempted to overexert themselves. This bioactive organic substance is very powerful.

The C C Pollen Company originally named the Morales formula *Rejuvenation,* but found this name confusing to the consumer. We now proudly market *24-Hour Royal Jelly* as formulated by Dr. Betty Lee Morales. This tableted formula is a powerful blend of 24-hour royal jelly, lypholized on-site, of course, with High Desert Honeybee Pollen, High Desert Bee Propolis, and natural Vitamin E. Betty Lee herself formulated our 24-Hour Royal Jelly. I know we do it right.

Bee Propolis

As you have already learned, propolis is a valuable natural healer and a very important preventive medicinal that works safely and naturally to strengthen the system. For apitherapeutical purposes, propolis is prepared in various forms, including granules, powders, soft and dry extracts, and liquid tinctures, which contain alcohol.

When freshly gathered, propolis is soft and sticky in warm weather, hard and brittle in cold weather. This brownish/greenish substance is a solid heterogenous mass which often includes many foreign bodies, not the least of which is its content of twenty to twenty-five percent beeswax. In order to end up with a propolis preparation as rich as possible in the biologically-active substances which give propolis its remarkable power, it's obviously necessary to start with a chuck of propolis as pure as possible, with the lowest possible percentage of wax, foreign debris, and any other materials which impair its quality.

The bees themselves select propolis from plants in their flying range which show the highest possible biological resistance. That secretion we see oozing from trees and leafbuds is essential to the defense of the tree. It has a marked biological activity which controls numerous phytopathogenic micro-organisms, fungi, and viruses which would otherwise destroy or inhibit healthy growth of the species. These secretions are particularly effective in holding back the development of competitive flora, which would otherwise develop and steal nutrients and growing-space from the trees themselves.

In spite of its scientifically-documented valuable properties, propolis is still the stepchild, as far as U.S. beekeepers are concerned. Overseas, especially in the Soviet dominated countries, propolis is sought after and plays an important role in Apitherapy

Clinics which treat various conditions with all the products of the beehive. Here at home, there are many giant American bee-keeping operations which harvest only honey, just as there are a growing number of large bee yards where both honey and bee pollen are the money-makers.

But there are just a few successful commercial harvesters of propolis in the United States. The best propolis comes from northern climes where poplar and conifer trees flourish. These trees and their leafbuds produce the highest quality propolis. To those in the know, this is the only propolis worth bragging about.

To obtain the highest possible percentage of active properties without the unwanted debris, propolis chunks must be deep-frozen, then ground. The resulting finely-ground propolis then must be filtered through an extracting agent to float out all foreign substances. The grinding process itself is very difficult. The hard sticky globs of fresh propolis can easily gum up the equipment. To side-step this problem, the grinding itself must be performed in two or more stages.

The first stage of the grinding process consists of cutting the propolis with mechanically-operated stainless-steel knives into granules of 20 to 30 mm in size. During the second stage, these granules are reduced to 3 to 4 mm in size. This machine employs a rapidly-revolving drum. As the drum revolves, the propolis granules are forced to pass across a plate fitted with very sharp knives. By adjusting the space between the blades ever closer together, the desired grind is accomplished.

If the propolis is to be tableted or encapsulized, the process stops here and the propolis powder goes to the end producer for incorporation into the finished product. This is the type of finely-ground fresh propolis that The C C Pollen Company uses in the *High Desert Bee Propolis* tablet and capsule formulae we offer. In this case, the 'High Desert' name signifies the quality of the product. The propolis we employ is harvested by the bees directly from northern conifers and the poplars that research shows are the most biologically-active and which are warranted to contain the highest quality and most powerful properties of any propolis product on the market.

Propolis is the strongest antibiotic found in nature. It has no toxic side effects, no contraindications, nor upper limits of ingestion. Unlike chemical antibiotics produced in a drug laboratory, the body does not build up a tolerance to this natural from the beehive or become accustomed to its effect. The ingestor will receive as much benefit from a bee propolis tablet taken at the last of his life as he gets from the first one he ever ingests. In regular use, propolis builds resistance to respiratory distress, flu, coughs and colds, and more. Propolis assists the immune system and does not inhibit its action, as lab produced antibiotics do.

Another CCPC product that makes me proud is our *Bee-Clear Skin Cream*. This cream has shown spectacular results even against disfiguring cases of long-standing chronic acne which resisted medical treatment, sometimes for many years. The formula consists of a High Desert Bee Pollen/Honey extract powered with 10 percent high-quality High Desert propolis. The whole is greatly potentiated with 24-Hour Royal Jelly.

This seems like a good place to introduce you to Kristi Perkins, a teenager who suffered embarrassment and humiliation because of the condition of her skin. In her own words, this is her story.

I, Kristi Perkins, hereby certify that I had the worst case of pimples and acne imaginable. My dad and grandfather took me around to many dermatologists, but no matter what the doctors tried, absolutely nothing did me any good. During the four-year period that I was affected, my face became scarred and pitted. No sooner would one pustule (that's what the doctor said they were) dry up than two others would come out. Then these new pimples would grow so huge they burst and the pus that came out just made more infection. My complexion was so awful that I often refused to go to school or even church.

My prayers were answered when my granddad brought me my first jar of Bee-Clear Skin Cream. I used this cream religiously, morning and night, according to instructions. I couldn't believe it, but by the time I used up the jar, all of my pimples and pustules were gone. It sure looked like my acne days were over.

But I still had scars. Some of the pits were very deep and looked red and nasty. Even though the acne was gone, I still hated to look in the mirror. Four years of fighting the condition had left me with ugly scars and marks on my face and neck.

But I had a hunch that Bee-Clear might even help fade away my scars. I asked my granddad to get me another jar. I kept using it. I went through that second jar and then the third. By the time I finished with the second jar, all the redness had faded away from my skin. By the time I used up most of the third jar, about fifty percent of my scars were corrected. By this, I mean that the severity of the scars and the depth of the scarring were reduced by half.

I'm still using Bee-Clear and it's still working great. I really think that if I keep using Bee-Clear for another six or eight months, maybe a year, all the scars on my face and neck will be gone.

Because I know only too well all the agony and humiliation I myself suffered with pimples and acne, I have told The C C Pollen Company to let my story be known. When my granddad got me Bee-Clear Skin Cream, it was the real answer to all my prayers and I'm so thankful. I sing the praises of Bee-Clear. I hope The C C Pollen Company publishes my story all over the world for the good of all young people elsewhere.

We know that Bee-Clear works almost miraculously to clear up even the worst cases of acne, but we can't guarantee that everyone will find that it fades scars and redness. Kristi's testimonial is heartfelt and very impressive and we are really happy for her, but the correction of scars is an individualized thing and depends on many factors. Still, anyone suffering from scarring might want to see what Bee-Clear will do for them.

Shopping for The Products of the Beehive

If you've been paying attention and have absorbed everything we've told you so far, you are armed with all the information you need to shop for the very highest-quality most-superior bee products. Don't shop on price. You only get what you pay for. The C C Pollen Company products are fairly priced.

Bee pollen is a miraculous food. Even the most inferior bee pollen is better than any of the manufactured food products you find in the supermarket. But I believe in having the best obtainable, and I think you do, too. As a general rule of thumb, the best quality bee pollen is domestic, not imported from the humid areas of the globe where excessive heat must be employed to sterilize and retard molding. Watch out for the foreign stuff.

There is only one exception to this rule. As we told you earlier, The C C Pollen Company is engaged in on-going correspondence with the Soviet Union. We are negotiating for the purchase of Caucasus Mountain bee pollen, the powerful bee pollen that plays such a large part in extending the lifespan of the mountain people in upper Russia. Our aim is to incorporate some of these very potent granules in the High Desert blend.

Whether you are shopping for bee pollen, royal jelly, or propolis, be very sure of your source. Purchase only from reliable well-established purveyors of beehive products who are in it for the long-term. There will always be manufacturers looking for a quick-buck who don't mind putting out inferior-grade products in an effort to make a profit. These types are counting on your not knowing the difference between good and bad. Most health-food store personnel will be able to advise you, if you're still in doubt.

It's hard to believe how much The C C Pollen Company has grown over the years. Quality creates its own market. In 1975, the company occupied a small corner of my offices and the staff numbered *one*. Now The C C Pollen Company has many hundreds of beekeepers who harvest for us, the in-house personnel numbers twenty-eight, and we occupy an entire suite of many individual offices. We are computerized and do business around the world. High Desert apiaries (bee yards) are now established in many states besides Arizona. Most of the health food stores in this country carry The C C Pollen Company products. Some pharmacies and supermarkets do, too. We are international now and market a heavy volume in many countries of the world.

Am I satisfied? For the moment, yes. We do it right. But the research continues and who knows what advances science might make in the next decade? I promise you, if new research shows a better way to harvest, produce, process, handle, or store beehive products, The C C Pollen Company will be the first to know. We won't drag our feet about putting better ideas into production either, no matter what cash outlay is required.

Looking back, hard as it may be to believe, this whole thing started out as a personal odyssey. I had no idea that what I discovered would lead to the founding of the largest bee pollen product producer in the world. But what I learned along the way was just too important to keep all to myself. I was sure that you needed to know, too.

I've taken you down that long road step-by-step. This book is the distillation of my twenty-year search for the best beehive products in the world. I'm happy to pass on the results of all my study and research.

Someone *you* know *needs to know.* If this is your first introduction to the truly miraculous and incredible health-giving products created by the industry of the bee, pass it on.

An ancient oriental phrase of great courtesy, accompanied always with the correct deep bow, consists of: "May you live 1,000 years." The Apiarian Lifestyle may be the key to the Chinese puzzle of the millennial lifestyle... living 1,000 years!

In the following chapter, which concludes this book, I'm going to let you in on the Apiarian Lifestyle that is keeping me young and healthy. It will work for you, too.

CHAPTER 14

THE APIARIAN LIFESTYLE
May You Live A Thousand Years - The Millennium

You know what a vegetarian is? As a broad category, strict vegetarians do not eat anything that has a heartbeat, including meat, dairy products and eggs. There's a subcategory that further differentiates a certain type of vegetarian. Lacto-ovo vegetarians do not eat animal flesh, but do take dairy products, signified by the term *lacto* (Latin for milk), and do eat eggs, signified by the term *ovo* (Latin for egg).

I am an apiarian, a descriptive term I coined myself to explain my lifestyle. I do eat certain types of dairy products, do eat certain kinds of eggs, and do eat certain *uncooked* meat. *Apiarian,* of course, come from *apiary,* which is where bees are kept, which in turn comes from *Apis mellifera,* the domestic honeybee which 'manufactures' all those miraculous products mankind prizes. I make the products of the beehive — bee pollen, bee propolis, royal jelly, honey and beeswax — *the* basic staples of my diet.

THE APIARIAN PHILOSOPHY

Apiarianism is a healthful and fulfilling lifestyle. It is based on ingesting the best nutrition, raw, uncooked and entirely natural — from all organic sources — which of course includes all the healthy products of the bees' industry, practicing the best form of exercise, enjoying the best sleep and rest patterns, total management of stress and, most important of all, a personal relationship with the Supreme Being, the Ruler of the Universe.

BASIC APIARIAN PRECEPTS

1. Apiarianism demands the most healthful totally-organic nutrition possible. Because it offers all the nutrients necessary for life, except air and water, High Desert Bee Pollen may be the only perfect food on earth. High Desert Honeybee PollenS and other products of the beehive are enjoyed with each and every meal every day.

2. The complete apiarian will engage in at least one hour of strenuous exercise five days per week. The exercise regimen should bring on a continuous healthy and cleansing sweat for the hour's duration of the exercise.

3. An apiarian will enjoy a regular sleeping pattern of 5, 6, or 7 hours of uninterrupted sleep each night. The successful apiarian will peacefully pass into the deepest 5th stage of slumber, the most healthy and restful sleep of all.

4. Apiarianism helps the individual completely manage any

stressful situation he encounters during the day. The fully-evolved apiarian will effortlessly transform daily stress from a destroying force in his life into a potentiating and building force.

5. True apiarianism cannot be fully experienced unless the individual has a personal relationship with the Supreme Being. No matter what the name the Supreme Being is called in his particular faith (God, Christ, Yahweh, Jehovah, or whatever), a high-level apiarian will have perfect faith.

ORGANIC NUTRITION

Don't Be Fooled: Don't be misled by the simplistic axiom: "All you need to do to consume all the nutrients your body requires is to eat balanced meals from the four (or five) basic food groups." This fairy tale might have been true once upon a time; today it is dangerous nonsense.

Why? If you've been paying attention, I think you already know why. Remember those U.S.D.A. studies which showed that no state in the U.S. still has all natural nutrients present in the soil? Then, too, there's all those poisonous agribusiness chemicals commercial food growers till in their fields. There's irrefutable proof that the food producers aren't doing it right:

a) The U.S. Department of Agriculture has determined that from 35 to 37 percent of the foods eaten by the average

American is manmade and can't legitimately be categorized in any one of the four basic food groups.

b)   In 1987, the U.S. Department of Agriculture surveyed the food intake of 21,000 average Americans to determine if they were consuming 100 percent of the Recommended Daily Allowance of ten essential nutrients. Not surprisingly, *not one person in the entire 21,000* was consuming a diet which provided the RDA of ten essential nutrients.

The only possible conclusion that can be reached from this disturbing study is the fact that the essential nutrients are not present in the foods in our supermarkets. Surely, if sufficient nutrients were available in our foods to permit consumption of the RDA of ten essential nutrients, at least 100, or 10, or even *one* person in the study of 21,000 would have tested positive on their RDA requirements.

The U.S.D.A. study proved that the average American family who shops supermarkets is eating a less than adequate diet for healthy functioning.

Processed Manmade Foods: "Never eat any food man has tampered with to make a profit." This truism is espoused by the super-great 95-year old Victor Earl Irons, the greatest fighter for our health freedoms that I know. By and large, any of the manufactured and processed so-called 'foods' advertised on television are no-no's. Virtually all of the foods so colorfully advertised on TV are manmade for one reason: to make someone a profit, not to build your health.

If the processed manufactured food products which are available in the supermarket do not provide the essential nutrients, and they do not, what's the solution?

Eat Organically-Grown Foods: You already know that the High Desert products of the beehive are organic powerhouses of nutrients. But what exactly are organically-grown foods? There are many definitions of such foods, but here's the truest definition I know:

Organically-grown foodstuffs are the foods cultivated in rich soil that contains an abundance of earthworms. If there's an abundance of earthworms in the soil, you can be certain the soil is organic and the produce grown in such soil can accurately be termed "organically-grown."

The reason for this conclusion is the fact that artificial chemical fertilizers, pesticides, herbicides, any poisons of this kind, drive the earthworms away. Earthworms are God's environmentalists. If the earthworms are not in the soil where foodstuffs are grown, you are getting a less than perfect nutrient-rich food.

The World's Number One Apiarian: I have appropriated the title 'World's Number One Apiarian.' Since I coined the term, I guess there's no one to challenge me just yet. The following list of foods are the best foods I know in each category, as follows:

1. Organically Perfect: High Desert Products of the Beehive

2. The Best of Meat: Raw Veal Liver

3. The Best of Fowl: Raw Fertile Eggs

4. The Best of Fish: Codliver Oil

5. The Best of Dairy: Raw Goat's Milk
    Raw Goat's Milk Cheese
    Raw Mare's Milk

6. The Best of Fruits: Raw Mangoes
    All Raw Organic Vine-Ripened and Tree-Ripened Fruits

7. The Best of Vegetables: Raw Carrots or
    Raw Carrot Juice
    Leafy Greens
    All Organically-Grown Vegetables

8. The Best of Grains: Millet

9. The Best of Cereals: Buckwheat, Rye, Oats

10. The Best of Nuts: Almonds

11. The Best of Seeds: Chi - Alfalfa
    Sesame - Pumpkin

12. The Best of Oils: Linseed Oil, Pumpkin Seed Oil

13. Pork: Forbidden

14. Shellfish: Forbidden

15. Coffee, Tea, Alcohol: Forbidden

16. Cola, all soft drinks: Forbidden

17. Tobacco: Forbidden

The Scavengers: Never eat any animal which feeds on decaying dead matter and the droppings of other animals. This category includes the pig, sole, and shellfish, such as crab, lobster, shrimp, and oysters. They grow plump by scavenging on the bottom of seabeds.

This category of animals is forbidden as food in the teachings of many religions. In addition, there is scientific research which shows man should not eat the meat of scavenging animals because man cannot possibly digest such foods; they knock man's metabolism out of kilter.

Goat Cheese: The apiarian eats raw uncooked, unpasteurized, unhomogenized goat cheese at breakfast. The Swiss-type goat cheese is recommended. The best source of goat cheese and goat whey, according to Dr. Bernard Jensen, the greatest healer and health authority who ever lived, is the Mt. Capra Cheese Company of Chehalis, Washington. (see Source Listing at the close of this chapter).

Dairy Products: Always eat all dairy products together at one meal, preferably breakfast. One to four ounces of goat cheese can be eaten with acidophilus goat's milk. Each apiarian must regulate his personal intake of dairy products to suit his particular lifestyle and ingestion requirements.

Fowl: Raw *fertile* eggs are the best foods from this group. The life cycle of the chicken or the duck or any bird is perpetuated by the egg laying that bird accomplishes. Each egg that is raw and fertile contains the life force of one living thing. If that egg is eaten raw, it is one of the best foods man can ingest.

I do not worry about the cholesterol in eggs. The Creator has never made any mistakes. He placed an abundance of lecithin in the yolk of the egg to emulsify all fats. It is only when eggs are cooked that the lecithin loses valuable properties and the cholesterol content becomes dangerous. Why?

Because lecithin is heat-sensitive. Heat destroys the lecithin in the egg. When the lecithin is damaged, there is no emulsifying agent to process the cholesterol in the egg. Heat destroys. Heat kills!

Fruit: All organically-grown fruit is good food, but must not be eaten until it is ripe and, preferably, vine-ripened or tree-ripened. Green fruit is difficult to digest and does not contain the nutrients necessary and beneficial for mankind.

To my way of thinking, the best of all fruits is the mango, commonly called "the king of fruits," not only because of its superior taste, but for its superior content of nutrients. The best source of mangoes is Starr Organic Produce, Inc. of Miami, Florida. (See Source Listing at the close of this chapter.) The watermelon closely follows the mango. The other fruits, if ripe, are eaten.

If you're not used to it, eating acidic (citrus) fruits can be upsetting to the stomach. Citrus fruits are the least desirable of all fruits and probably should be avoided. Start adding fruits to the menu slowly until you can comfortably enjoy one fruit meal daily during the summer months when the sweet harvest is vine-ripened or tree-ripened and fresh.

Enjoy Whole Fruits: The apiarian will not be satisfied to merely drink the juice, but will eat the whole fruit, taking care to chew each bite thoroughly. Fruit juices can interfere with the metabolic processes. As a rule of thumb, bypass fruit juices and enjoy nature's bounty in its nutrient-rich whole form.

If you insist on drinking juices, remember to 'chew' them. (More about that a little later.) The apiarian 'drinks' his solids and chews his liquids diligently until they are entirely saturated to the maximum with the digestive enzymes present in his saliva.

Vegetables: All the vegetables are edible foods for an apiarian if they come from organically-enriched soils. Juiced vegetables are recommended. The green leafy vegetables are especially good. Cruciferous vegetables (the cabbage family), which includes broccoli, have been shown to offer astounding cancer preventive properties. The orange vegetables provide beta-carotene, which the body uses to manufacture vitamin A. Beta-carotene is another documented cancer preventive that belongs on the menu. When I juice my vegetables, I use the Champion Juicer (see Source List at the close of this chapter).

By now it probably won't surprise you to learn that bee pollen contains twenty-times more beta-carotene than carrots by weight.

Meat: Raw veal liver is the best food in the meat category. Whenever a lion or tiger kills an animal, the first part of the flesh that predator consumes is the liver of his kill. I believe that the lion or tiger knows more about nutrition than any man walking on earth. Instinctively, the lion or tiger knows the liver of his prey is the most nutritious and consumes it first because it is the most invigorating food and contains the most-needed nutrients.

I stop every morning on my way to the office to buy very fresh raw veal liver from Raeys Grocery at the corner of East Camelback Road at 40th Street. Raeys handles Coleman organic beef, which is raised cleanly (without chemicalized feed or anti-biotic injections) in the Rocky Mountains near Saguache, Colorado.

Fish: Grandmother was right when she routinely spooned a dose of codliver oil into the mouth of every member of the family every day. In spite of their shudders, all dutifully swallowed the fishy-tasting oil. However, the next generation had it easier. By then codliver oil was available in 'football-shaped' soft-gel capsules that were washed down with a swig of water. But capsules are a poor second choice. Because I believe it to be the best food in the fish category, I still take codliver oil, the liquid and not the capsules. I swig down a mouthful once or twice a week. The best codliver oil comes from V.E. Irons in Natick, Massachusetts. (See Source List at the close of this chapter.) I order regularly.

The Essential Fatty Acids: Chemically-altered dietary fats are all forbidden. Over half (57 percent) of the fats in the American diet comes from commercially processed fats and oils, such as vegetable oils, margarines, salad dressings, and shortenings. All the nutrients have been processed out of these 'dead' non-nutritive oils; most are hydrogenated (or partially hydrogenated) and contain alien metabolites; many contain harmful chemicals, especially those bottled in plastic. Hydrogenated and partially-hydrogenated fats, in just about every manufactured food product in the supermarket, are impossible for the body to process properly and lay the foundation for the diseases of fatty degeneration, including heart disease and cancer. These 'dead' artificial dietary fats have been clinically shown as harmful to the body.

The essential fatty acids, linoleic and linolenic, are called *essential* because the body can't synthesize them from any other nutrient or combination of nutrients. Linoleic and linolenic fatty acids are required every day by many internal systems for healthy normal functioning. For life support, the essential fatty acids must be supplied to the body every day. The body attempts to compensate for a fatty acid deficiency, sometimes for many years. When a serious illness strikes, a nutrient deficiency is seldom pinpointed as a contributing factor and often escapes unnoticed.

Linseed (flax seed) oil is acknowledged to be the world's most abundant source of the essential fatty acids. The research scientists of the world use unrefined linseed oil for determining the properties of the fatty acids. Studies show dramatically that linseed oil can be considered a proven preventive and active therapeutic agent. For example:

Polish scientists have shown that the fatty acids in linseed oil destroy cancer cells without harming the vital white blood cells of the immune system. In Britain, medical detectives showed that even when fed a grossly high-fat diet, subjects protected by linseed oil were free of the harmful elements present in the blood when fats can't be processed by the body. Australian researchers demonstrated that hypertension (high blood pressure) was reduced in subjects supplied with the essential fatty acids regularly.

The strongest documentation of all comes from Dr. Johanna Budwig, Germany's premiere biochemist. Dr. Budwig proved that the blood of seriously ill and diseased persons always exhibits very low levels of linoleic acid. She found that healthy blood always contains the essential fatty acids and quality protein; diseased blood does not. Without the vital combination of the essential fatty acids and sulphurated proteins, the production of hemoglobin (oxygen-carrying red blood cells) is impaired. Cells and tissues suffer from oxygen starvation.

In over a decade of clinical application, Dr. Budwig has been successfully treating victims of the diseases of fatty degeneration (even terminal cancer patients) with a dietary therapy consisting of unrefined linseed oil and protein-rich low-fat cottage cheese. She has put into practice what laboratory studies prove. Once the body is provided with the essential fatty acids and other required nutrients, the body can very often work incredible internal corrections and restore itself to health. Scientists, medical researchers, and biochemists worldwide justifiably praise Dr. Budwig as a healer of heroic proportions.

You'll find several brands of linseed oil in health-food stores, but be careful. Some are not true cold-pressed unrefined oils, no matter what the label may claim. For reasons known only to themselves, U.S. government guidelines say that an oil may be called 'cold-pressed' if no *external* heat is applied in the processing. But the giant screw presses commonly used in processing oils build up friction-generated temperatures of close to 500°. These so-called 'cold-pressed' oils are nutritively deficient.

The best of the oils are from BioSan Pharmacals. Major health food stores carry them and it's worth your while to search them out. The best is *C-Leinosan Linseed Oil*, a liquid gold sunshine with a fresh taste that analyzes out to an impressive 62.9% linolenic acid and 14.52% linoleic acid content. C-Leinosan is a true cold-pressed unrefined linseed oil from the first pressing of the seeds. For those who prefer premeasured convenience, the company also puts out soft-gel *C-Leinosan Linseed Oil Capsules* containing the same golden oil.

BioSan also offers *Pumpkin Seed Oil* (43% linolenic, 16% Linoleic), *Canola Oil* (12% linolenic, 21% linoleic), *Sunflower Oil* (low in linolenic, but powerful in linoleic and with natural vitamin E), and *Safflower Oil* (irresistibly buttery, 74% linoleic, but just a trace of linolenic).

Because studies have shown that chemicals used in the manufacture of plastic containers have a way of leaching into the contents, I very much appreciate the fact that all the imported BioSan oils are decanted into pharmaceutical-quality amber glass bottles. These nutrient-rich oils with their essential content of the essential fatty acids are better than the best any other supplier has to offer.

Incidentally, High Desert Bee Pollen contains both linoleic and linolenic essential fatty acids in relative abundance, as well as ALL other essential nutrients.

Drink Pure Water: Never drink water from a public water supply. Municipalities artificially chlorinate and fluoridate the water that comes from your tap. Chlorine kills cells, injures hemoglobin (red blood cell) production, and interferes with blood pressure.

Fluoride is a poisonous byproduct of aluminum manufacture and is used as a rat poison. It is a documented fact that persons drinking fluoridated water have a higher death rate from all causes, cancer in particular, than those drinking pure water. These facts have been scientifically confirmed in worldwide research.

To be certain of perfectly pure water, the only purifying system which works perfectly is *reverse osmosis.* Because pure water is so vital to your life and health, you might want to consider purchasing a reverse osmosis home purification system which fits onto your kitchen faucet. (See the Source List for the best water purifier around.) In this method of purification, tap water is forced through a semipermeable membrane. The microscopic holes in the semipermeable membrane permit the passage of only hydrogen and oxygen, all harmful chemicals, contamination and pollutants are separated out and flushed down the drain into the sewer where they belong. The result is an unlimited flow of pure H_2O, perfectly pure water.

Virtually all water purification systems denude the water of minerals. Jeffrey Bland, Ph.D., concluded that approximately 25 percent of the total mineral intake of mankind comes from the water we drink. Therefore, I recommend you fortify your water with MiVita Mineral Water (see Source List) at the rate of a tablespoon or more per gallon.

Liquifying Your Food: Most people eat entirely too fast, barely tasting their food before the next bite follows. To have perfect digestion and assimilation, the good apiarian chews his food until the solids have become liquified before swallowing. This is a very difficult challenge to master, but perfect health is difficult to achieve without taking the time to liquify the solid bites of food you put in your mouth. (Some people call this *Fletcherizing*, which means chewing your food 30 times before swallowing.)

You may find this process difficult to turn into a healthy habit, but if an overweight apiarian will not swallow any solid food until he has it completely liquified, he will notice that he will start losing weight in a consistent and systematic way and will gradually achieve his perfect weight. It is a medical fact that twenty minutes must pass, on average, before your stomach signals your brain that you have eaten enough. That rule applies whether you are shoveling in massive amounts and swallowing rapidly, or systematically liquifying each bite.

Eat slowly. After each bite, put your fork or spoon back on your plate. Continue chewing until that bite has completely liquified. Follow this method with each bite and very soon you will find you have developed another life-extending habit.

Chew Your Liquids: When an apiarian drinks his goat's milk, or any other liquid, he is advised to swish each sip around in his mouth and 'chew' it from 8 to 15 times to completely saturate the liquid with the digestive juices present in saliva.

Chewing of liquids begins the digestive process so necessary when an apiarian is trying to achieve perfect digestion and assimilation.

Perfect Elimination: This is not a very tasteful subject, but it is important. Regulating the digestive tract to foster perfect elimination, evidenced by healthy feces, is often bypassed by nutritionists and other health authorities. Checking your feces is the best way to tell what's going on internally. Here's what to look for:

Perfect fecal matter will be an inch or inch-and-a-half in diameter and approximately 12 to 15 inches long. Fresh healthy feces will float. Generally speaking, evacuated feces will be connected. However, expect to find the matter broken in two or three pieces, as it may come apart on hitting the water in the toilet bowl.

Healthy feces will be of a yellowish or brownish color. Fecal matter should not smell offensive. At most, the smell should not be repulsive. A slightly sour odor indicates the presence of hydrochloric acid and is normal in healthy feces.

Consider this: The bloodstream of the body can be no cleaner than what you deposit in the bowl. If your intestines are full of putrifying matter, or if your feces are not healthy (hard, dry, fractured, runny), then your blood is less than perfect. You can gauge the condition of your blood by the floating fecal matter in your toilet bowl. Everyone should strive for perfect fecal matter in order to have perfect blood.

Acidophilus goat's milk is alive with millions and millions of acidophilus bacillus, the friendly bacteria. Lactobacillus has been identified as a powerful enemy of undesirable bacterial strains. This friendly bacteria is normally present in a healthy body, but is quickly wiped out by antibiotics and hormone therapy. Fortunately, it's possible to re-establish an acidophilus bacillus colony. I do it by drinking my fortified goat's milk.

If you don't find the clabbered goat's milk I enjoy so much to your liking, the poor second best way to supply your body with this helpful bacteria is to take a *L-Acidophilus Plus* capsule or two every day. These capsules from Fountain of Health might be just what your body needs to clean up a yeast infection or intestinal contamination. Everything from chronic diarrhea, gastrointestinal upsets (with accompanying gas attacks and flatulence), common vaginal yeast infections (lactobacillus controls the candida organism which causes yeast infections), low energy levels, to canker sores and fever blisters (herpes simplex) have yielded to L-Acidophilus treatment.

Each L-Acidophilus Plus capsule offers you an impressive 500 mg of pure organically-produced lactobacillus acidophilus culture with pectin (organic fiber), but no unwanted additives. These caps are a welcome natural addition to the American pharmacopeia. If I can't convince you to drink my clabbered and doctored raw goat's milk, remember this name.

Drinking goat's milk provides the digestive and intestinal tracts of the apiarian with billions of bacterium which happily take up residence on the walls of the intestines in the best manner possible. The ingestion of the fortified goat's milk first thing in the morning serves as an excellent breakfast. In spite of the daily injection of these friendly live spores, it may take the beginning apiarian from six months to a year to achieve his desired goal of perfect elimination, shown by perfect fecal matter.

By examining the stool each morning quite closely, the apiarian will notice that little-by-little the fecal matter is progressing toward perfection, showing that digestion and assimiliation are improving with each passing day.

Do It Now: When peristalsis begins and your body signals that your bowels require emptying, never wait. Always answer the call immediately. Bowel elimination is best accomplished at nature's urging. Evacuation is more thorough when the first urge arises.

One reason why the so-called 'primitive' peoples of the

world, including those in the Caucasus Mountains of the USSR, Hunza Land, Vilcabamba in Ecuador, and Tibet enjoy such good health is because they are completely uninhibited in their bodily functions. When nature calls, they may even make a deposit by the side of the road and no one thinks them crude or rude. Evacuating the bowels is a natural healthy function.

EXERCISE

Exercise Extends The Lifespan: It has been scientifically documented that exercising regularly increases longevity, and enhances the quality of life as well. This fact has been confirmed in worldwide studies so many times that it is impossible to refute. I myself work out with weights, swim, skip rope, and run, although there are some drawbacks inherent in a running regimen.

On November 6, 1988, I ran in the New York Marathon for the first time and completed the distance of 26 miles, 385 yards and two feet. Noel Johnson (see Chapter 6), the 90-year old marathoner who gave his autobiography the descriptive title of *A Dud at 70 - A Stud at 80,* holds the North American continent record for senior marathoners. Noel Johnson is probably *the* super human being in the entire universe. He always betters his time in his marathons. Thanks to High Desert Bee Pollen, Johnson seems to grow younger each year!

In his book, Noel swears he owes his return to sexual potency one hundred percent to High Desert Bee Pollen. This book is available from Plains Corporation (see Source List at the close of this chapter). At 88, Johnson completed the 1987 New York Marathon and is the oldest person on record in the Western Hemisphere to run a complete marathon — and finish on his feet. The man is a rock.

When running the marathon in 1988, I became acquainted with Manning Wein of Van Nuys, California. At 86 years of age, he is runner-up to Noel Johnson. Wein qualifies as the second-oldest marathoner of record.

The beginning apiarian who has not been exercising on a regular basis must see his doctor to make sure his physical condition will permit him to engage in a daily exercise program. If the doctor gives the OK, an exercise regimen can commence. All authorities stress that a beginner should start at a slow pace and work up to his optimum level.

A word of caution is in order here. Nearly everyone who begins exercising is overenthusiastic and pushes himself beyond healthy limits at first. Starting out with a walk/jog program is advisable. As your strength and confidence build, ease into running. If you can only manage to run 50 steps at first before feeling tired, that's all right. Stop. The following day, you may run 60 steps before pooping out.

The apiarian is smart enough not to overdo any type of exercise until his body has become accustomed to an exercise regimen. Nathan Pritikin once told me that it took him five years to work up to running an hour as fast as he was able every day. He revealed he was afraid of having a heart attack during the entire time.

We believe five years is too long to 'ease' into an exercise program. But we do advise that you take at least a year of gradually escalating running before you try to run all-out for an hour.

Skipping Rope: Boxers routinely skip rope to develop their leg muscles and enhance the balance and cordination they need to dance around the ring. The most strenuous single exercise I know is skipping rope (with feet together) on a fast continuous basis. This exercise accelerates the heart rate and causes the entire body to pulsate and gives a maximum workout.

Running: Next best is running *UP*stairs or *UP*hill. Running on the level is probably the type of exercise that suits most physically-active people. I myself run all out as fast as I can for one hour three days per week, Mondays, Wednesday, and Fridays. On Tuesdays and Thursdays, I work out with weights. I also swim laps five evenings per week.

Let's face it. Running is *boring.* That's why a lot of people enthusiastically take up running, only to drop it after a month or two. I've worked out some tricks that eliminate the boredom of running alone. Try my ideas and you won't get bored.

Run the same path every morning. Carry a stopwatch and time yourself as you pass certain designated landmarks along the way. You'll be surprised at how exhiliarating and encouraging it is to find you've cut a second or two off your previous time as you speed past the yellow fireplug in the middle of the block, then reach the big tree in the park, On the homestretch, hustle around the corner where the gray house with the black shutters is and give yourself a mental cheer on finding you're three seconds ahead of your previous time. You get the idea.

Remember, you aren't competing with anyone but yourself. Of course, once you get really fast, you might want to enter a 10 K or run a marathon to test yourself against some real competition. But that isn't the goal of the apiarian's exercise program. What the apiarian aims for is his personal best, running as close to his maximum capacity as possible while still sustaining the pace for the entire hour.

I thoroughly enjoy competing with myself. I like pumping uphill and working up a sweat. For me, running is the greatest. But there's another form of exercise that give tremendous physical results without such hard work.

Rebounding: A rebound exercise device is a personal-sized home version of a trampoline. The best are round, about three feet in diameter, and stand nine inches high. Because it is very resilient and won't sag or bag, the best bouncing surface is Permatron.

Rebounding combines the forces of acceleration and deceleration to fool the cells of the body into believing they are being subjected to increased gravity. And that's the secret of the rebound's success.

Every cell in the body adjusts immediately to its environment. When our astronauts were traveling in space at zero gravity, they lost bone density and muscle mass very quickly. Swiss scientists took blood samples from U.S. astronauts and Soviet cosmonauts and subjected these weakened cells to an increase in G-Force. The cells responded by becoming stronger than they were under normal gravity and the body benefited by a dramatically strengthened immune system. NASA has established that rebounding is 68% more efficient than running.

When you step up onto the pad and begin, you'll notice that you feel heavier at the bottom of the bounce when you are in the deceleration mode. That's the increased G-Force that challenges all the cells in the body to become stronger. Since NASA's test of rebounding, all our returning astronauts rebound to overcome the effects of space travel.

The real beauty of rebounding is that it can be custom-tailored to the age and condition of the individual. Unlike running, which requires real physical stamina, no one is too old or too infirm to benefit from rebounding. Even a patient in a wheel chair can rest his feet on the bouncing surface while a partner does the bouncing. The effect will travel from the soles of the resting feet throughout the entire body.

The best rebounder around is *The Dynabound*, engineered by Albert E. Carter. This one won't let you down in mid-bounce. Carter is acknowledged internationally as the world's foremost authority on rebound exercise. He is the author of *The New Miracles of Rebound Exercise* and *The Cancer Answer*. When it comes to rebounding, Carter's qualifications are of the highest order. He does it right. For more information on *The Dynabound*, contact New Dimensions Distributors. The address and phone numbers are shown on the Source List at the close of this chapter.

TO SLEEP, PERCHANCE TO DREAM

REM Sleep: REM, short for Rapid Eye Movement, signals that the sleeper is dreaming and has entered the fifth-stage of deep sleep. Fifth-stage slumber, or REM sleep, is the most healthful and restorative of life energies. The contribution that sound deep sleep plays in keeping us well and energetic is often overlooked. The sleep that comes in the fifth stage is such restful sleep that it is actually rejuvenating.

Unfortunately, many people never receive the full restorative benefits of deep sleep. They are restless, sleep fitfully, and remain in the third level of sleep the entire night. These are the people who wonder why they always awaken grouchy and still tired.

The best way to coax your body into progressing naturally into fifth-stage slumber is to initially become completely relaxed. Regardless of what motive or method or regimen you adopt to accomplish this, complete relaxation of the entire body is what sets the stage for healthy REM sleep.

You cannot enter fifth-stage slumber unless your stomach is empty. Never eat four hours before retiring. Seventy-five percent of your entire blood supply goes to digest food in your stomach. You want that seventy-five percent of your blood repairing body tissue while you're sleeping, not digesting food.

People who regularly progress through the fifth-stage sleep deeply and awaken refreshed and raring to go. These people need less sleep than others because their bodies are benefiting completely from their slumbers each night, as nature intended.

Once complete relaxation has been achieved, deep-breathing from the abdomen will assist the apiarian to drift off into dreamland and progress into fifth-stage slumber quite naturally. This may not happen the first time you try it, but it will happen in time. Once you experience the full effects and restful benefits of deep sleeping, you will marvel at the difference you feel upon awakening in the morning.

The restorative and rejuvenating benefits of fifth-stage slumber are incalculable. Believe it.

Bee Sleepy: If you need help in falling asleep, C C Pollen Company has a tablet called Bee Sleepy® which works wonders and is not a drug — it's a food.

SEXUAL FUNCTION

The Life Force: Sex is a driving life force that is mishandled by most people. Because of the way the male body reacts, it seems logical to assume that the Creator probably meant man to have sex the first thing in the morning.

When awakening in the morning, the man is rested. He normally wakes with an erection because he hasn't voided his urine all night. His wife is rested. They are lying together side-by-side in bed. And that's the time to have sex. The apiarian thinks man should have sexual intercourse every day the first thing in the morning. With the help of the products of the bee, there's no reason why this regimen should not continue throughout life. The Apiarian Lifestyle insures it.

MANAGING STRESS

The Stressful Lifestyle: In the hectic pace of the modern world, stress is unavoidable. A loved one is seriously ill. We fight a traffic jam on the way to work. The boss is a bear. A thorny decision is required to resolve a problem and sometimes, no matter how we decide, someone is left disgruntled. The car needs repair. The kids are cranky. Our mate is cross. There's too much that needs doing and not enough time. Rush, rush, rush. Wrong, wrong, wrong.

Slow down. Relax. Here again, deep abdominal-breathing is an excellent combatant of destructive stress. So is exercise. Work off that surge of adrenalin in a hard workout. Quiet meditation is an another fine way to eliminate stress and promote relaxation.

Stress is part of life. Stress can be destructive, or it can be beneficial. Whether it is harmful is largely up to you. Once a person makes up his mind to take things as they come and handle the stress in his life calmly, the daily challenges to be faced can become invigorating, instead of enervating.

You must learn to accept circumstances as they arise. Change for the better those you can; accept those you can't alter. Always strive to live and let live; be philosophic. By next week, today's destructive stress will be only a dim memory, if we treat it as such.

PERFECT FAITH

A Personal Matter: We do not believe perfect health can be achieved without a personal relationship with the Supreme Being. Deep personal faith helps everyone function better in every department. Faith can overcome and eliminate stress.

President Dwight D. Eisenhower said of himself: "I must be a Christian."

Eisenhower revealed that being a good Christian required about 10 percent of his money, about 10 percent of his time, and enjoined him to do the right thing at all times, which he said he felt he should do anyway. Eisenhower confided that the alternative, being a nonbeliever and to be mistaken, was so horrible, he couldn't afford the risk.

If the alternative of being a nonbeliever is eternal hell, every apiarian must be a devout follower of his personal religion.

All faiths acknowledge there is only one Supreme Being. Christians call the Supreme Being God. Other religions have other names for Him. No one knows for sure just how the hereafter is constructed or what it encompasses.

There's one great problem.

If an apiarian doesn't live an exemplary life here on earth, his chances of enjoying the hereafter will necessarily be curtailed or reduced or even eliminated altogether. Here again, no one knows for sure.

One thing an apiarian can be guaranteed: A sinful-living carousing gluttonous person on earth will not be rewarded in the hereafter.

A WEEK IN THE LIFE

What I've given you so far in this chapter are general guidelines. Everyone will adapt the lifestyle to suit his personal time-table. I'm not a doctor. I can't write out a prescription for you to follow, but I can tell you exactly what works for me.

My apiarian lifestyle evolved over a period of years and underwent some fine-tuning along the way. Yes, it was difficult in the beginning. It takes strong physical and mental self-discipline to live healthy, but the rewards are great. With the hope that others might be encouraged to make some changes for the better in their lives, here's a review of the regimen I've been practicing for perhaps fifteen to twenty years.

MY EVERYDAY DAILY REGIMEN

In the dawn of time and down through the centuries, man was awake and active during the sunlight hours. Man rested and slept during the dark hours of the night. That's the way our bodies were designed to operate by the Creator.

But, as artificial lighting became common, the cycle changed. We discovered how important the daylight hours are to health during the Industrial Revolution. As more and more families left the farms and began working under artificial lighting in factories, the adults were afflicted with osteomalacia, a softening of the bones; they battled constant rheumatic pains in the limbs, spine, thorax and pelvic region, and suffered an all-pervasive general weakness. The children living in the urban sprawl under the sun-dimming smoke belched out by the factories developed rickets.

All these conditions are caused by a severe deficiency of Vitamin D. The skin produces Vitamin D on exposure to sunlight. Science solved that particular problem by putting Vitamin D in milk. Rickets is all but unknown today.

But there's a growing body of studies which shows that most artificial lighting is harmful to health. Fortunately, there is a man-made light source that mimics the sun. All the electric fixtures in my office and my home, even the spotlights around the grounds, are fitted with Luxor Full-Spectrum lights. These lights are the closest manmade light source we have to sunlight and are very beneficial health-wise. You might want to consider Luxor's 'manmade sunlight' for your home or workplace. The benefits are very real. I even carry a 185 watt Duro Test light globe in my B-4 bag which I use in hotels and motels when I travel. In fact, I am writing this paragraph in the Sheraton Hotel in New Port Richey, Florida under the light given by my 'traveling' Duro Test light globe.

There's considerable research which concludes that we are born with an internal biological clock set in accordance with dawn and dusk. The more nearly we can adapt our lifestyle to correspond to our biological clock, the healthier we will be. If we rise at dawn and are active during the daylight hours, the more beneficial our waking hours will be, and the more beneficial our darkness hours of rest and relaxation will be.

Therefore, an apiarian should discipline his mind to awaken each morning sometime between 4 and 6 a.m., depending on the length of the day. If 5 o'clock is targeted as the year-around time of awakening, the internal time clock will become attuned to this time and we will automatically wake up at 5 o'clock.

I usually awaken naturally each morning around 5:00 a.m. I don't use an alarm clock. I don't think it's healthy to be jolted awake artificially by a harsh noise when the body isn't ready to rise.

Immediately upon awakening, I take my temperature, then descend to the first floor and enter the bathroom off my exercise room. The next thing I do is void my urine. After voiding, I weigh myself. At 5'9" tall, I allow my weight to fluctuate from 119 to 129 pounds. If my weight rises to 130 or more, I immediately go on a two-day water fast and lose 4 or 5 pounds and then resume my regular eating habits.

I believe the time to correct weight gain is when that first pound over the acceptable maximum is gained. If you weigh yourself daily, preferably at the same approximate time, it's easy to modify your lifestyle to eliminate unwanted pounds.

You might think I'm underweight. You would be wrong. In fact, I did not always weigh even this much. For many years,

I deliberately kept my weight between 105 and 109 pounds, and then between 109 pounds and 119 pounds. However, my wife nagged me about my skinny appearance. I made a deal with her that I would gain 10 pounds if she would stop fussing at me to eat more. I gained the 10 pounds at her request. I now maintain the higher weight level in accordance with her wishes and peace reigns at home.

The best rule of thumb for the most perfect health is to eat all foods the way the Creator made them. . . originally. The less you eat, on balance, the healthier you're probably going to be. It was the Duchess of Windsor who said, "You can't be too rich nor too thin." Science has confirmed the back half of that statement. Studies show that consuming fewer calories and maintaining a lean body helps extend the lifespan.

There is considerable high-quality research in medical literature which concludes that the less you eat, the longer your lifespan.

In experimental studies, fish that "fasted" every other day (they were fed only every other day) lived twice as long as the controls who were fed daily. Other lab animals (rats and mice) given low-calorie low-volume diets enjoyed increased longevity of 90 to 120 percent over animals given the usual rat chow. A medical doctor at U.C.L.A. Medical School fasts two days per week and confidently expects this regimen will lengthen his lifespan. Members of some religious orders routinely fast every fifth day; others fast every Sunday, and so on.

I believe the correct way to extend your lifespan by

controlling your weight is to:

1. Attain your ideal weight, whatever it may be, by
2. Gradually reducing your food intake to the point where you experience a very slow natural weight loss, then
3. *Slightly* increase your food intake to maintain lean-body weight equilibrium.
4. As a rule of thumb, you can probably safely judge that your nutrient intake at this point represents your ideal food intake.

I can only conclude that the American custom of eating three meals every day is a quick ticket to the morgue. For 71 years, I myself have eaten three small meals every day. Yet my body resists putting on fat and I have not gained excessive pounds. The way our bodies process food is a perfect example of how magnificently we have been constructed.

As I write this chapter, I am experimenting by eating only breakfast and a combined lunch/dinner between 2:00 p.m. to 3:30 p.m. in the afternoon. I have been following this routine for eight weeks and I have not lost a pound. Does that mean that I have been eating too much and too often all these years? It sure looks like taking only two meals per day can be declared the perfect diet pattern for the Apiarian! So be it!

Here are some general guidelines for calculating your perfect weight: For the large-boned person, multiply your height in inches by two; the resulting figures shows your perfect weight. For the average adult, multiply your height in inches by two, and subtract 10 percent. For a small-boned person, multiply your height in inches times two, and subtract 20 percent.

Immediately after my weigh-in, I record my daily weight and body temperature in a ledger which I keep handy in a drawer in my downstairs bath. After recording these readings, I chug-a-lug 32 ounces of room-temperature Bee-Dew® Water (see page 364 for how to prepare). Within one minute of ingesting the water, peristalsis begins. Chug-a-lugging a quart of water usually triggers the colonic valve, insuring a healthy and complete emptying of the bowels.

Next, I dry-brush massage my face, scalp, and body, going twice over every body part. I use a fabric brush, a rubber pronged plate, and a rough loofah glove. I brush from top of my head to the tip of my toes twice-over every morning. Dr. Bernard Jensen has analyzed typical discarded skin cells which slough off during a brushing of this type. His tests show an almost 100 percent content of uric acid.

Dry-brush massaging compensates for man wearing clothes. Since the skin is the largest organ of the body and the one which absorbs life-giving nutrients and excretes toxins, it is beneficial to keep the skin in good working order. Immediately after enjoying my stimulating dry-brush massage, I shave with my Schick electric razor. After shaving, I refill my glass quart water bottle with Bee-Dew® water in readiness for the drinking to come the next day.

I then go to the refrigerator I have outdoors by my swimming pool and fill an empty half-gallon goat's milk container with 16 ounces of my previously prepared clabbered fortified goat's milk, my 'Breakfast Bacillus' (see page 365 for how to prepare). To this mixture, I add two heaping tablespoons of High Desert bee pollen, two heaping tablespoons of crushed lecithin granules, two raw fertile eggs, three squirts of High Desert Bee Propolis Extract, or six crushed 500 mg High Desert Bee Propolis tablets (if and when the High Desert Bee Propolis Extract is not available), and one tablespoon of C-Leinosan Linseed Oil. I pop on the top and shake everything quite thoroughly as I return to my downstairs bathroom.

I draw sufficient hot water to fill the washbowl. I put the container of fortified clabbered goat's milk in the hot water, holding it in place with a rubber band around the faucet. The hot water will gradually warm up the mixture to body temperature (98° F.), which is the ideal temperature for ingesting anything and everything.

Exercise Regimen: Monday - Wednesday - Friday:

Now I'm ready for the day's exercise. On Monday, Wednesday, and Friday, my exercise of choice is running. After suiting-up, I go outside and engage in about 15 minutes of yoga warm-up exercises. I do alternate toe touches 100 times, run in place for five minutes, and skip rope as fast as I can with both feet for three minutes. (See page 340).

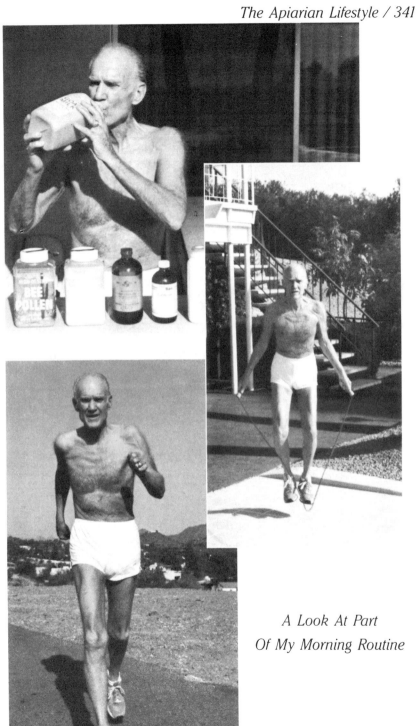

*A Look At Part
Of My Morning Routine*

After these warmups, I'm ready for my hour's run. I pick up my digital stopwatch and my exercise computer and proceed to the top of the road in front of my house prepared to run from 11 to 15 laps, depending on the season, how I feel that day, and how early I awakened that morning.

I engage my stopwatch, set the control of my exercise computer to monitor my heartbeat, and set off. I run at a pace that keeps my heart beating 170 beats per minute or more all during the course of my one hour run. I run full-out as fast as I can for one hour. I run every Monday, Wednesday and Friday at approximately the same time each morning.

Once in a great while, I stay up late the previous Sunday evening and do not retire until midnight or even later. On these rare occasions, I may not awaken at my usual time of between 4 and 5 o'clock, but sleep to 6 or even 7 in the morning. When these occasions occur, I may only run four laps on my regular course. I tell you this to demonstrate that even the best routines should occasionally be sensibly adjusted to conform to circumstances. However, irrespective of time constraints, I never run less than four laps, which times out to approximately 20 minutes. According to Dr. Ken Cooper, at least twenty minutes of continuous running is required for the cardiovascular system to benefit.

All authorities agree that the proper equipment is important. I personally prefer high-quality New Balance shoes for all my running.

With my exercise computer strapped to my wrist and

monitoring my heart rate, I run at a pace calculated to achieve a heartbeat of 170 or more per minute throughout the run. On my last lap, I step up the pace to achieve a heart rate of 180 beats or more for the first half of that lap. On the last half of the last lap, I run full out attempting to force my heartbeat to 200 beats per minute or more during what is approximately a 2-½ minute period.

All during my run, I am always trying to beat my personal "world record" time. I find that I must compete with myself while running or the process of running alone becomes so boring and monotonous that the temptation to quit is very real. When I compete with myself and try to establish a new "world record" for myself every Monday, Wednesday, and Friday, the competition keeps me alert and eliminates the usual boredom of running alone.

When I hit the finish line, I am perspiring profusely. In the summer, spring and fall, my running shorts and heavy socks are soaking wet with perspiration. Summer temperatures in Phoenix routinely top out at over 110 degrees. Even with our blessed dry air and lack of humidity, that's scorching hot. During the hottest days of summer, I have trouble seeing because of the perspiration running down my face and trickling into my eyes. I have to wear a sweatband to keep the sweat out of my eyes.

After finishing my one hour run, I walk down the hill behind my house to my backswing. This circular device is designed to counteract the constant downward pull of gravity the body is subjected to by upending the body and reversing the field for a period of time. I fasten myself to the backswing and invert myself, ending up head down and feet in the air perpendicular to the ground. I stay in this upside-down position for one minute. At the end of the minute, I right myself with head skyward and feet to the ground. I count from one to eleven while in an upright position. At the count of eleven, I reverse myself again.

I do the backswing inversion 11 times, staying inverted approximately 53 seconds out of each minute and upright for approximately 7 seconds. This inversion and righting forces the blood to the head and extremities 11 different times. It was under the guidance of Dr. Paavo Airola, the dean of health writers, that I developed this backswing routine. (See page 344).

The good, clean, pure healthy red blood cruising throughout the veins and arteries after running for an hour is the best, most healing and repairing blood I'll experience all day long. This hemoglobin-rich oxygenated blood is forced to the brain, the eyes, the head, the stomach, the heart and all vital organs of the body with the most purifying cleansing, and healing effect at this time every day that I run.

After eleven minutes of inversion therapy, I spend five minutes on my *Bee-Taller*™- *Gro-Taller*® course to straighten out and elongate my spine. Sales Inc. International offers a regimen which will cause your height to increase. Whether this increase in height comes from "growing taller," or whether it comes from straightening out the kinks and stretching the spine and neck is beside the point.

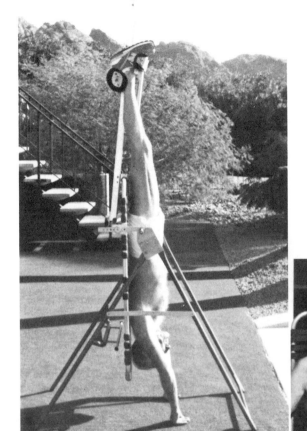

Ready To Flip

Strapped In
The Backswing

Hanging Around

I do 11 sets, remaining
upside down for
53 seconds out of
each minute

Sales Inc. International emphasizes you will *Bee-Taller* if you follow instructions. In fact, Sales Inc. guarantees it.

The cost of the course is $2,000 per inch of increased height. Sales Inc. guarantees you will "grow" at least one inch, or your money will be refunded.

However unfair it is, it is a sorry fact that height, more than ability or any other factor, plays a large part, perhaps the largest part, in how an individual is judged — by women, by men, by employers, even by acquaintances and friends.

Height even plays a large part in how you see yourself!

If you're interested in more information, the Source List includes Sales Inc. International's address .

Enjoy the High Life. You can *Bee-Taller.* Sales Inc. guarantees it.

After following the *Bee-Taller* regimen for five minutes, I take my shower. Because soap destroys the necessary acid mantle of the skin, I wash with water only. I use soap only once a month on my birthdate, the 26th. Washing and cleansing the face or neck or body with soap or commercial skin cleansers is counter-productive. During the many millions of years of man's early existence, soap didn't exist. Soap is a relatively recent 'invention' of the past few centuries.

Washing with these unnatural preparations removes the naturally occurring skin oils and protective skin secretions provided for us at the time of Creation. Only when scrubbing with water can't remove visible dirt or stains should soap or cleaning compounds be used, and then only very infrequently.

Once I'm clean, I turn the water as hot as I can stand it

for a count of 11, then cold for another count of 11. I alternate between hot and cold three times, ending with a cold spritz. I owe thanks to Dr. Bernard Jensen for teaching me this invigorating routine.

Exercise Regimen: Tuesday - Thursday:

On these alternate days, I lift weights for an hour, concentrating only on the back muscles. Thanks to the late great Bob Hoffman, founder of the York Barbell Company of Pennsylvania, I no longer try to lift to my maximum of heavy weights. Great strength is not necessary for my lifestyle. I don't believe overtraining and developing bulging muscles is healthy. This effect would add nothing to the quality of my life. Therefore, I do more repetitions with light weights. My aim is merely to perspire freely and keep the muscles of my back toned and in good shape. I don't want to carry an excess *ounce* of fat or muscle, let alone a *pound!*

Each extra pound of flesh is equipped with veins and capillaries, and the heart is required to service those additional passageways. It has been determined that each pound of excess body weight a person carries (whether fat or muscle) forces his heart to pump his entire blood supply an *extra mile* every year. And, if you're hauling around an extra five pounds, the heart labors to service an *extra five miles* of passageways every year.

You never see any overweight people of 100 to 125 years of age. Think about it. Body fat is a killer! Beware!!

During the course of these back exercises, I have a bar which I place across my shoulders. I extend my arms and clasp each end of the bar, bend over, and alternately touch my left and right toes 101 times. I do four sets of 101 toe touches during my weight lifting exercise.

I also do 42 chins on my chinning bar. I used to think my chinning ability was extraordinary in my age group. Then I discovered that the world's record for a 70 year old man was 155 chins. I no longer talk about my chinning accomplishments.

I have been lifting weights for a least 25 years. Consequently, I pretty well know how my body reacts to this type of exercise. I find I can miss working out with weights or miss chinning for as long as a week and still pick up where I left off by achieving the maximum reps and chins I did the week before. By the same token, if I miss ten days, I can feel my strength receding. The longer between workouts, the greater the strength loss.

If you want to gain great strength and muscular development in a hurry, weight lifting targeting each muscle group should be performed every other day. If you want to become toned and conditioned and slowly gain strength, lifting weights twice a week will do it for you.

As soon as I have dried off, I pull on my boxer shorts. A word of explanation is in order here. Because the experts say that jockey-type shorts are injurious to the male sex organs, I always wear boxer shorts. Jockey shorts (and too-tight jeans or pants) constrict the testicles and hold the penis in an unnatural position pressed against the body, thereby raising the temperature of the male organs. That's not the kind of 'hot and bothered' I want to be. Studies show that this unhealthy confinement of the testicles and penis can be a contributing factor to unsatisfactory sexual performance and impotence. Always wear boxer shorts.

Now I'm ready for my Breakfast Bacillus, my fortified 'doctored' goat's milk. It's been nicely warmed to body temperature by immersion in the hot water bath in my wash bowl. But first I check my ledger to remind myself what my body temperature registered that morning. Broda Barnes, M.D. informed me that his lifelong research on the action of the thyroid gland had convinced him that 98 degrees is the ideal body temperature. When body temperature falls below 98 degrees, the thyroid needs a nudge.

This is a matter of individual judgment, but I take one grain of Armour Dessicated Thyroid if my temperature is below 98 degrees. If my temperature registers between 97.0 and 97.5, I ingest two grains of dessicated thyroid. If my temperature is exactly 98 degrees or higher, I take no thyroid.

If I am taking thyroid that morning, I chew the tablet well and then take two large mouthfuls of the goat's milk mixture, swishing it throughout my mouth before swallowing. This is tantamount to 'chewing' your liquids and insures complete disgestion and assimilation.

At this time, I also take three 400 I.U. Vitamin E capsules, Betty Lee Morales Signature Brand, (see Source Listing.) These vitamin E capsules are a concentrated mixture of all eight natural tocopherols. But I burst the caps with my teeth and chew away until I am certain all the E oil has been expelled. I do not swallow the gelatin caps, but spit them out when I'm sure I have extracted all the tocopherol vitamin E. Then I take another two mouthfuls of the fortified goat's milk and 'chew' it well before swallowing.

I take vitamin E on a regular basis because health authorities say that the only two ways to elevate your high density lipoprotein (HDL) levels are (1) by ingesting vitamin E, and (2), by strenuous exercise. Researchers at the University of Oregon have found that it is all but impossible to have a heart attack if your HDL levels total 75 or greater.

Research has shown that if your HDL count is 50 percent or more of your LDL levels, heart attacks are virtually impossible.

After ingesting my fortified clabbered goat's milk and whatever tablets or capsules I am taking that particular morning, I check my eyes. Hanging on one wall in my exercise room, I have the standard eye chart as used by opthalmologists. You know, the one that has the big "E" at the top. I measure the accuracy of my eyesight on the chart every morning. Any time I find that my eyesight has slipped from a perfect 20/20, I immediately take steps to remedy the situation, as you will see.

However, unless I have been straining my eyes exceedingly by long periods of close work or by forcing them to adjust to the screen of our computers for a long period, my eyesight is excellent. It is shocking to find that over half the people in the U.S. require artificial correction of their eyesight in the form of glasses or contact lenses when the solution is so simple. I attribute my 20/20 eyesight to a product and the special accompanyng regimen I have developed called *Bee 20/20*™. I am living proof that the failing eyesight so common in the aged need not be. Using Bee 20/20 and following the Bee 20/20 regimen every morning has dramatically strengthened and protected my eyes. I want to retain my 20/20 eyesight for life.

In radial keratotomy, the eye operation so much in vogue right now, the surgeon removes an elliptical sliver from the eyeball to restore the correct shape. It is this reshaping of the eyeball which corrects near-sightedness and far-sightedness and restores clear vision. The good news is that you need not resort to such a risky, drastic, expensive surgical procedure.

It has been determined scientifically that the shape of the eyeball changes under assault by nutritional deficiencies, stress, pressure, exercise, illness, shock or trauma. The Bee 20/20 system takes all these factors into account. It consists of a special nutrient-rich all-natural eyewash, a drink fortified with beehive products, and an educational booklet. The booklet explains how the eye works, tells what nutrients the body requires to strengthen and correct eyesight, and provides a series of strengthening eye exercises (illustrated) which really do work, as well as the appropriate eye-relaxing exercises.

Bee 20/20 is so effective it even comes with a *moneyback guarantee*. When the Bee 20/20 regimen is faithfully followed, the system has been amazingly successful for individuals having vision of 20/30 up to 20/2000, those with such dim vision they have been declared legally blind. Of course, Bee 20/20 is not a 'quick-fix' surgical procedure. With the legally blind, the system might take a year or two before vision is completely restored.

The Bee 20/20 system is not sold on the open market. The complete system is available by mail at a cost of $49.00, which includes a 30-day supply of eyewash and the fortified drink, plus the booklet of monthly instructions. Refills consist of the eyewash and drink, but not the booklet, and are available at a reduced cost of $29.00. By sending your check or credit card information, you may order from The Escrow Company. The address is shown on the Source List at the close of this chapter.

After completing the Bee 20/20 regimen, I splash on Brut or Polo or Obsession shaving lotion (my wife likes these scents), get in my Trans Am and drive to my office, usually arriving between 8 and 9 a.m.

GIVE US THIS DAY OUR DAILY BEE POLLEN

My Apiarian Menu: Along about 10:00 or 11:00 in the morning, I munch three or four 130 mg High Desert Honey/ Vanilla tablets or have a President's Lunch bar, sometimes two. Lately, I have given up eating President's Lunch bars. They taste so good they sometimes ruin my appetite for the next meal! (I guess that's one reason why they work so well in a weight-loss program.) I know from personal experience why President Reagan calls these bars "meal replacements."

During the summer, except for Sunday, my lunches and

dinners will not vary much. Between noon and 1:00 p.m., depending on work flow, I have lunch. During summer, which begins with a vengeance in Arizona around May 1st and ends around October 1st, I eat some type of fruit with a handful of the sweet/tart always delicious raw High Desert Bee Pollen granules. I usually take one heaping teaspoonful of High Desert granules, take a juicy bite of fruit, and chew these two all-natural foods together, masticating well for good digestion.

I try to eat only organically-grown fruit that's in season at the time. Ideally, the fruit will have been ripened on the vine or tree. During the course of the summer, I eat a variety of fruits, everything from grapes to mangoes. Generally speaking, when mangoes are in season and the taste is best, I will eat mangoes to the exclusion of all other fruits. Not only do I think mangoes have the best taste, but I believe them to be the most healthful of all fruit.

My next choice is watermelon, closely followed by tree-ripened peaches and pears from the mountains of Colorado and Arizona. I often enjoy a salad of fresh greens with an all-natural poppyseed and honey dressing. In season, I eat raw corn-on-the-cob. It is a pleasure to nibble off those sweet kernels bursting with sun-warmed juices.

In the afternoon, usually around 2:30 to 3:30 p.m., I will eat two, three, even four or five, of the Pollenergy 520 tablets. Sometimes I will eat the Pollenergy 1500 tablets. Often, I will munch several President's Lunch bars, especially if I want to forego dinner. I really do not have a set 'afternoon snack' regimen. I operate more on impulse.

I try to take my second and last meal of the day as close to 5:00 pm as possible. No matter what the season of the year, my 5 o'clock supper or dinner, call it what you will, is High Desert Bee Pollen by the spoonful, with choice fruit in the summer and vegetable juices, raw veal liver, and green leafy vegetables during the winter. My afternoon meal is when I ingest one, two, or three *24-Hour Royal Jelly* tablets on a regular basis. Accordiing to all that documented scientific research, royal jelly is the most sexually stimulating and rejuvenating food available to man. For the reasons expounded in Chapter 10, I am well satisfied that my High Desert 24-Hour Royal Jelly is the finest most biologically-active royal jelly obtainable. I will take no more food until the following morning at breakfast.

The following material is a verbatim reproduction of a fax (telefacsimile) sent to one of our overseas distributors to explain the vital differences between ordinary liquid royal jelly and our biologically-active *24-Hour Royal Jelly:*

Liquid Royal Jelly vs Lyophilized 24-Hour Royal Jelly

For years we handled the liquid Royal Jelly. In fact, I personally used to buy one pound of Royal Jelly on the 1st day of every month. I would eat at least a teaspoonful at a time. I did this for years until Dr. Betty Lee Morales found out what I was doing.

Dr. Betty Lee Morales was generally and widely recognized as the greatest female health authority that has ever lived. Unfortunately, she died late last year in an automobile accident. During her lifetime she sold more Royal Jelly than any other person. She was the leader of the great Royal Jelly craze in California, Hollywood and the world right after World War II and lasting into the late 1950's and early 1960's. This is the time the claims began to get wild for Royal Jelly and the F.D.A. shut down all importation of Royal Jelly, including hers.

Nevertheless, she still has had more experience and knows more about Royal Jelly and Bee Propolis and other products from the beehive than any other person.

She convinced me that the Royal Jelly the queen bee eats is not the liquid Royal Jelly I was eating. The queen bee eats the 24-Hour Royal Jelly.

As you probably know, it is almost impossible for a consumer to eat Royal Jelly that isn't at least 30 to 90 days old. 24-Hour Royal Jelly may be 50 times more biologically active than that Royal Jelly that is 30 days old.

You should have your Japanese people find out when the liquid Royal Jelly they are eating is harvested from the beehive. I imagine you will be surprised at the long time span between harvest and their consumption.

Further research by Dr. Betty Lee Morales led her to conclude that placing bee pollen and bee propolis in the tablet of 24-Hour Royal Jelly would potentiate the Royal Jelly. She also discovered that Vitamin E, the natural form, (D-Alpha Tocopheral Succinate — the most stable form for tablets) also potentiated the 24-Hour Royal Jelly.

The 24-Hour Royal Jelly we manufacture is the formulation given to us by Dr. Betty Lee Morales. When we first issued this tablet we called it Rejuvenation® but then decided to just call it 24-Hour Royal Jelly because there were too many letters in Rejuvenation to be read on the small bottle.

In reviewing the label I see that we left off the Dr. Betty Lee Morales trademark of formulation by her. The next time we redo labels we will add the following, "formulated by Dr. Betty Lee Morales."

When a queen bee in the beehve dies or swarms and leaves

the colony, etc., the beehive is without a queen. The remaining bees select a random female bee and feed her nothing but water and Royal Jelly throughout the balance of her life. The nurse bees make the Royal Jelly from bee pollen in the colony. The bee pollen permits the nurse bees to manufacture the 24-Hour Royal Jelly — not the ordinary liquid Royal Jelly consumed by most consumers — causing the following almost unbelievable results:

1.   Permits the queen bee to emit a pheromone so strong it causes all the other bees in the colony to literally work themselves to death for the benefit of the colony. There may be more than 100,000 bees in that colony.
2.   Permits the queen bee's body to grow 150% to 200% larger than the other female bees in the colony.
3.   Permits the queen bee to be pregnant and continue to remain highly fertile with one impregnation for 5, 6, 7 and even 8 years.
4.   Permits the queen bee to lay during season more than her body weight in eggs every day and that may be more than 2000 eggs per day — each one fertile.
5.   The female bees in the colony have a life expectancy of about 35 days. The queen bee after eating 24-Hour Royal Jelly extends her life expectancy to 5, 6, 7 and even 8 years.

24-Hour Royal Jelly makes these changes and not ordinary liquid Royal Jelly.

24-Hour Royal Jelly is the greatest rejuvenating food in the world.

24-Hour Royal Jelly is the greatest sex stimulant for both male and female in the world.

The 24-Hour Royal Jelly manufactured by The C C Pollen Company and potentiated by the High Desert® Bee Pollen, the High Desert® Bee Propolis and the natural Vitamin E as formulated by Dr. Betty Lee Morales, must be considered the best rejuvenation food and the best sex stimulant known to man.

Although the Arizona climate is very kind in winter, I do miss my fresh tree-ripened fruits. Although my intake of High Desert products never varies no matter what the season, during the winter months, my menu changes. I take one, two, three, or four ounces of goat's cheese with caraway seeds with my Breakfast Bacillus. As I mentioned earlier, this cheese is shipped to me from the Mt. Capra Goat Farm. As you have probably figured out by now, my respect for Dr. Bernard J. Jensen is boundless. Dr. Jensen calls this cheese " the finest in the world" and I agree.

Instead of lunching on fruit, during winter I eat a great variety of vegetables, eaten raw and juiced by my own hand. I go to my favorite source for organically-grown produce. There I select one of every type of lettuce offered, excluding only Iceberg head lettuce which is nutritionally lacking. Anything and everything that looks fresh and appealing goes into my shopping basket, including my number one choice, carrots, but also brocolli, kale, radishes, onions, cabbage, jicama and on and on.

I take about 16 to 20 ounces of freshly juiced vegetables for lunch and dinner. About half of the juice is fresh carrot, with the other half a mixture of fresh greens and other vegetables in season. When it is not too bitter, celery is a favorite addition. Unfortunately, it seems that the last few years the celery has been thick-ribbed and very bitter tasting. I don't know why, but speculate that the farmers may be overwatering to produce a heavier crop, or perhaps the celery has been grown in non-organic soil lacking important minerals.

Get ready for a shocker. During the winter months, I used to eat from 4 to 6 ounces of raw liver at lunch and dinner every day. Now I take my raw liver only once in the afternoon. I try to eat only the most valuable foods in each food group in their most natural form. I rationalize that the tiger or lion and all carnivores instinctively know more about nutrition than modern man. When one of God's meat-eaters kills his prey, the choicest and most nutritionally valuable bit is eaten first. The first piece a carnivore goes for is the liver. Because I speculate that commercial meat producers will have less time to bastardize the liver of veal than of a more mature animal, I always eat very young organically-grown 'baby beef' or veal liver.

Don't try eating raw meat unless you are certain you have good digestion and assimilation capabilities. Over the years, I have accustomed my body to eating raw foods, including raw liver. For those unable (or unwilling) to eat raw veal liver, it's easy enough to find dessicated raw veal liver in powdered or capsule form.

The experts warn that raw meat can contain harmful bacteria which are killed by cooking. Horse feathers! I view this statement as just another 'old wive's tale.' I have been eating raw liver for over fifty years. The so-called health authorities who say the poisons of the body are lodged in the liver just don't know what they are talking about. The poisons of the body are lodged in the blood.

It's hard to believe today, but the whole civilized world once "knew for a fact" that the tomato was a poisonous fruit. This wrong thinking continued for decades, until someone was brave enough to eat one. The same type of false thinking today is what causes the "authorities" to say that body poisons are lodged in the liver.

I have demonstrated to my personal satisfaction that my high ingestion of High Desert bee pollen protects me from injurious microbes, air pollution, electrical pollution, harmful rays and radiation dangers.

Perhaps the greatest nutritional sin in the world is eating cooked foods, especially cooked protein. This may well be the primary cause of all degenerative disease. Sooner or later, the American consumer is going to wake up to the fact that the primary cause of so much ill health is the consumption of foods which have had the nutrients cooked away. Another nutritional mistake is the heavy consumption of saturated-fat foods and dairy products, including pasteurized and homogenized cow's milk (even the non-fat type), ice cream, cheeses and so on.

I normally work all day long and leave the office around 8:00 p.m. in the evening. Upon arriving home, I retreat to my downstairs bathroom where I exercise my gums, put mineral oil in my ears, get into my swimming shorts and go to my back-yard swimming pool.

I usually swim 50 laps in my pool, which is 50 feet long. I don't know why I don't swim 53 laps, which would total a mile, but I never have. I never heat my swimming pool. After my swim, I strap on a 20 pound-belt, put on my snorkel equipment, and climb into my therapy pool, which is automatically heated to

110 degrees. Breathing through my snorkel, I stay completely submerged for seven minutes, then swim a lap in my unheated pool, and return to the heated therapy pool for another seven minutes. I do this three times and end by swimming two more laps in my swimming pool. This water therapy and swimming routine has been gained from Paul Bragg. Bragg was an early crusader in the health food movement and is a strong advocate of the natural way of life. (See page 360.)

After this invigorating regimen, I return to the house, take a shower, go in my den and read the evening paper. By this time, it's about 11:00 p.m. and I retire shortly thereafter. I sleep soundly until I awaken naturally sometime between 4:00 and 6:00 a.m. the next morning. When I awaken, of course I start a new day.

Saturday: Saturday is not exactly a day of R & R for me. Although I don't exercise or work out, I follow my usual wakeup regimen before going into the office, enjoy the same menu as the day before, and return home around dusk. If you're getting the idea that my business affairs keep me very busy, perhaps too busy, you are right!

Sunday: The Sabbath is a day of worship and rest. We are Episcopalian and attend St. Barnabas of the Desert in Paradise Valley, Arizona. St. Barnabas celebrates Mass and offers communion the first and third Sundays of each month. At this time, we partake of the new wine and bread. The service we usually attend commences at 9:00 a.m. and ends around 10:30 a.m.

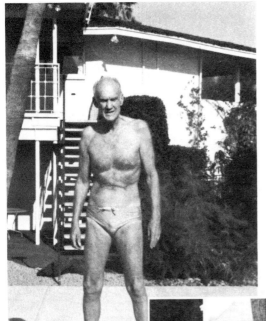

My Wet Workout

Ready to Swim
A Fast 50 Laps
In The Pool

Dive! Dive!

With 20-Lb. Belt
And Snorkel, I'm Ready
For The Therapy Pool

After worship, we often breakfast with friends at the Camelback Inn Country Club during the summer and the Hilton Hotel in the winter. My breakfast consists of whatever fresh fruit is being served. I know I would be better off with raw goat's milk, but no restaurant on this planet, at least none I know about, offers raw goat's milk.

It's not possible for the dedicated apiarian to dine out properly! I travel considerably, as my business takes me many places, both in the U.S. and around the world. For example, I am writing this particular section of the book on November 3rd, 1988, the Friday night before the New York City Marathon in the Sheraton Inn in New York City.

Without doubt, a lot of business 'socializing' takes place over a meal, so sometimes I must partake. Many restaurants now offer selected packets of herbal teas. It's always possible to order an 'undressed' green salad, my favorite is spinach, or a vegetable plate. Of course, I always carry a supply of High Desert products. Although I don't travel on Air Force One, my travel rations always include a box or two of President's Lunch bars, High Desert 130 mg Honey/Vanilla Wafers, and High Desert Bee Pollen granules. No matter where affairs of state take him, President Reagan makes sure he has his High Desert Bee Pollen and those delicious President's Lunch bars to sustain him.

Quarterly: I closely monitor my body every day without thinking too much about it. I've been doing it for so long that I can usually tell approximately what my internal chemical balance is by the way I feel.

Still, forewarned is forearmed. For this reason, I have a hair analysis done quarterly to make sure the mineral levels in my body are in the normal or appropriate ranges. I almost never find an excess of any mineral in my body, but I have very occasionally been low in some trace element. When this occurs, I simply step up my intake of High Desert Bee Pollen for ninety days until it's time for another hair analysis. If that analysis shows that all minerals are once again within healthy ranges, I revert back to my usual daily intake of High Desert to maintain optimum levels.

I also have a blood test done quarterly, instructing the lab to be sure to read my high density lipoprotein levels. My normal cholesterol reads between 110 and 134. My triglycerides levels usually fall between 50 and 65. I had my cholesterol levels tested at the National Health Federation convention in Pasadena, California on January 21, 1989. My blood serum cholesterol was 128, a little higher than usual.

I personally monitor my resting heart beat every morning, which runs from about 40 to 45 beats. I occasionally take my own blood pressure and find it is generally about 120 over 60.

These measurements are considered too low by orthodox medical practitioners. Still, I believe they are near perfect for an apiarian who is careful with his diet and who exercises regularly.

Before giving you some general guidelines on such readings, I must acquaint you with an experience I had at the Nevada Clinic for Preventive Medicine in Las Vegas. Dr. Betty Lee Morales told me about the Nevada Clinic and said I should go through their diagnostic procedures. I did. At the close of the tests, Dr. Fuller Royal remarked that my readings were all "so low." He said I either had "cancer of the blood" (leukemia), or something had gone haywire and they would have to reprogram their instruments.

The doctor explained there was only one type electronic microscope that was powerful enough to "see" cancer cells in the bloodstream. This microscope was in the laboratory of Dr. Arnold Schenk, Ph.D. M.D., a medical doctor working in Tijuana, Mexico. I wasn't worried, mind you. I knew I did not have leukemia. I knew my apiarian lifestyle had me well protected. But I was curious. I made the trip to Dr. Schenk's facility. He drew blood, made a slide and examined it closely under his very costly and extremely powerful electronic microscope. There were no cancerous cells hitching a ride in my blood.

When Dr. Royal was informed of the results, he acknowledged that he would be required to reprogram his diagnostic instruments.

Keeping in mind that I am not a medical doctor and that the guidelines I am giving next are based only on my own experience, it seems to me that a person in perfect health will exhibit the following readings.

(1) Blood cholesterol: 110 - 135

(2) Triglycerides: 55 - 65

(3) High density lipoproteins: 75 - 100 (or more)

(4) Resting heart rate: 35 - 45

(5) Blood pressure: 120 over 60

HOW TO PREPARE

What follows next are my personal recipes for preparing Bee-Dew Water and my Breakfast Bacillus. I am hopeful that many of you will take the time to prepare these electrically-charged and fortified golden elixirs that I have found so beneficial.

BEE-DEW® WATER

1. Put one teaspoon of Bee-Dew concentrate and one teaspoon of *Elixir,* the High-Desert Honeybee Pollen extract, in a clean empty gallon jug.
2. Place a D Cell in the funnel through which you will pour the water into the gallon container.
3. Add water. We draw water from a deep well over 650 feet underground to be assured of clean, pure water with no additives of any kind. Pour the water over the D Cell and let it mingle with the High Desert Extract.

A word of explanation is in order here. D Cells are specially formulated in such a way as to capture solar energy. Any liquid poured over D Cells becomes supercharged as the liquid absorbs some of the sun's own energy. Plants fed D Cell charged water grow faster, larger, and healthier than plants given ordinary water. They are more productive, too.

About ten or fifteen years ago, I purchased a large number of D Cells from the inventor, a licensed pharmacist. I have enough D Cells on hand to last me and my family until the millennium. For your own supply of D Cells, contact 81-year old Joe Dun Sloane; his address is given in the Source List at the close of this chapter.

Once the apiarian's body becomes accustomed to the early morning ingestion of this specially-prepared Bee-Dew water, this charged mixture will trigger a healthy and continuing evacuation of the intestines and lower colon. The healthy effects of this regimen will be apparent in short order.

BREAKFAST BACILLUS

Here's your shopping list. You will need to purchase 4-½ gallons of raw, unpasteurized, unhomogenized goat's milk, a 14 ounce box of Eugalan Topfter, a pint of Continental Acidophilus Bacillus, and Mt. Capra Dairy Whex (see Source List), plus 28 ounces of raw unprocessed honey.

To prepare a healthy breakfast feast, have a large stainless steel pan (with lid) ready to receive the ingredients.

First: Put the jar holding the 28 oz. of raw honey in a bowl of hot (not boiling) water. While you are following the next steps in the procedure, the honey will warm. Allow the honey to reach about 100° in temperature. It should feel slightly warmer than body temperature.

Second: The goat's milk and Eugalan Topfter powder are combined. The Eugalan Topfter powder tends to cake, To minimize this effect, pour a cup or so of the goat's milk in a blender and add about ⅓ of the box of Eugalan Topfter. Blend thoroughly and pour the mixture into the stainless steel pan. Continue in this manner until the entire box of powder has been thoroughly blended into the milk. Add the remainder of the goat's milk to the Eugalan Topfter/milk mixture in the pan and stir thoroughly.

Third: Add the pint of Continental Acidophilus Bacillus and blend completely.

Fourth: Add the warmed honey to the goat's milk and other ingredients. By now, the honey will have liquified and will be easier to blend. Stir well to distribute the honey throughout the entire mixture and encourage it to become a part of the blend.

Fifth: Put the lid on the pan and allow the bacillus mixture to remain undisturbed until the blend clabbers and the cream forms a solid crust on top. At room temperature, clabbering will take place in from 36 to 48 hours. In summer, the process can be hurried by placing the pan in the sun. Normally, clabbering will take place in from 24 to 36 hours.

When clabbering has occurred, take a spoon, break the crust, and reincorporate the coating into the mixture. You can hurry the process by scooping the mixture into a blender. Whirl for three to four seconds to blend thoroughly.

Sixth: Have ready six empty clean ½ gallon goat's milk containers. Add one heaping tablespoon of Whex to each container. Then pour sufficient of the clabbered blend into each container to reach the indentation where the handle begins on the bottle. You must allow sufficient headroom for the mixture to continue working. Once the containers are filled, shake thoroughly to incorporate the tablespoon of powdered Whex into the mixture.

Place the filled containers in the refrigerator, but DO NOT COVER. This very powerful mix continues working. If you cap the bottles, as fermentation continues, the gases will pop the top and the mixture will spill over into the refrigerator.

Check on the bottles every time you open the fridge to make sure all is well. If the mix threatens to rise over the top of the bottle, give it a good shake and decant part of it into another half gallon container.

When the mix is ready for the refrigerator, it's ready for breakfast. Take out one bottle and shake it thoroughly to redistribute the honey and make sure all ingredients are well blended.

As I told you earlier in the text, each morning I pour out one pint. To this pint of mix, add:

1. Two raw fertile eggs, beaten, and
2. Two heaping tablespoons of fresh raw High Desert Bee Pollen granules, and
3. Two heaping tablespoons of lecithin granules, and
4. Three squirts of High Desert Bee Propolis extract (or six crushed 500 mg High Desert Bee Propolis tablets,) and
5. One tablespoon of C-Leinosan Linseed Oil.
6. Warm in hot water,
7. Shake vigorously and enjoy your Breakfast Bacillus feast.

This mixture assures you will never develop an ulcer. Don't forget to chew this liquid powerhouse of nutrients. Take one mouthful at a time; swish it around in your mouth; chew 11 times before swallowing to insure that the digestive enzymes present in saliva are thoroughly incorporated into the mouthful.

The ingestion of this Breakfast Bacillus goat's milk following your drink of Bee-Dew will reinhabit your digestive tract with friendly bacteria. When your digestive tract reaches the saturation point with the friendly acidophils bacillus bacteria, the digestive tract will begin to function perfectly.

IN CONCLUSION

I am convinced my high ingestion of High Desert Products of the Beehive and the foregoing Elixirs, plus my vigorous lifestyle, have all played an important part in keeping me young and healthy.

In this chapter, I have told you how I achieved perfect health and am living the millennial lifestyle. Along the way, I've mentioned several acceptable (but not perfect) alternatives to the severe regimen I personally follow. I know that most people will not have the will-power needed to self-discipline themselves in order to follow the Apiarian Lifestyle every day in every way for the rest of their lives.

However, if you want to approach perfect health and enjoy a dramatically extended lifespan, I'm guessing that you almost certainly need to make some big changes in your lifestyle.

Whether you opt to put raw veal liver on your menu or not, you do need to eat as much of your food uncooked as possible. Try never to eat cooked protein. I am convinced that cooked protein is the most serious cause of the growing incidence of the degenerative diseases so common to Westernized nations. Remember, High Desert Bee Pollen offers more protein than beef, cheese, or eggs of equal weight, and that high-quality protein is *uncooked* protein. When you are eating sufficient bee pollen, your body will not lack for the essential amino acids that comprise protein.

When is the best time to start living healthy? It doesn't matter how old (or young) you are, *the best time to start is right now!!!*

If you need an incentive, perhaps you should give some thought to how much longer and how much healthier you want to live. Do you want to live twenty more years? Fifty more years? Two hundred and fifty more years? In what condition? The quality of life you enjoy is even more important than your biological age. I have known individuals of twenty-five who were dragged out and apathetic, and I have known grand oldsters of ninety-five who greet each day with eagerness and boundless energy. You decide.

Do you want to run a marathon? You can, you know – if you want to. I ran the New York City marathon in November in company with Manning Wein, a youngster of 86. And Noel Johnson (you read about him in Chapter 6) runs several marathons every year. He brings home the gold, too. Noel Johnson – the super superman – will be 94 years young his next birthday, which isn't far off!

Healthwise – you can attain almost any degree of perfect health you desire – if you have the self-discipline it requires!

You probably have a pretty good idea of what changes you

need to make in your lifestyle to achieve better health for a longer period of time.

I suggest you read and reread this chapter on The Apiarian Lifestyle again and again. Perhaps on the fifth or sixth reading, you should jot down the changes you *need* to make, which you feel you *can* and *will* make, in your own life. Add to this list every so often to try to obtain perfection. Be persistent. Discipline yourself. You really can improve your health and increase the odds in your favor in life's sweepstakes.

The single most important change you can make in your life is the ingestion of High Desert Bee Pollen products. I offer myself as living proof that this is the first giant step toward better health and extended longevity.

Take that first step. Better health and extended longevity are yours for the doing.

I am convinced you can enjoy better health — yes, *super health,* even *perfect health* — if you have the determination and self-discipline necessary to eat and drink only what is best for you, to *do* what is best for you. When you think about it, to give yourself less than the best is suicidal.

Start this very minute! You will be the better for it!

All major health food stores carry the High Desert Products of the Beehive and the other fine products I've told you about. To make it even easier for you to get started living the Apiarian Lifestyle, I have compiled a list of sources for you. The list even includes two firms which will provide you with beekeeping equipment, plus the bees you need to populate a hive, if you want to 'grow your own' beehive products.

Beekeeping is one of the most ancient and most-honored professions in the universe. I'm proud to report that not only do I head up C C Pollen Company, probably the largest harvester and producer of beehive products in the world, but I'm also a beekeeper myself. (See page 372). I have several hives tucked away on the outskirts of the grounds around my home. And, yes, I work those hives personally. Once you know what you're doing, tending your colony is very relaxing. I enjoy it. . . a lot.

I carry on an extensive correspondence with like-minded individuals all over the world. I would be pleased to hear from any reader who has benefited by taking High Desert products or from reading this book. You may write to me c/o Plains Corporation, 4343 E. Keim Drive, Paradise Valley, Arizona 85253-3928. I know what the Apiarian Lifestyle has done for me. I expect it will do the same for you, even in modified form, so I am looking forward to a substantial increase in my correspondence.

I completed this manuscript in the Holiday Inn at the Pasadena Convention Center, Pasadena, California, and put "finis" on it in midair on the America West flight back to my homebase in Phoenix, Arizona in time to enjoy the Super Bowl game in Miami, Florida on television.

It's been a pleasure visiting with you via the printed page. The next time you're buzzed by a bee when you're out in the garden, don't forget to say 'thank you.' Without the pollen-carrying honeybee, life as we know it would cease to exist.

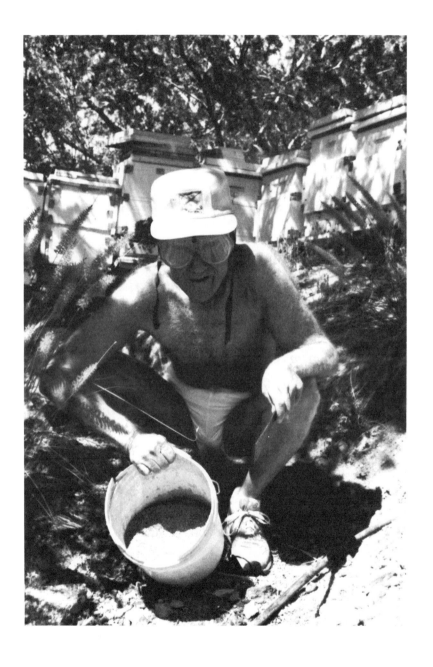

To your bee pollen health and bee pollen wealth, naturally. May you live a thousand years, prosper in perfect health, and enjoy the millennium with me!

> Royden Brown
> Phoenix, Arizona
> June 26, 1917 - June 26, 2917

OTHER GREAT BOOKS FROM HOHM PRESS

Natural Healing with Herbs, $16.50 post paid (pp)
Food Enzymes: The Missing Link to Radiant Health, $6.75 pp
Intuitive Eating, $18.50 pp
Ten Essential Herbs, $13.50 pp
Herbs, Nutrition and Healing (4 cassettes), $47.00
Energetics of Juicing (2 cassettes plus 48-page booklet), $21.50
Food Enzymes (3 cassettes plus 80-page book), $47.00

Mail Check or Money Order payable to Hohm Press to:

> Hohm Press
> P.O. Box 2501
> Prescott, Arizona 86302

FOR YOUR CONVENIENCE
The Source List

There's nothing more frustrating than not knowing where to find something you need. To make it easy for you to contact various sources for more information on the healthy products we cite in this book, to request a catalog, or for the items themselves when you can't locate them on the shelves of your favorite health-food store, we have compiled a handy list of ready references for you:

HEALTH-ORIENTED PRODUCTS
High-Desert Products of the Beehive
Bee Pollen - Bee Propolis - Royal Jelly
Free Pamphlet
The Scientific Study of Bee Pollen
C C Pollen Company
3627 E. Indian School, Suite #209
Phoenix, AZ 85018-5162
Call Toll-Free Nationwide:
1-800-950-0096

BioSan Unrefined Seed Oils
The Dynabound Rebound Exerciser
Phone for prices/catalog:
New Dimensions Distributors
16548 E. Laser Drive
Fountain Hills, Arizona 85268
Toll-Free Nationwide: 1-800-624-7114
In Arizona (602) call: 1-837-8322

World's Best Goat Cheese & Whey
Mr. Capra Goat Farm
279 S.W. 9th Street
Chehalis, Washington 98532
1-206-748-4224

Codliver Oil
V.E. Irons, Inc.
P.O. Box 296
89 North Avenue
Natick, Massachusetts 01260
1-617-653-8441

Organic Fruit (Mangoes, Etc.)
Starr Organic Produce, Inc.
Box 561502
Miami, Florida 33256
1-305-262-1242

Continental Acidophilus
Eugalon Topfter
Most good health food stores and natural food groceries

SELF-CARE HEALTH BOOKS
How To Live The Millennium
The Bee Pollen Bible
Plains Corporation
4343 E. Keim Drive
Paradise Valley, Arizona 85253-3928
Credit Card orders:
Call 1-800-950-0096 Toll Free

Miracles of Rebound Exercise
The Cancer Answer
Extend Your Life A Through Z
A.L.M. Publishers
9412 E. Cortez
Scottsdale, Arizona 85260
Toll-Free Nationwide: 1-800-367-3981
In Arizona (602) call: 1-837-9813

Honeybee Pollen and the New You
Mr. Bee Pollen Himself
The Golden Pollen
Mr. Bee Pollen, Inc.
7360 E. Acoma Drive, No. 3
Scottsdale, Arizona 85260
1-602-998-3958

The Living Proof
I Found The Fountain Of Youth
Noel Johnson
1370 Beryl Street
San Diego, California 92109
1-619-272-6243

HEALTH AIDS:

D-Cells
Joe Dun Sloan
6315 Middleton Street
Huntington Park, California 90255
1-213-589-4128

MiVita Mineral Water
Lynne B. Johnston
122 S. Sirrine Street
Mesa, Arizona 85210
1-602-969-7207

BEES & BEEKEEPING EQUIPMENT
Dadant & Sons, Inc.
Hamilton, Illinois 62341
1-217-847-3324

A.I. Root Company
P. O. Box 706
Medina, Ohio 44258
1-800-289-7668

Pollen Traps
The Plains Corporation
4343 E. Keim Drive
Scottsdale, AZ 85253-3928
Telephone 800-950-0096

HEALTH PRODUCTS
Boxer Shorts
Men's Department Stores
Dilliards Department Store
7014 E. Camelback Road
Scottsdale, AZ 85251
Telephone 602-949-5869

Raw Veal Liver
Most Meat Markets displaying
Coleman's Meat Sign
Reay's Ranch Market
Camelback & 40th Street
Phoenix, AZ 85018
Telephone 602-954-0584

Reverse Osmosis Equipment
Jensen Enterprises
Rte. 1, Box 52
Escondido, CA 92025
Telephone 619-749-2727

Raw Unprocessed Honey
Most Health Food Stores
Crockett Honey Co.
1880 E. Buchanan Street
Phoenix, AZ 85034
Telephone 602-254-2371

Stop Watch
Most Jewelers
Best Products Co.
1900 N. Scottsdale Road
Scottsdale, AZ 85257
Telephone 602-994-9401

Exercise Computer
Heart Monitor
Hermans Sporting Goods
3107 E. Indian School Road
Phoenix, AZ 85018
Telephone 602-955-5831

Oral Thermometer
Most Drug Stores
Crandall's Pharmacy
4832 N. 40th Street
Phoenix, AZ 85018
Telephone 602-955-3280

Desiccated Veal Liver
Free of all drugs from Agentina or
New Zealand
Most Health Food Stores
Arizona Health Foods
4224 N. 19th Avenue
Phoenix, AZ 85015
Telephone 602-265-7494

Vitamin E
Betty Lee Morales, Ph.D
Eden Ranch
Box 370
Topanga Canyon, CA 90290
Telephone 213-455-2065

Bee 20/20™
The Escrow Co.
4343 E. Keim Drive
Scottsdale, AZ 85253-3928
Telephone 800-950-0096

Champion Juicer
D. Scott
122 S. Sirrine Street
Mesa, AZ 85210
Telephone 602-969-7207

Fertile Eggs
Most Health Food Stores
Arcadia Health Food Store
3724 E. Indian School Road
Phoenix, AZ 85018
Telephone 602-955-5480

Weight Lifting Equipment
York Barbell Co.
Box 1707
York, PA 17405
Telephone 717-767-6481

Weider Products & Equipment
Most Sporting Goods Stores
Sears & Montgomery Ward
Joe Weider Health & Fitness
21100 Erwin Street
Woodland Hills, CA 91367
Telephone 800-423-5590

Back Swing-Barbells
Max Huberman
Natural Health Foods & Barbells
4981 Market Street
Youngstown, OH 44512
Telephone 216-788-7295

Fruits & Vegetables
Your Roadside Stands and Farmers
Markets are the most likely to have
Organically Grown Fruits and
Vegetables

New Balance Shoes
Runner's Stores

Electric Razor
Mine is a Schick but they are out of
business. Suggest a Schick-type at
larger electric razor sellers.

Bee-Taller™ Course
Gro-Taller Course
Sales Inc. International
4613 N. 31st Place
Phoenix, AZ 85016
Telephone 602-381-3100

Water Energizer
Patrick Flanigan
Sedona, AZ 85291

Lecithin & Beehive Products
Most Health Food Stores
Feel Rite Health Foods
13107 Shaker Square
Cleveland, OH 44120
Telephone 216-561-6047

Full Spectrum Light Globes
Duro-Test Corporation
9 Law Drive
Fairfield, NJ 07006
Telephone 800-289-3876

Goat's Milk
Most Grocery Stores having Health
Foods Sections

Loofah Glove-Skin Brush
Rubber Pronged Plate
Most Larger Well-Stocked Health Food
Stores

Armour Desiccated Thyroid
Unfortunately, the FDA has declared
Thyroid a drug; therefore, you will need
to go to your MD or Dentist and get a
prescription to take to the Drug Store
for your Thyroid

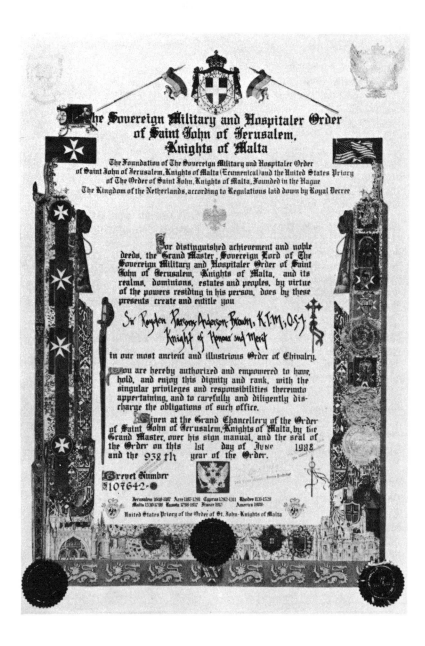

The Sovereign Military and Hospitaler Order
of Saint John of Jerusalem,
Knights of Malta

The Foundation of The Sovereign Military and Hospitaler Order
of Saint John of Jerusalem, Knights of Malta (Ecumenical) and the United States Priory
of The Order of Saint John, Knights of Malta, Founded in the Hague
The Kingdom of the Netherlands, according to Regulations laid down by Royal Decree

For distinguished achievement and noble deeds, the Grand Master, Sovereign Lord of The Sovereign Military and Hospitaler Order of Saint John of Jerusalem, Knights of Malta, and its realms, dominions, estates and peoples, by virtue of the powers residing in his person, does by these presents create and entitle you

Sir Royston Parsons Anderson-Brown, KTM, OSJ

Knight of Honour and Merit

in our most ancient and illustrious Order of Chivalry.

You are hereby authorized and empowered to have, hold, and enjoy this dignity and rank, with the singular privileges and responsibilities thereunto appertaining, and to carefully and diligently discharge the obligations of such office.

Given at the Grand Chancellery of the Order of Saint John of Jerusalem, Knights of Malta, by the Grand Master, over his sign manual, and the seal of the Order on this 1st day of June 1988 and the 938th year of the Order.

Brevet Number
107642

Jerusalem 1048-1187 Acre 1187-1291 Cyprus 1292-1311 Rhodes 1311-1529
Malta 1530-1798 Russia 1798-1917 France 1917 America 1939-

United States Priory of the Order of St. John, Knights of Malta

EPILOGUE
By Bruce R. Brown

When my dad started writing this book, he had no idea that a very high honor was in store for him. In September of 1988, Royden Brown was made a Knight of Malta for his philanthropic work and pioneering efforts in the bee pollen industry. When I proposed he tell you about his knighthood, he disagreed with me, saying, "I don't want to toot my own horn." Royden Brown is a humble man. It took a lot of persuasion on my part before he would agree that I could add this Epilogue.

As a history buff, I'm not ashamed to say that it thrills me to know that my dad is now part of the long history of The Sovereign Military and Hospitaler Order of Saint John of Jerusalem, Knights of Malta. Most historians agree that this ancient order was established in 1048, although some put the date as early as 1023, and still others say it was not actually founded until the 1100s.

The origin of the Hospitaler Order was a hospital in Jerusalem set up to treat sick pilgrims coming to the Holy Land. After the crusaders conquered Jerusalem in 1099, a Roman Catholic monk named Gerard, the hospital's superior, founded hostels in Provencal and some of the Italian cities on the route to Israel. Grateful crusader knights healed of wounds suffered in battle bestowed a portion of their estates on the Order; other altruistic knights never returned to their homes, but stayed behind to assist in the work. In this way, the Order grew into a wealthy and powerful body dedicated to the combined task of tending the sick and poor, while the crusading knights continued waging war on those they viewed as 'unbelievers.'

The Order established hospital centers throughout almost all of Europe and developed into a mighty force, gaining many victories while building up wealth and much power. It was during the Middle Ages that the Hospitalers became a Federation of many national societies, instead of the original single Order, and flourished in many countries.

When Jerusalem fell to those they called the 'infidels' in 1087, the Order moved their operations to Acre. The sovereign principalities established by the crusaders came to an end when Acre was lost in 1291. The Hospitalers then migrated to Cyprus, which was as close as they could safely stay to the Holy Land, and prayed for its Christian reconquest. The monks and knights continued their work tending to the pilgrims, the poor and the sick. In 1309, the Order acquired Rhodes, built yet another hospital and ruled the island as an independent state, soon becoming a naval power in the eastern Mediterranean. In spite of legendary feats of heroics on the part of the Hospitaler Knights, the Ottoman Turks vanquished Rhodes in 1522.

In recognition of their good works, the Spanish emperor Charles V gave the Hospitalers possession of the island of Malta in 1530. The valiant knights reached the height of their power on Malta, withstanding violent Ottoman attacks. They increased their naval strength and maintained an advanced hospital at the same time. As a sovereign power, the Knights of Malta finally appeared to be ensconced in a secure, permanent home, but it was not to be. In 1798, Napoleon took Malta and the Knights were dispersed throughout Europe.

It was then that Emperor Czar Paul I of Russia became Grand Master in place of the Roman Catholic Grand Master, Ferdinand von Hompeach. Czar Paul I established a new Grand Priory of the Order in Russia for non-Catholics, and the Prostestant Orders came into being. Under Queen Victoria, the Prostestant Orders were established in England in the 1830s. The prestigious St. John's Ambulance Corps. is part of the Order yet today. In Europe, the individual Prostestant Orders merit honors for distinguished service as well. The Catholic Order continues its solid hospital activity throughout the world.

Although the Order no longer exercises territorial rule anywhere, it continues its humanitarian tasks in many parts of the modern world. Today, the Royal Protector and Grand Master of the Hospitaler Knights is King Peter II; the Sovereign Heads of the Protestant Orders include Queen Elizabeth II of England; Queen Wilhelmina of the Netherlands; Prince Wilhelm Karl of Germany and Gustav V, King of Sweden. The Roman Catholic Grand Master is Prince Angelo de Mojana. Prince Angelo resides in Rome.

In the United States, the Ecumenical Order of the Knights of Malta is under Grand Master Prince Robert von B. Khimchiach-vili, head of the family House of Badische. In keeping with the non-discriminatory traditions of the U.S., the Order is open to all faiths. The prestigious honor of Knighthood is given strictly on merit, and is not based on religion, race or creed.

It is true that Royden Brown is a good man in the best sense of the word. He has always been ready to lend a helping hand to those in need. His charity work has been done quietly, behind the scenes, so to speak. He has never sought recognition or wanted praise, although he has been laboring in the vineyard of the Lord his entire life. True to Malachi's admonition in the Bible, a tenth of his riches is tithed to the church. My sister and I were taught this holy obligation at a very young age.

In the grand tradition of the Hospitaler Knights, my dad has long been dedicated to improving the health of the American consumer. His way is through the God-given nutrients found in the beehive. Royden Brown stands tall as a pioneer in the bee industry. Yes, there were a number of bee pollen products on the market before my dad got involved. These products were sold with vague claims of pollen's health-promoting benefits. But Royden Brown alone is responsible for *documenting* the incredible properties of all the hive products, with emphasis on bee pollen. He's the one who went overseas and searched out the scientific research that substantiated bee pollen's miraculous powers.

In the early years, just about everything serious that was written on the products of the beehive came from his pen. Before long, others marketing bee pollen started 'borrowing' freely from his work to sell their own products. I remember that dad's staff was furious over this outright plagiarism. They were proud of the quality of High Desert products and incensed that his material was being used to sell inferior goods. My dad remained unruffled. "It's more important to get the word out," he said. "The people should know the facts, no matter who publishes them. The consumer will find High Desert. Our quality will sell itself, you'll see." The history of the company has proved him right.

The 940th Anniversary of the Order of St. John — Knights of Malta — was observed in New York last year. The year 1988 not only marks the 940th year of the Order, but the 77th anniversary of its founding in America and the 11th year of its Ecumenical Charter.

Although my dad, now Sir Royden, was knighted by Prince Robert in an informal investiture, the formal ceremony took place with suitable pomp during the anniversary festivities in New York. To read the history of the hundreds of years of the Hospitaler Knights in their valorous passage through the ages is an inspiration. I am overwhelmed to know that my father's work qualifies him to be in such distinguished company.

BIBLIOGRAPHY

Bee Pollen

L.J. Hayes, Fr. R.A. Baldensnerger, *Bees Sterilize Pollen By Means Of A Glandular Secretion Which Is Antagonistic to Tumors:* L'Ariculteur haut-rhinois, Guebwiller, Germany, 1958.

W. Robinson, U.S.D.A., Agricultural Research Administration, *Delay in the Appearance of Palpable Mammary Tumors in C3H Mice Following the Ingestion of Pollenized Food:* Journal of the National Cancer Institute, Vol. 9. No 2, October, 1948.

F.A. Soliman, A. Soliman, *Gonad Stimulating Potency of Date Palm Pollen Grains:* Physiology Department, Cairo University, Gisa, Egypt, October, 1957.

Y. Solberg, G. Remedios, *Chemical Composition of Pure & Bee-Collected Pollen:* Agricultural University of Norway, Chemical Research Laboratory, Oslo, Norway, May, 1980.

Dr. L. Louveaux, Director, *Apiarian Research Station at Bures-Sur-Yvette:* Insitut National de Recherches Apicoles (National Institute of Apiarian Research) Nice, France, September, 1974.

Gunther Vorwohl, M.D., *Pollen and Honey:* Germany

New Apitherapy Research on Honey, Propolis, Pollen & Royal Jelly, 2nd International Symposium on Apitherapy: Apimondia Publishing House, Bucharest, Rumania, 1976.

M. Nilsson, Ragnar Ryhage, E. von Sydow, *Constituents of Pollen:* Acta Chemica Scandinavica, Vol. 11, 1957.

I. Osmanagic, D. Biljenski, N. Mavric (Yugoslavia), *Therapeutic Effects of Melbrosin in Irradiation Diseases:* Apimondia, Bucarest, Rumania, September, 1978.

Prof. Drs. L. Pokrajcic, I. Osmanagic, *Treatment with Melbrosin of Dysmenorrhoea in Adolescence:* Endocrinological Department of the University Clinic for Women, Medical Faculty, Sarajevo, Yugoslavia.

Prof. T. Inada, M.D., T. Kitagawa, M.D., M. Miyakawa, M.D., Tobishi Pharmaceuticals, *Use of Cernilton in Patients with Prostatic Hypertrophy:* Acta Urologica Japonica, Vol. 13, No. 6, Tokyo, Japan, June 1967.

Drs. E. Palos, Z. Voiculescu, C. Andrei, *Comparative Studies Concerning Biochemical Characteristics of Beebread as Related to the Pollen Preserved in Honey:* Agronomic Institute, Faculty of Zootetchnics, Rumania.

A Summary of Clinical Tests Concluded with Bee Pollen and Other Substances: Naturheilpraxis, Germany, 1977.

F.E. Todd, O. Bretherick, U.S. Department of Agriculture, Bureau of Entomology, *The Composition of Pollens:* Journal of Economic Entomology, Vol. 35, June 1942.

Prof. Dr. Alberto Chattas, *Administration of Biological Pollen Products to the Undernourished:* Universidad Nacional de Cordoba, Faculty of Medicine, Chair of Pediatrics, Cordoba, Spain.

Chuck Badone, *Bee Pollen Making Impact at Turf Paradise:* Turf Paradise News, Phoenix, Arizona 1988.

R. Breslin, et al, *Observations of the Effect of Pollen in the Nutrition of Pregnant Cows and their Progeny:* Yugoslavia.

G. Calcaianu, F. Cozma, *Treatment with Bee Products of the Behaviour Troubles in Young People in the Period of Puberty & Teen-Age;* Apitherapie Second Symposium, Rumania.

Bienenzell-Gesellschaft m.b.H., Argestorf/Hann, *On The Track of Life's Secrets:* Germany.

M. Poljak-Blazi, M. Hadzija, M. Slijepcevic (Institute of Microbiologia, Ljubljana, Yugoslavia), *Impact of Pollen on the Immunological Reactions of Test Mice:* Apimondia, Bucarest, Rumania, September, 1978.

Effects of Melbrosia in Cases of Reduced Sexual Potency: Gynacological Clinic, University of Sarajevo, Yugoslavia.

P. Hernuss, M.D. et al, *Pollen Diet as an Adjunct of Radiation Therapy in Gynecological Carcinomas;* Germany.

Paul Uccusic, Bee Medicine: *The Healing Virtues of Pollen, Royal Jelly and Propolis & Their Applications:* Facultas, Publishers of Medicine & Pharmacology, Vienna, Austria, 1981.

T.J. Sawicka, P. Laszczyca, kB. Smylla, Z. Jethon, *Metabolic Adaption of Muscles to Exercise, Vibration & Raised Temperature Under the Influence of Cernitins,* Chair of Human Psysiology & Ergonomics, Faculty of Biology, Silesian University, Katowice, Poland: *Acta Physiologica,* February, 1984.

M. Boracic, et all, *Effect of Pollen in the Diet on the Fertility & Sexual Organs of Laboratory Mice:* Yugoslavia.

R.J. Maughan, BSc, PhD., S.P. Evans, BSc., *Effects of Pollen Extract Upon Adolescent Swimmers:* British Journal of Sports Medicine, Vol. 16, No. 3, September, 1982.

F. Pratviel-Sosa, F. Percheron, National Center for Scientific Research, Faculty of Pharmceutical & Biological Sciences, Rene Descartes University, Paris, France, *The Sophorosides of Flavonols from Certain Pollens:* Phytochemistry, Paris, France, 1972.

John Feltman, *A Nutritional Shield Against the Arrows of Stress:* Prevention Magazine, September, 1976.

Gh. Salajan, Gh. B. Baltan, *Influence of Maize Pollen on Ovulation: Results of Incubation & Biological Value of Hen Eggs:* Rumania.

Prof. Drs. I. Osmanagic, I. Bukvic, N. Mavric, *Melbrosin in The Treatment of Menopausal Troubles:* Symposium International d'Apitherapie, Portoroz, Yugoslavia, September, 1978.

R. Chauvin, Apicultural Research Station of the Ministry of Agriculture, Bures-Sur-Yvette, Sein-et-Oise, France, *On The Physiological & Therapeutic Effects of Various Pollen Extracts:* La Revue de Pathologie Generale et de Physiologie Clinique (Review of General Pathology & Clinical Physiology), PACHOMHY, Paris, France, No. 687, April, 1957.

The Hive Products for Food, Health & Beauty, International Symposium on Apitherapy: Apimondia, Madrid, Spain, 1974.

Betty G. Morales, *Energy Galore:* Organic Consumer Report, Eden Ranch, Topanga, California, July, 1980.

Yoshio Kai, M.D., Department of Urology, Showa University School of Medicine, *Clinical Experience with Cernilton By Means of Double Blind Test:* Tobishi Pharmaceuticals, Tokyo, Japan, March, 1968.

The Anti-Bacterial Substances of Pollen Collected by Apis Mellifica L: Apimondia Symposium IV.

L.N. Standifer, Apiculture Research Branch, Entomology Research Division, Agricultural Research Service, U.S.D.A., Tucson, Arizona, *Some Lipid Constituents of Pollens Collected by Honeybees:* Journal of Apicultural Research 5(2), 1966.

M. McCormick, *The Golden Pollen - Nature's Unique Force of Life:* Third Edition, 1984.

Dr. Delia Dello Preite, Cosmetic Research Department PIANA, *The Use of Bee Products in Cosmetology:* Revue francaise d'apiculture, Bologna, Italy, September, 1976.

R.R. Bell, E.J. Thornber, J.L.L. Seet, M.T. Groves, N.P. Ho, D.T. Bell, *Composition & Protein Quality of Honeybee-Collected Pollen:* School of Community Health, Western Australian Institute of Technology, Bently, Western Australia, Department of Botany, University of Western Australia, Nedlands, Western Australia: American Institute of Nutrition, May, 1983.

Dr. Aleksandar Jankovic, *Bee Products As Food & Medicine:* Institute of Microbiology, Ljubljana, Yugoslavia.

Agronomic Institute, Faculty of Zootechnics, Cluj-Napoca, Rumania, Maize Pollen - *Biostimulator & Supplementary Protein Source in the Feeding of Poultry:* Zeitschrift fur Tierphysiologie, Tiernahrung und Futtermittelkunde (Periodical for Animal Physiology, Animal Nutrition & Fodder Science), Vol. 39, Germany, December, 1983.

Robert Delperee, *The Secrets of the Life of Bees:* The Royal Society of the Naturalists of Mons, Belgium & Borinage, France, General Assembly, No. 10, Vol XLIV, 1961.

University Professor Dr. Izet Osmanagic, *Clinical Testing of Melbrosia on Women Suffering from Climacteric Syndrome:* Endocrinological Department of the University Clinic for Women, Medical Faculty, Sarajevo, Yugoslavia, May, 1972.

Rune Cederlof, *A Statistical Evaluation of the Results of A Clinical Investigation of Cernilton:* A.B. Cernelle, Stockholm, Sweden, April, 1964.

Gunther Vorwohl, *Pollen & Honey:* Apiarist Convention, Sontra, October, 1976.

R. Borneck, *The Products of the Hive:* Informations techniques due Directorat des services veterinaires francais, 60/63, Paris, France, 1977.

Prof. M. Ohkoshi, Drs. N. Kawamura, M.D., I. Nagakubo, M.D., Clinical *Evaluation of Cernilton in Chronic Prostatitis:* Japanese Journal of Clinical Urology, Vol. 21, No. 1, 1967.

M. Walker, D.P.M., *Honeybee Pollen & Other Products from The Beehive:* Freeland Communications, Stamford, Connecticut, 1984.

Drs. V. Bejan, N. Oita, C.C. Araman, I. Humita, *The Effects of Aerosols with Bee Honey on Chronic Exudative Asthma-Creating Bronchitis:* Yugoslavia.

Alin Caillas, *Pollen - A Pharmaceutical Product:* L-Abeille de France et l'apiculteur, #568, Paris, France, January, 1974.

C.E. Alken, Prof., M.D., Professor of Urology, Homburg/Saar, Germany, G. Jonsson, Head of the Urology University Clinic, Lund, Sweden, L. Rohl, Prof., M.D., Associate Professor of Urology, Heidelberg, Germany, *Clinical Trials of Cernilton in Chronic Prostatitis:* University Clinics of Homburg/Saar, Germany, Lund, Sweden, Heidelberg, Germany. Published Heidelberg, Germany, March, 1966.

S.L. Vinci, M.D., P.A., *Research on Honeybee Pollen:* Gynocology & Female Diseases Clinic, Ft. Myers, Florida.

M.J.F. Arroyo, (Madrid, Spain), *Effect of Bee Pollen (Water & Lipid Extract) on the Prolificity & Teratogency of Test White Mice:* Wissenschaftliche Bulletin der Apimondia, 1974.

A. Ceplak, M. Matpasic, *Contribution to the Study of the Antiviral Effect of Apikompleks during An Influenza Epidemic:* Symposium III International d'Apitherapie, Yugoslavia, 1978.

Propolis

J. Crisan, V. Cioca, A. Morffi, O. Burducea, N. Cajal, R. Repanovici, *Effects of Propolis Extract on Surface Antigen B of Hepatitis Compared to Some Chemical Agents:* Apiacta. An International Technical Publication of Apicultural & Economic Information, Vol. XIV, 1979.

A Remarkable Hive Product: Propolis - Scientific Data Concerning Its Composition, Properties & Use in Therapeutics: Apimondia Publishing House, Bucharest, Rumania, 1978.

Dr. Felix Murat, Propolis - *The Eternal Natural Healer:* English Edition, 1982.

Robert Delperee, *The Secrets of the Life of Bees:* The Royal Society of the Naturalists of Mons, Belgium & Borinage, France, General Assembly, No. 10, Vol XLIV, 1961.

New Apitherapy Research on Honey, Propolis, Pollen, & Royal Jelly, 2nd International Symposium on Apitherapy: Apimondia Publishing House, Bucharest, Rumania, 1976.

Paul Uccusic, *Bee Medicine: The Healing Virtues of Pollen, Royal Jelly and Propolis & Their Applications:* Facultas, Publishers of Medicine & Pharmacology, Vienna, Austria, 1981.

Drs. S. Bunta, B. Podrumac (Yugoslavia), *Anti-Inflammatory Effect of Propolis:* Apimondia International Symposium on Apitherapy, Portoroz, Yugoslavia, September, 1978.

Dr. L. Louveaux, Director, *Apiarian Research Station at Bures-Sur-Yvete:* Insitut National de Recherches Apicoles (National Institute of Apiarian Research) Nice, France, September, 1974.

R. Borneck, *The Products of the Hive:* Informations techniques du Directorat des services veterinaires francais, 60/63, Paris, France, 1977.

Dr. R.I. Anastausi (Rumania), *Effect of Propolis on Pseudomanas Aeruginosa. In Vitro Experiments:* Apimondia International Symposium on Apitherapy, Portoroz, Yugoslavia, September, 1978.

The Hive Products for Food, Health & Beauty, International Symposium on Apitherapy: Apimonida, Madrid, Spain, 1974.

Dr. Delia Dello Preite, Cosmetic Research Department PIANA, *The Use of Bee Products in Cosmetology:* Revue francaise d'apiculture, Bologna, Italy, September, 1976.

B.A. Aliev, *Local Utilization of the Products of the Bees:* Propolis in Otorhino-Laryngology, 1968.

E.L. Ghisalberti, P.R. Jefferies, R. Lanteri, *Potential Drugs from Propolis. Mass Spectometry in Drug Metabolism:* Plenum Press, New York, New York, 1977.

R. Hill, *Propolis - The Natural Antibiotic:* Thorsons Publishers Limited, Wellingborough, Northamptonshire, England, 1977.

J. Cizmarik, J. Trupl, *Effect of Propolis on Yeasts:* Apitherapie First Symposium, Czechoslovakia.

Dr. Aleksandar Jankovic: *Bee Products As Food & Medicine,* Institute of Microbiology, Ljubljana, Yugoslavia.

G. Calcaianu, F. Cozma, *Treatment with Bee Products of the Behaviour Troubles in Young People in the Period of Puberty & Teen-Age:* Apitherapie Second Symposium, Rumania.

Dr. C. Cakov, *Propolis in Medical Practice:* Apiacta. An International Technical Publication of Apicultural & Economic Information, Vol. XIV, 1979.

Royal Jelly

Effect of Melbrosia in Cases of Reduced Sexual Potency: Gynacological Clinic, University of Sarajevo, Yugoslavia.

Dr. A. Saenz (Montevideo, Uruguay), *Biology, Biochemistry & The Therapeutic Effects of Royal Jelly in Human Pathology:* Pasteur Institute, Paris, France, July, 1984.

University Professor Dr. Izet Osmanagic, *Clinical Testing of Melbrosia on Women Suffering from Climacteric Syndrome:* Endrocrinological Department of the University Clinic for Women, Medical Faculty, Sarajevo, Yugoslavia, May, 1972.

M. Zabey, *The Reasons for Using Royal Jelly by Mouth:* Vivre Jeune (Live Young), Switzerland, 1958.

Dr. Aleksandar Jankovic: *Bee Products As Food & Medicine,* Institute of Microbiology, Ljubljana, Yugoslavia.

Robert Delperee, *The Secrets of the Life of Bees:* The Royal Society of the Naturalists of Mons, Belgium & Borinage, France, General Assembly, No. 10, Vol XLIV, 1961.

Prof. Drs. I. Osmanagic, I. Bukvic, N. Mavric, *Melbrosin in The Treatment of Menopausal Troubles:* Symposium International d'Apitherapie, Portoroz, Yugoslavia, September, 1978.

Dr. I. Dobrovoda (U.S.S.R.), *Psychoneuroses & Royal Jelly with Complement False Euphoria:* Czechoslovakia III. 46.

H.W. Schmidt, M.D., *Royal Jelly in Diet, Prophylaxis & Therapy:* German Medical Association, Leipzig, Germany, 11:911-912, October, 1956.

G. Calcaianu, F. Cozma, *Treatment with Bee Products of the Behaviour Troubles in Young People in the Period of Puberty & Teen-Age:* Apitherapie Second Symposium, Romania.

Dr. Yves Donadieu, *Royal Jelly:* France, August, 1984.

Dr. Ivo Pavlisk, *An Experimental Treatment of Bronchial Asthma with Royal Jelly:* Tschekoslowakischer Badeort, Luhacovice, Czechoslovakia.

Drs. E. Maly, M. Pacenovska, D. Jarcuskova, *Diseases Successfully Treated with Royal Jelly:* Dermatology-Venereal Clinic of the Medical Faculty of Safarik University at Kosice, Czechoslovakia, 111/5.

P. Peichev, N. Atanasov, R. Beleva-Stoikova, *Effect of Royal Jelly on the Oxygen Consumption & Activity of Adenosine-Triphosphatase in Guinea Pig Tissues:* Bulgaria.

G.F. Townsend, W.H. Brown, E.E. Felauer, B. Hazlett, Departments of Apiculture & Chemistry, Ontario Agricultural College, Guelph, Ontario, and Department of Therapeutics, University of Toronto, Toronto, Ontario, *Studies on the In Vitro Antitumor Activity from Royal Jelly Against Transplantable Mouse Leukemia:* Canadian Journal of Biochemistry & Physiology, Vol. 36, 1961.

Dr. L. Louveaux, Director, *Apiarian Research Station at Bures-Sur-Yvette:* Insitut National de Recherches Apicoles (National Institute of Apiarian Research) Nice, France, September, 1974.

The Hive Products for Food, Health & Beauty, International Symposium on Apitherapy: Apimondia, Madrid, Spain, 1974.

Dr. J. Matuszewsky, E. Kaczor, *Investigations on the Biomechanism of Royal Jelly:* Poland

Pual Uccusic, *Bee Medicine: The Healing Virtues of Pollen, Royal Jelly and Propolis & Their Applications:* Facultas, Publishers of Medicine & Pharmacology, Vienna, Austria, 1981.

Dr. Med. Hans Haferkamp, *Gelee Royale:* Germany.

Dr. B. de Belvefer, Prof. M. Gautrelet, *The Action of Royal Jelly on the Adrenal Gland:* France, 111/41.

Dr. Delia Preite, Cosmetic Research Department PIANA, *The Use of Bee Products in Cosmetology:* Revue francaise d'apiculture, Bologna, Italy, September, 1976.

Dr. Madelein Molnar-Toth, Chief Physician Unified Hospital, District of Marghita, Crisana Region, Rumania, *The Effect of Royal Jelly on Nursing Infants: Dystrophic, Convalescent & Immature:* Commission on Apiarian Pathology, Rumania, August, 1965.

Honey with Royal Jelly & Medicinal Herbs: Apifit 3

Activity of 10-Hydroxydecenoic Acid from Royal Jelly Against Experimental Leukaemia & Ascitic Tumors: Nature, Vol. 183, May, 1959.

Hans Weitasser, M.D., *Royal Jelly in Dermatological Cosmetics:* Medizinische Kosmetick, Germany.

R. Borneck, *The Products of the Hive:* Informations techniques du Directorat des services veterinaires francais, 60/63, Paris, France, 1977.

Prof. Drs. L. Pokrajcic, I. Osmanagic, *Treatment with Melbrosin of Dysmenorrhoea in Adolescence:* Endocrinological Department of the University Clinic for Women, Medical Faculty, Sarajevo, Yugoslavia.

New Apitherapy Research on Honey, Propolis, Pollen, & Royal Jelly, 2nd International Symposium on Apitherapy: Apimondia Publishing House, Bucharest, Rumania, 1976.

General

ABC & XYZ of Bee Culture: A.I. Root Company, Medina, Ohio, 1980.

The Hive & The Honey Bee: Dadant & Sons, Hamilton, Illinois, 1975.

Encyclopaedia Britannica, 15th Edition: Benton, Chicago, Illinois.

Columbia Viking Desk Encyclopedia, 2nd Edition: Columbia University Press, New York, New York.

Taber's Cyclopedic Medical Dictionary, 12th Edition: F.A. Davis Company, Philadelphia, Pennsylvania.

The Encyclopedia of Common Diseases: Rodale Press, 1976.

Food Chemicals Codex: National Academy of Sciences Publication No. 1406, Washington, D.C., 1966.

Chemicals Used in Food Processing: National Academy of Sciences Publication No. 1274, Washington, D.C., 1965.

Toxicants Occurring Naturally in Foods: National Academy of Sciences, Washington, D.C., 1973.

Recommended Dietary Allowances: National Academy of Sciences, Washington, D.C., 1980.

Beekeeping in the United States: U.S. Department of Agriculture, Agriculture Research Service, Agriculture Handbook No. 335.

Composition of Foods: Raw, Processed, Prepared: Agriculture Handbook No. 8, U.S. Department of Agriculture, Washington, D.C., 1963.

Nutritive Value of American Foods in Common Units: Agriculture Handbook No. 456, U.S. Department of Agriculture, Washington, D.C., 1975.

Diet, Nutrition & Cancer Prevention - A Guide to Food Choices: U.S. Department of Health & Human Services, National Institute of Health Publication No. 85-2711, Washington, D.C., 1984.

Scientific Study for Research of Health Foods & Their Benefits for Mankind - The Honeybee Pollen Story: Plains Corporation, Scottsdale, Arizona, 1988.

Harvesting Honeybee Pollen - Standard Operating Procedure for High Desert Bee PollenS Beekeepers: Plains Corporation, Scottsdale, Arizona, 1983.

Killion, Gene, Move Your Colonies With Care: *The American Bee Journal,* Hamilton, Illinois, Vol. 122, No. 12, December 1982.

Rudolf Steiner, *Nine Lectures on Bees,* (Dornach, Switzerland, 1912), Translated from the German: St. George Publications, New York, 1964.

Bernard Jensen, Ph.D. Clinical Nutrition, *Food Healing for Man:* Bernard Jensen Publications, Escondido, California, 1983.

Naum Ioyrish, *Bees and People:* MIR Publishers, Moscow, U.S.S.R.

U. Erasmus, *Fats & Oils - The Complete Guide to Fats and Oils in Health and Nutrition:* Alive Books, Vancouver, British Columbia, Canada, 1986.

N. Johnson, *A Dud at 70 - A Stud at 80 and How To Do It:* Plains Corporation, Scottsdale, Arizona 1982.

A.E. Carter, *The New Miracles of Rebound Exercise:* ALM Publishers, Phoenix, Arizona, 1988.

A.E. Carter, *The Cancer Answer:* ALM Publishers, Phoenix, Arizona, 1988.

H.A. Hunter, *Extend Your Life, The Handbook of Natural Healing A Through Z:* ALM Publishers, Phoenix, Arizona, 1987.

SUMMARY – BEE POLLEN vs. ALLERGIES

Leo M. Conway, M.D., Medical Allergist reports:

1949	6,200	cases treated with Pollen
1872	60,000	cases treated and documented with Pollen
1981	100,000	cases treated with Pollen, estimate

With the following miraculous results:

1. Complete relief from allergy symptoms.
2. Absolute safety.

   Whereas deaths have been reported from hypodermic injections of pollen, there has never been any ill effects from oral taking of pollen (except for slight temporary reactions producing symptoms).
3. Flexible dosages.
4. Low cost.

   The cost of oral pollen to the patient is one-third to one-half of that given by hypodermic.
5. Colds.

   Also from a paper written by Dr. Conway, "Pollen Allergy," printed in "Southern Medicine and Surgery," Charlotte, N.C. Vol. 105, No. 1, January 1943, he asks the question, "Could colds be allergy? Even though one does not present the apparent symptoms and signs of pollen allergy it is possible that there is an invisible reaction due to these dusts which leaves us susceptible to the virus, supposedly operative in causation of colds. It was accidentally discovered that patients in whom pollen allergy was controlled were free from colds during the season in which they had been frequently afflicted theretofore.

6. Sinus conditions.

   Further investigation revealed that many patients who had had sinus conditions were singularly free from involvement following successful treatment of their allergy by oral method.

7. <u>NO ILL CONSEQUENCES HAVE RESULTED.</u>

8. 94% of all were completely free of allergy symptoms.

9. 6% were partially relieved. Of these 6% not one strictly followed directions.

10. All who had taken the antigen for three years of control have since been able to remain free from all allergy symptoms – no matter where they lived.

11. Same for food allergy, regardless of diet.

12. Ever increasing control of sinus conditions, asthma cases and hay fever, following the control and elimination of allergies.

13. "Cure."

    Results achieved are the nearest to a permanent "cure" ever obtained in medical practice.

INDEX for THE WORLD'S ONLY PERFECT FOOD

INDEX for THE WORLD'S ONLY PERFECT FOOD

INDEX for THE WORLD'S ONLY PERFECT FOOD

INDEX for THE WORLD'S ONLY PERFECT FOOD

INDEX for THE WORLD'S ONLY PERFECT FOOD

INDEX for THE WORLD'S ONLY PERFECT FOOD

INDEX for THE WORLD'S ONLY PERFECT FOOD

INDEX for THE WORLD'S ONLY PERFECT FOOD

INDEX for THE WORLD'S ONLY PERFECT FOOD

INDEX for THE WORLD'S ONLY PERFECT FOOD

INDEX for THE WORLD'S ONLY PERFECT FOOD

INDEX for THE WORLD'S ONLY PERFECT FOOD

INDEX for THE WORLD'S ONLY PERFECT FOOD

INDEX for THE WORLD'S ONLY PERFECT FOOD

INDEX for THE WORLD'S ONLY PERFECT FOOD

INDEX for THE WORLD'S ONLY PERFECT FOOD

THE DYNAMIC TRIO™ IS THE WORLD'S BEST MULTI-VITAMIN & MINERAL DID YOU KNOW ?

1. Multi-vitamin/mineral tablets and capsules are the 1st, 2nd, 3rd and 4th leading sales products in nearly every health food store and,
2. In nearly every vitamin section of nearly every supermarket, grocery store, drug store, etc., etc., and,
3. Also the 5th, 6th and 7th leading sales producers in a good many other?
4. What is the world's best multi-vitamin/mineral?
5. Who makes the world's best multi-vitamin/mineral?
6. The Dynamic Trio consisting of High Desert® bee pollen, High Desert® propolis and High Desert® 24-Hour® royal jelly from CC Pollen Co. is the answer to both questions.
7. Where is your proof??? High Desert® proof follows:

THE DYNAMIC TRIO™ BEE POLLEN PROPOLIS ROYAL JELLY	OTHER SOURCES OF VITAMINS					
	All food stores	All super- markets	All grocery stores	All drug stores	All multi-level companies	All other
1. Nearly all vitamins are coal tar based made from petroleum or are synthetic.						
NO	YES	YES	YES	YES	YES	YES

We refuse to believe crank case oil, motor oil or petroleum belongs in the four great food groups. Under no circumstances will we knowingly eat crank case oil, motor oil or petroleum – and neither should you!

2. Always natural, probably the most natural of all and a live food.						
YES	NO	NO	NO	NO	NO	NO
3. Contains all known essential nutrients, all essential vitamins and minerals thus far found essential <u>Every Day</u> by the National Research Council in a live state.						
YES	NO	NO	NO	NO	NO	NO
4. Contains all enzymes originally bestowed by God.						
YES	NO	NO	NO	NO	NO	NO
5. Live enzymes content elevated to the highest level of activity.						
YES	NO	NO	NO	NO	NO	NO

THE DYNAMIC TRIO™ BEE POLLEN PROPOLIS ROYAL JELLY	OTHER SOURCES OF VITAMINS					
	All health food stores	All super-markets	All grocery stores	All drug stores	All multi-level companies	All other

6. Bombarded with the best ions in an Adam & Eve environment.

| YES | NO | NO | NO | NO | NO | NO |

7. Capable of sustaining life.

| YES | NO | NO | NO | NO | NO | NO |

8. Oldest food on earth, and God made, and never man made.

| YES | NO | NO | NO | NO | NO | NO |

9. Scientifically blended from worldwide sources.

| YES | NO | NO | NO | NO | NO | NO |

10. Contains many millions of parts.

| YES | NO | NO | NO | NO | NO | NO |

11. Only food that will dapple a 1200 lb. thoroughbred race horse.

| YES | NO | NO | NO | NO | NO | NO |

Dappling means perfect health balance and makes champions out of "also rans."

12. Contains the reproductive part — the strongest part — of all flowers, vegetables and fruits.

| YES | NO | NO | NO | NO | NO | NO |

13. Contains all known essential amino acids, and all known essential free amino acids, and all essential fatty acids.

| YES | NO | NO | NO | NO | NO | NO |

14. Agrees with the FDA and most of orthodox medicine's admonition to get your vitamins and minerals from the food you eat.

| YES | NO | NO | NO | NO | NO | NO |

15. Formulation of isolated chemicals.

| NO | YES | YES | YES | YES | YES | YES |

16. Contains mega doses of chemical vitamins which may cause contra-deficiencies in other nutrients.

| NO | YES | YES | YES | YES | YES | YES |

17. Contains mega doses of minerals which may cause contra-deficiencies in other nutrients.

| NO | YES | YES | YES | YES | YES | YES |

18. Contains drug-like quantities of chemical nutrients that some say become dangerous toxic poison drug substances like drugs.

| NO | YES | YES | YES | YES | YES | YES |

19. Most mentioned food in the Bible – 68 times.
20. First food given the risen Jesus Christ after the Resurrection.
21. THE CONCLUSION YOU SHOULD MAKE – THE DYNAMIC TRIO™ IS UNQUESTIONABLY:
    1. THE BEST OF ALL FOODS
    2. THE MOST WHOLESOME OF ALL FOODS
    3. THE MOST NUTRITIOUS OF ALL FOODS
    4. THE BEST MULTI-VITAMIN OF ALL
    5. THE BEST MULTI-MINERAL OF ALL
    6. THE CLOSEST TO LIFE ITSELF
    7. MAY BEE AND PROBABLY IS THE KEY TO YOUR BEST
       HEALTH!!
22. THE SUBTLE CONCLUSION:
    1. If you are not feeding your family the DYNAMIC TRIO - you
       are short-changing your family <u>Every Day</u>!
    2. If you are not feeding yourself THE DYNAMIC TRIO you are
       short-changing yourself <u>Every Day</u>!
Now that you know — you will move to, or should move to,
a higher plane of health than ever before and

Not only bee healthier, but
BEE MORE SATISFIED
BEE MORE CONTENTED
and, best of all
BEE HAPPIER THAN EVER BEFORE

23. Absolute money back guarantee:
Do you want to feel better?
CC Pollen Co. absolutely, irrevocably and unconditionally, guar-antees you will feel better - we don't care how healthy you are - you will feel better - after you have consumed the first order of the Dynamic Trio or we will refund your money - no questions asked!

    The government says it is best to get your nutrients from food. We agree. The problem for the average supermarket shopper — all of those nutrients are not available in the supermarket and there is only one food that contains every essential nutrient - live - and that is the Dynamic Trio™.

    If you feel better you will bee happier.

    You have everything to gain — (feeling better) and, your hap-piness - nothing to lose.

WORLD'S ONLY PERFECT FOOD BOOK

What do you mean when you say The World's Only Perfect Food?

I define a perfect food as that food that contains every nutrient thus far found essential by the National Research Council and that food that still has some part of the food that cannot be detected yet by existing chemical analysis. This part of the food that cannot be analyzed yet, I speculate, contains those essential nutrients which will be declared essential sometime in the future.

In other words, that food made by the Creator which contains every essential nutrient thus far known essential and some part of the food which cannot be analyzed, is a perfect food.

High Desert bee pollen fits this definition perfectly.

Mountain High bee pollen fits this definition perfectly.

C C Pollen Co. has been saying this for the best part of three decades and no one has challenged this statement.

Here is another thought:

There has been no research ever done worldwide on how little of any nutrient a human needs for perfect health when that person ingests a food that has all the essential nutrients present at the same time.

It is like a chain. As long as all the links in the chain are in place, the chain has strength. If one link is missing, the chain is broken. So is your health.

We do know that all nutrients in all foods are present in that food or in any food in quantities so small they are invisible to the naked eye; but, when they are in unheated fresh organic food, they are almost always totally assimilable and assimilated. When they are chemicals made by man such as isolated vitamins and isolated minerals or man-made combinations of vitamins and minerals such as a multi-vitamin or a multi-mineral tablet or capsule, we know that the body initially resists digesting these chemicals because they are man-made and not Creator made.

It goes without saying, you are better off trying to achieve perfect health by ingesting foods that contain all the nutrients thus far found essential for perfect health.

EAT RIGHT
OR DIE WRONG

NOTICE TO PRESIDENT BILL CLINTON
AND
FIRST LADY HILLARY RODMAN CLINTON
CONGRESS
THE CITIZENS OF THE UNITED STATES
AND
ALL THE CITIZENS OF THE WORLD

The following additional sections have been added to The World's Only Perfect Food Book, hoping someone reading these sections will become horrified and outraged that more than 1,600,000 Americans are dying every year needlessly and will be able to bring this country to its senses:

1. February 18, 1993 fax to First Lady Hillary Rodman Clinton telling her husband may be well on the way to developing throat and voice cancer and if he does, he will probably die.

2. January 5, 1993 fax to First Lady Elect Hillary Clinton telling her that the CC Pollen Co. food cures from the bee-hive will correct, eliminate, and, therefore, cure her husband's allergies, sinusitus, and voice and throat problems. This fax is a 25 page fax.

3. April 24, 1992 letter to the Ford Foundation. This letter offers the Ford Foundation the opportunity to correct, elim-inate, cure, and permanently cure nearly all degenerative diseases. The Foundation was not the least bit interested.

4. Attached is an exhibit to the April 24, 1992 letter to the Ford Foundation was a summary of the 32 Investigational New Drug applications and the 100 New Drug Applications to sell human products which contain the cures for virtually all degenerative diseases.

5. Exhibit B attached to the FDA IND's gives a definition of the primary, secondary, and third indications, and the stated effectiveness and the actual safety of the CC Pollen Co. cures from the beehive.

6. The CC Pollen Co. food cures from the beehive for virtually all degenerative diseases can be simply stated as absolutely safe with an effectiveness approaching 100%.

7. The CC Pollen Co. axioms that are always true can be simply stated as follows:

   If a CC Pollen Co. food cure will cure one, it will cure all or nearly all with an effectiveness approaching 100%.

   If a CC Pollen Co. food cure will not cure one, two, three, or four, it won't cure any if the patient is correctly diagnosed.

8. March 9, 1992 fax to the American Association for retired persons giving them the opportunity to place a public health benefit announcement in their newsletter to save 100,000 American lives every year. No answer was ever received. They are not interested.

9. April 20, 1992 fax to Prudential Life Insurance Co. giving them the opportunity to save more than 1,600,000 American lives every year, with an expenditure of only $16,000.00 total. They were not interested.

10. August 5, 1992 letter from the FDA to the Renaissance Laboratories mouthing the standard FDA line that all drugs must go through the ridiculous, idiotic, ludicrous clinical investigations required for their dangerous, toxic, poisonous drugs.

11. The 15 faxes in response to that letter, beginning with the first response dated August 25, 1992, addressed to the FDA with carbon copies to the President, Vice President, two Arizona Senators, the Chairman of the FDA Senate Oversight Committee, and the Chairman of the House FDA Oversight Committee, and a carbon copy to Utah Senator Orrin G. Hatch, telling these people and the world at large the CC Pollen Co. absolutely safe and absolutely effective food cures from the beehive would save more than 1,600,000 American lives annually - if these 7 most powerful

men would force the FDA to release these safe food cures.

What happened?

Nothing.

No one in government seems to care, or is too stupid to realize, the cures for all degenerative diseases is the answer to the health care monster. Health care, of course, is misnamed. We are talking about disease care not health care. M.D.s know nothing about health and prevention. The M.D.s treat the results, the effects, and never the causes.

The disease care crises, which we call the health care crisis, is really frightening. If the United States of America does not wake up real soon, the United States will be destroyed.

The health care crisis is insane. President Clinton is aware of these costs. He has said in the recent past the following, and we quote from newspaper reports:

1. "Health care is a joke."
2. "Health care costs will bankrupt this nation this decade unless something is done."
3. "Health care kills fiscal responsibility."
4. "Health care costs prevent a balanced budget and is the major cause of the deficit."
5. "Health care costs are growing at an alarming geometrical progression."

The President of the United States could not be more correct.

President Clinton is talking about the effects. He has not gone to the cause.

What is the cause? Health care that always treats - never cures.

Answer: Cure the degenerative diseases - do not treat anymore.

The U.S. M.D.s are only treating these degenerative diseases – not curing them. The M.D.s who are treating the degenerative diseases are giving these patients dangerous, toxic, poisonous allopathic drugs licensed by the FDA. These drugs never cure, they only treat. They cause dangerous, toxic, poisonous side-effects that destroy the patient's health, cause sudden death, and compound the disease - the very disease the M.D.s are treating. More often than not, dangerous, toxic, poisonous drugs will cause other symptoms that eventually kill the patient.

When is the United States going to wake up?

When is the United States going to come to their senses?

When are we going to say we have had enough?

When is some thoughtful person, hopefully the President, going to say, we must have the cures? The treatments are destroying the United States. We can no longer treat, we most cure.

We can't turn to the licensed, allopathic M.D.s in the United States because they know absolutely nothing about cures. These M.D.s are experts in drugs, disease, and death, but are totally ignorant of cures and health. The FDA does not know anything about the cures of degenerative diseases.

We hope First Lady Hillary Rodman Clinton will read these words and come to the conclusion she can no longer rely on the uninformed and ignorant religion of modern medicine, nor the misguided medical schools, nor the misdirected research community - all that only treat degenerative diseases and never cure! Only compound and destroy.

When we really think about it:

Who in their right mind would take any dangerous, toxic, poisonous drug for anything?

There is not one American that has ever been deficient of any dangerous, toxic, poisonous drug of any kind.

When are we going to wake up?

When is the United States going to come to their senses?

When are we going to say we've had enough?

We want the cures, the treatments are going to destroy the United States.

Renaissance Laboratories filed with the United States Food and Drug Administration 32 Investigational New Drug applications and 32 New Drug Applications to sell the food products of the beehive that will virtually eliminate all degenerative diseases with the FDA 2 years ago. These 32 IND's/NDA's contain the cures – we said cures not treatments – for virtually all the degenerative diseases affecting mankind.

These IND's/NDA's address and present the cures, not treatments, for every killer degenerative disease and all of the prevalent degenerative diseases such as Alzheimer's disease, arthritis, senility, memory loss, chronic fatigue syndrome, impotency, etc., etc.

The author hopes someone will read these added sections and say, if the information presented herein is true, why has the FDA covered up these cures of all degenerative diseases for 2 years?

Anyone who is an FDA watcher will know why. The FDA will fight the cures from the beehive to the death. They do not want to change the status quo.

In conclusion:

The author believes this book someday, somehow will have a serious reader who will come to the conclusion the President should force the FDA to license the 32 NDA's filed by Renaissance Laboratories for the cure - not treatment - of virtually all degenerative diseases to save 1,600,000 American lives every year.

To do otherwise would be criminal neglect.

CC Pollen Co. has had most of these cures for over a decade. That means more than 16,000,000 Americans have needlessly lost their lives for want of these cures.

The FDA doesn't care if 160,000,000 Americans die. They will never, never license the food cures from the beehive to save American lives - voluntarily!

FAXES TO FIRST LADY HILLARY RODHAM CLINTON

Even before Bill Clinton was elected President, after the first newspaper article came out about his allergies and sinusitis and his voice and throat problems, I tried to get the information to him that he need not suffer from these three degenerative diseases. CC Pollen Co. had the absolute GRAS safe cures and permanent cures of these conditions. CC Pollen Co. had these cures for 13 or 14 years but I was unable to get this information through to the President. I even sent the information to his mother. She did exactly opposite to what I told her. She gave it to the Secret Service and, of course, neither the President nor the First Lady ever saw it. The Secret Service destroyed the information and the product I sent.

I gave the following fax and the 24 additional page exhibits to Representative Bill Richardson from New Mexico to hand to the President the next time he saw him. He promised me faithfully – he said he would see the President in two weeks (the week of March 1st, 1993) and give him these faxes. Like all of the other attempts to get the message to the President he never received this information. I even donated $1,000 to Bill Richardson's campaign fund hoping he would follow through and hand the information to the President like he promised but, obviously, that never took place.

The following is an exact copy of the first six pages of this 24 page fax which was initially sent to First Lady Hillary Rodham Clinton at the White House:

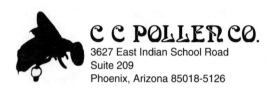

C C POLLEN CO.
3627 East Indian School Road
Suite 209
Phoenix, Arizona 85018-5126

FAX: (602) 381-3130
Telex: 559-834
Cable: CCPOLLEN

Phone: (602) 957-0096

February 18, 1993

From: Royden Brown
Chairman of the Board

FAX: 202-456-6244
First Lady Hillary Rodham Clinton
The White House, Washington, D.C.

Your husband may develop throat and voice cancer and die.

Every person I have ever known who has had voice and throat problems and hoarseness like your husband, concurrent with and complicated by allergies, has developed cancer and died. The last one was Bob Swanson, president of Del Webb Corporation.

Your husband may not have much time left. He may have cancer now. At least, I can assure you, he could be well on the way to developing cancer.

However — Cancer can bee avoided.

And cured, if begun.

Your husband's voice and throat problems can be cured - once and for all.

So can his allergies.

So can his sinusitis.

But you must act now…today!

After hearing your husband's courageous and absolute wonderful address and his hoarseness last night - I am compelled to tell you — exactly what I *know* is going to happen.

I predict your husband will bee diagnosed with cancer before his first term in office is over - unless he is cured!

The following 24 page fax should convince you beyond doubt — the CC Pollen Co. GRAS safe food cures from the beehive will *cure* and permanently *cure* your husband's three diseases — safely!

If there is the slightest doubt in your mind - you can contact your head of the Office of Unconventional Medicine in your National Institute of Health in Bethesda, Maryland, telephone 301-496-3152 Dr. Jay Moskowitz, Jr. Dr. Jay Moskowitz, Jr. knows and will verify the CC Pollen Co. Food Product X66 will cure allergies, asthma, hay fever, sinusitis, chronic obstructive pulmonary diseases and, most likely, will cure your husband's voice and throat problems.

By-the-way, if your husband really wants an FDA Commissioner that will help you *cure, not treat,* the U.S.A's health care catastrophe and crises - Dr. Jay - 2 -

- 2 -

Moskowitz may be and probably is your husband's best choice. You could not pick a better FDA commissioner than Dr. Jay Moskowitz.

The very fact that he is a Ph.D. and not an M.D. would bee your husband's signal to the world - he is honoring the voter mandate *for change!*

If your husband wakes up and stops being mesmerized by the medical establishment and decides to *cure* and not treat degenerative diseases in the USA, all of his problems, both personal and national, will be solved in the first term of his office and this country will enter a millennium of prosperity and happiness never previously known.

C C POLLEN CO.

3627 East Indian School Road
Suite 209
Phoenix, Arizona 85018-5126

FAX: (602) 381-3130
Telex: 559-834
Cable: CCPOLLEN

Phone: (602) 957-0096

January 5, 1993

From: Royden Brown   FAX: 501-682-1382
Chairman of the Board   First Lady Elect Hillary Clinton

It has been widely publicized President Elect Bill Clinton suffers incurably and miserably from three chronic degenerative diseases:

1. Allergies
2. Sinusitis
3. Voice and throat problems.

Renaissance Laboratories filed two Investigational New Drug Applications (IND) and two New Drug Applications (NDA) with the U.S. FDA two years ago containing the CC Pollen Co. food cures from the beehive having the following indications or cures of degenerative diseases:

1. IND & NDA 37318
   Indications or cures for:
   Allergies, asthma, hay fever, sinusitis, chronic obstructive pulmonary disease and like conditions.

2. IND & NDA 37336-2
   Indications or cures for:
   Hoarseness, raspy voice, sore throat and mouth, mouth and throat infection, and inflammation and like conditions, including lost voice.

Both of these cures have a risk benefit ratio of:

RISK: Zero…absolute zero or as close to absolute zero as is possible. Both carry less risk than any drug ever licensed by the FDA.

BENEFIT: 100% or as close to 100% as is possible. Much greater benefit than any drug ever licensed by the FDA.

Both of these cures have a GRAS safety. GRAS is an abbreviation or acronym for the phrase…generally recognized as safe…found in the U.S. Code of Federal Regulations, Section 21, Parts 170.30.

Both of these cures have an efficiency rating:

EFFICIENCY: 100%

EFFECTIVENESS: 100% or at least approaching 100% effectiveness. Both are more effective than any drug the FDA has ever licensed.

Renaissance Laboratories has been unable to reach President Elect Bill Clinton to cure his three degenerative diseases. It would bee a shame for President

Elect Bill Clinton to continue to suffer from these devastating diseases when the sure, absolute safe cures are available for his use...but he is unaware of their availability.

We call on you as a patriotic American to get this message to President Elect Bill Clinton before he leaves Little Rock to be inaugurated. To have a President of the United States inaugurated, suffering from three degenerative diseases, would be disastrous to the great public relation image of the United States worldwide. You must help.

How do you know I am telling the truth? Here is the absolute proof:

I use the phrases:

"Sure and absolute cures"

"Risks/benefits...zero/100%

"GRAS safe and 100% effectiveness"

knowing when I filed these two IND's and two NDA's on behalf of the CC Pollen Co.cures from the beehive two years ago, I must tell the truth, the whole truth and nothing but the truth or be guilty of a federal felony. I personally signed both of these IND's and both of these NDA's. Please see and re-read the reverse side of the U.S. FDA Form 1571 and the FDA Form 356H for both, which more aptly describe this burden faxed hereinafter to *always* tell the truth to the U.S. FDA on all filings. And, you can rely on the fact I am in my right mind, a responsible U.S. citizen of 75 years with the following background:

Graduated with a BS Degree in Accounting from the University of Colorado in 1938.

Pilot RCAF, RAF, and UASAAC in Europe during WWII for 5 plus years.

Owner and president of four Colorado banks.

Retired to Phoenix, Arizona.

Now own ranches in AZ, CO, NM and TX, and

Chairman of Renaissance Laboratories and CC Pollen Co. and 11 other corporations.

You know I am telling the truth.

The penalty for lying is too great to endure.

We have done everything we can do to bring to the attention of President Elect Bill Clinton the cures, the absolute and positively safe cures of his three degenerative diseases...to no avail, we can't reach him.

It is now up to you!

God bless and keep you and President Elect Bill Clinton during his eight years in office.

Copy of both of the FDA IND Forms 1571 and the FDA NDA Forms 356H follow.

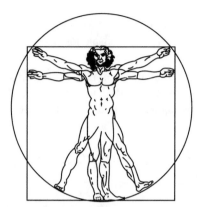

THE SAFETY AND EFFECTIVENESS OF THE DRUG X66

We extract from FDA Regulations the general FDA measures of safety and effectiveness, as follows:

"Reasonably safe

"Minimal risk

"Both are acceptable to the FDA

"Risk/Benefit Ratio

"Even though a drug has adverse side effects — sometimes death — if the benefit to the patients is great enough, the FDA will still license the drug even though the drug is only effective 51% of the time."

RL has no quarrel with the FDA operating guidelines — these guidelines are ideal for dangerous toxic poison drugs, but not for safe foods !

RL says the drug X66 is:

1. *Safety:*
   Absolutely safe - or as absolutely safe as any drug can be — *safer for human ingestion than any drug the FDA has ever licensed.*

2. *Effectiveness:*
   100% effective - *more effective than any drug the FDA has ever licensed.* 100% effectiveness is guaranteed by the responsible manufacturer.

3. *Proof:*
   The drug X66 has been ingested by humans over a 10-year period in the United States and in many countries. A great deal more than 50,000 persons have ingested this drug. Since no accurate records have been kept. RL can only estimate the numbers who have ingested this drug to be 50,000 persons more or less.

4. There has never been one report — not one — of anyone ever reporting any toxic discomfort, problem, adverse reaction, contraindication or otherwise with the drug X66.

- 2 -

5. The manufacturer of this drug is now having marvellous luck in having patients ingest all 66 tablets of the bottle at one time. They believe the drug is preventative. It appears the 66 tablet dose prevents the reoccurrence of the symptoms in more than half of the people - an unbelievable result. Drug X66 is probably the only drug ever that the manufacturer is having patients ingest the entire bottle at one time to give additional benefits of being preventative. A true testimonial to the safety of this drug and to the absence of problems with over-dosage.

6. The ingredients in the drug X66 are only foods - none of which have been extracted to try and find the active ingredients; therefore, none of these ingredients have any toxicity - but are as safe as safe foods.

7. CC Pollen Co., the responsible manufacturer of the drug X66, is instructing the Publishers of the Physicians Desk Reference to list the new drug X66 as follows:

   1. Contraindications.................................none
   2. Warnings.......................................none
   3. Precautions....................................none
   4. Adverse reactions..............................none
   5. Over-dosage....................................none - even if occurs the patient is not at risk
   6. Human safety for ingesting.....................absolutely safe and riskless - or as absolutely safe and as riskless as any food substance can be
   7. Effectiveness..................................100% - absolutely guaranteed 100% effective by manufacturer

All manufacturers of drugs tend to know more than any other party about the safety and effectiveness of their drugs.

8. The publishers of the Physicians Desk Reference informed RL they have never listed a drug where the manufacturer has no listed side effects and who guarantees in writing 100% effectiveness.

9. The manufacturer reports in the previous ten years of ingesting their product, many pregnant lactating females and their 3 and 4 yr. old asthmatic children suffering from all extremes of allergies, asthma, hay fever, sinusitis, chronic obstructive pulmonary disease and like conditions, have ingested this product.

   The manufacturer reports the product is ground to a powder and mixed -

- 3 -

with honey and water to permit these babies to take the tablets. Surprisingly, CC Pollen Co. reports in every instance thus far of which they know, these babies are free of their symptoms before they finish drinking this mixture.

10. An associated company of the manufacturer has been feeding thoroughbred race horses the formula of the drug X66 for four or five years to cure the allergies of these thoroughbred horses. Some of these thoroughbred race horses are worth $5-10 million, and even a few, $20-25 million. Had there been any problem with this product, the owners of these expensive animals would have been in touch with this company and sued them, that is for sure, if the horse had ever suffered ingesting this product.

11. Additionally, the company reports this product has been absolutely guaranteed to be effective for allergies in horses and there has never been a request for a refund because the product was ineffective.

12. The strongest proof of all-empirical proof —
    Since CC Pollen Co. has never paid a single product liability insurance claim of any kind during their entire existence, Renaissance Laboratories believes this fact alone is the best proof possible the CC Pollen Co. food products — all of them, including the drug X66 — are as safe as water and, probably, should be judged as completely safe and, perhaps, even absolutely safe for human consumption.

CONCLUSION:

We quote from the FDA guidelines, "general considerations for the clinical evaluation of drugs" published by the FDA, as follows:

"The guidelines must not be used to force new compounds into their mold as the fruit of original ideas may be lost. History is replete with discovery that could not have been made if the investigation was constrained by established methods.

"A person may also choose to use alternate procedures even though they are not provided for in the guidelines."

We must not worship the regulations and sacrifice the cures!

We know for certain these insidious conditions are causing deaths in the United States. No one knows for sure how extensive and how many are dying because there is no cure yet on the market for these conditions.

RL says the FDA can be instrumental in RL savings as many of these American lives as is possible with the drug X66.

RL has presented the FDA with positive proof the drug X66 will correct, elimi-

- 4 -

nate and cure allergies, asthma, hay fever, sinusitus, chronic, obstructive pulmonary disease and like conditions, the fifth leading cause of death in the USA and the world — proof of 100% effectiveness.

The foregoing proof appears to be positive proof of the safety of X66 for human ingestion and far exceeds the previous FDA requirements for the conventional prescription drug safety.

The foregoing proof appears to be positive proof the effectiveness of drug X66 for human ingestion and far exceeds the previous FDA requirements for the conventional drug's effectiveness.

The herein proof of safety and effectiveness of drug X66 warrants the FDA granting an immediate FDA license for RL to sell the drug X66 both as a pharmaceutical drug and as an over-the-counter drug.

RL so requests the FDA for permission to immediately, temporarily provide this drug for the health and welfare of Americans - the sooner the drug is made available - the more American lives will be saved. 100,000 Americans die every year for want of food product X66.

THE FORD FOUNDATION LETTER

You would have thought the Ford Foundation with $7 billion in assets would have been interested in eliminating degenerative disease and, in the process, save 1,600,000 American lives every year, but that is not the case. The letter we sent them under date of April 24, 1992 follows:

Additionally, this identical letter was addressed to every other Foundation in the United States having total assets of $100 million or more and many of those having less.

With this letter to the Ford Foundation and the many foundations, Renaissance Laboratories included the following:

1. March 9, 1992 Fax to Horace B. Deets, Executive Director of American Association of Retired Persons
2. April 20,1992 Fax to Prudential Life Insurance
3. Summary of 32 FDA IND/NDA containing the cures for virtually all degenerative diseases
4. CC Pollen Co. facts that are always true
5. Final comment

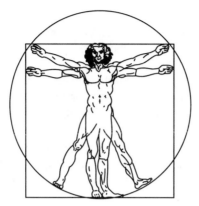

April 24, 1992

Barron M. Tenny
Vice President
The Ford Foundation
320 E. 43rd St.
New York, NY 10017

                  Re: The Correction, Elimination,
                            Cure and the *Permanent Cure of*
                            Nearly All Degenerative Diseases

Dear Sir or Madam:

Renaissance Laboratories is offering the Foundation the opportunity to do more good for mankind than has been done thus far by all other foundations worldwide. No one has ever before cured the first degenerative disease - we are offering you the *opportunity to cure nearly all degenerative diseases!*

THIS OPPORTUNITY IS THE OPPORTUNITY OF THIS MILLENNIUM - yes, this is the opportunity of all times!! Do not delay!

Since Renaissance Laboratories is presenting The Foundation with, perhaps, the best of all opportunities to be the greatest of all "do-gooders," the opportunity to do the greatest good of all time for American public health, limiting considerations such as:

           1.   Area of funding
           2.   Annual giving
           3.   Specific purposed
           4.   Etc., etc.

should be waived and set aside to permit The Foundation to truly fulfill to the ultimate the hopes and aspirations of the founders of The Foundation.

Restraints of The Foundation because of area, application of funds, type and kind of investigation, etc, become insignificant when The Foundation has the opportunity to fund the *CURES* of degenerative diseases - each a miracle!

-2-

Renaissance Laboratories is seeking a benefactor - a true philanthropist - a "do-gooder in the very best sense," which we know you are, to contribute $2 million to fund the final 1,000 patient randomized, controlled, double-blind with placebo, cross-over clinical investigations (herein "clinical investigations") of each of the CC Pollen Co. new drugs to be presented to the FDA to support and as proof for drug licenses to *cure* - not treat - *yes, permanently cure* all the major degenerative diseases of mankind with non-toxic, High Desert® beehive food cures from CC Pollen Co. - all of which are GRAS safe.

GRAS is an acronym, an abbreviation, for the phrase and definition…"generally recognized as safe"…found in the Code of U.S. Federal Regulations, Section 21, Part 170.30.

Renaissance Laboratories has filed 32 Investigational New Drug Applications (IND's) with the FDA, having more than 100 indications in and for the curing of degenerative diseases and conditions.

The Foundation can furnish the funding for one or more clinical investigations The Foundation choose at an estimated $2 million each.

Renaissance Laboratories is enclosing a summary of the 32 IND's filed with the FDA for your examination.

As The Foundation knows, conventional medical wisdom says all the degenerative diseases are incurable. They are incurable with the drugs allopathic, modern M.D.s use in their practice. There are probably over 700,000 M.D.s in the United States. Not one of these M.D.s has come up with the first cure of a degenerative disease. Harvard Medical School. John Hopkins Medical School, the Mayo Clinic and the FDA have never come up with any cures of degenerative diseases.

CC Pollen Co. has - for all major degenerative diseases!

Enclosed is the recent fax Renaissance Laboratories sent to Prudential Life Insurance Co. only to learn their charter forbids funding medical research. Nevertheless - this fax outlines how a mere $16 million could wipe out degenerative diseases as we presently know them, and actually usher in the Golden Millennium of disease-free, long life.

$16 million would save approximately 41,272,148 American lives over the next 17 years. We compute as follows:

1994 - 2010 - 17 years x 1,604,244 American lives saved annually = 27,272,148 saved American lives by the year 2010.

Alzheimer's Disease lives saved by the 2010 = 14,000,000 plus, or a total of lives saved = approximately 41,272,148, or every approximate 39¢ saves an American life perhaps, the greatest bargain ever.

- 3 -

To prove to The Foundation, Renaissance Laboratories does have these cures of degenerative diseases, Renaissance Laboratories suggests the proof commence with the curing of the fifth leading cause of death in the U.S.A. and worldwide - chronic obstructive pulmonary disease, allergies, asthma, hay fever, sinus and like conditions, which takes about 100,000 American lives each year, about 225 lives everyday.

Renaissance laboratories realizes The Foundation will not want to spend the $2 million to do the CC Pollen Co. clinical investigation of the fifth leading cause of death in the United States and worldwide unless The Foundation feels certain the cure will be obtained. Renaissance Laboratories knows this hesitancy will be present at the commencement of each $2 million funding of the clinical investigations. Therefore, Renaissance Laboratories suggests the following arrangement could be employed prior to the funding of the $2 million dollars for the clinical investigation for each cure for degenerative disease.

The Foundation or some third party selected by The Foundation selects a small number of persons chronically and hopelessly ill with the degenerative disease to be investigated. Renaissance Laboratories will give the CC Pollen Co. beehive food cure for that degenerative disease to those selected persons. When that small number of selected persons is cured of their degenerative disease and restored to normal, The Foundation will advance the $2 million funding to Renaissance Laboratories to immediately commence the randomized, controlled, double-blind with placebo, cross-over clinical investigation of that degenerative disease under study - knowing full well the sought after cure will be obtained.

Back to the cure of the fifth leading cause of death in the U.S.A. and worldwide.

The present drugs for treating chronic obstructive pulmonary disease, allergy, asthma, hay fever, sinus and like conditions are at best only treatments - never cures! At worst, these drugs destroy the immune system of the patient, create complications and cause other diseases. The horrible side-effects of the present drugs are published in the Physicians' Desk Reference - and make very chilling reading. It's time a cure for these diseases is brought forth.

CC Pollen Co. has this sought after cure.

In fact, CC Pollen Co. has been curing these diseases for 12 to 13 years and has been successful with thousands and thousands of persons.

Here is the proof CC Pollen Co. has the cure - in September and October of 1990 CC Pollen Co. randomly summoned, by insertion of an advertisement in the local newspapers, 119 persons in off the streets of Phoenix, Arizona with these diseases and gave them the drug, Bee Allergy Free - Asthma Bee Gone in front of television cameras. All were cured of these conditions ingesting 12

- 4 -

tablets total. CC Pollen Co. made a 23 minute summary film showing a representative sample of the 119 people in their diseased state taking the tablets, showing the look of disbelief coming over their faces when they realized their symptoms were leaving and were gone and then showing them 6 months later.

One 76 year old retired pharmacist from Philadelphia, Pennsylvania, who retired in Del Webb's Sun City, informed us he was born with allergies and developed chronic obstructive pulmonary disease right out of pharmacy school and has been plagued with it ever since. He said he has suffered 26 life-threatening seizures where he had to be hospitalized in order to breathe and 23 life-threatening seizures where the doctor had to open his breathing passage or he would have suffocated. This gentleman came in with his wife and before he finished taking the first 12 tablets, his symptoms disappeared completely and he was permanently cured - his symptoms were permanently gone and have not reoccurred to this date. All the 119 are available for recall and cross-examination should you wish.

The changes in these people in the intervening 6 month period of time is unbelievable. No one before has ever been able to show persons cured of these conditions and then show them 6 months later because no one else in the world has ever been able to cure these diseases - not Harvard Medical School, the Mayo Clinic, the FDA, the 700,000 M.D.s in the U.S. - no one in the world has been able to cure the fifth leading cause of death except CC Pollen Co. When you view this film, the changes in these men and women are so startling and so great as to be almost unbelievable, which we describe as follows:

1. How much more relaxed and at ease these people looked in the after-pictures.
2. How much more self-satisfied and comfortable they appeared in the after-pictures.
3. How much happier they all appeared in the after-pictures.
4. How much more beautiful they all appeared in the after-pictures.
5. How much more energetic they all appeared in the after-pictures.
6. How much younger - a great deal younger they all looked in the after-pictures.

CC Pollen Co. also did another successful 185 patient study of these same diseases January 11-12, 1992 with the Bee Allergy Free - Asthma Bee Gone food tablet.

Dr. Smith, Dr. H.C. Romero and Morris Tinterrow, M.D., Ph.D., were in attendance at this trial and demonstration. The report of this 185 patient trial and demonstration has been submitted to a Peer Review Journal for publication. Dr. Tinterrow believes he will have this paper completed and presented in May. As soon as we have a copy, we will send you a copy and we will send you a copy of the published report.

-5-

These moving pictures are proof positive you can reverse the aging process for those persons who have been life-long sufferers of these diseases. The toll on health and the energy these diseases take from each suffering patient is great.

This film is also proof positive the Bee Allergy Free - Asthma Bee Gone tablets do cure these diseases.

A copy of this film called, "Bee Allergy Free - Asthma Bee Gone" is enclosed for your viewing.

When this drug, Bee Allergy Free - Asthma Bee Gone, is made available to the American public and these diseases are eliminated, how great the beneficial effect will be upon the overall health of most Americans might be immeasurable.

Renaissance Laboratories is aware The Foundation may like to have some additional assurance and a guaranty the Bee Allergy Free - Asthma Bee Gone drug will indeed cure chronic obstructive pulmonary disease, allergies, asthma, hay fever, sinus and like conditions with either 100% effectiveness or with an effectiveness approaching 100%. Renaissance Laboratories proposes the following specific informal study will assure The Foundation the Bee Allergy Free - Asthma Bee Gone drug will cure chronic obstructive pulmonary disease, allergies, asthma, hay fever, sinus and like conditions (for ease of reference, "Allergies" herein) with an effectiveness approaching 100%. This trial study is outlined as follows:

1. The Foundation or some party selected by The Foundation chooses a small number of severe, advanced, hopeless allergy patients - say, two, three, four, five or fifty or whatever number - to test the CC Pollen Co. food cure, soon to be called a drug upon licensing after an informal study supervised by The Foundation.
2. Allergy patients can either come to Phoenix, Arizona, or Renaissance Laboratories will go to wherever The Foundation selects to conduct the study.
3. Renaissance Laboratories will instruct the patients how to be cured.
4. All will come to the meeting place at the same time the first thing in the morning. They should not have any food or drink except for water during a minimum of eight hours. The Bee Allergy Free - Asthma Bee Gone should be taken on an empty stomach.
5. All must be experiencing some symptom of their diseases (otherwise they will not know when they are cured). As you know, most allergy patients have severe symptoms the first thing in the morning before breakfast.
6. All will be seated and instructed to commence ingesting 12 of the Bee Allergy Free - Asthma Bee Gone tablets every 15 minutes until their symptoms are gone.

-6-

7. Most will have their symptoms disappear upon the ingestion of 12 tablets.
8. All will have their symptoms disappear before ingesting 60 tablets and probably 48 will be the maximum.
9. When the symptoms disappear for all in the informal study, they are cured, probably for the first time in their lives.
10. The time span for these cures will probably be less than an hour for all patients and most will be just a few minutes.
11. When all patients in the informal trial are cured of their allergies. The Foundation will advance the $2 million in funding to Renaissance Laboratories to immediately commence this 1,000 patient clinical investigation.

Renaissance Laboratories would work with The Foundation one-by-one to cure the other degenerative diseases of mankind.

Renaissance Laboratories would be more than happy to entertain any other suggestions and arrangements The Foundation might wish.

Since time is of the essence, Renaissance Laboratories would appreciate receiving The Foundation's response to these suggestions to participate in these many most worthwhile clinical investigations at the earliest possible moment.

Renaissance Laboratories wants to thank The Foundation for its consideration. Renaissance Laboratories predicts The Foundation will find their great contributions to these clinical investigations will be the most satisfying and the most rewarding of any ever undertaken by The Foundation in its entire existence.

Again, please accept our thanks for The Foundation's consideration and Renaissance Laboratories is looking forward to the great help The Foundation can give in eliminating degenerative diseases as we know them.

Very truly yours,
RENAISSANCE LABORATORIES
Royden Brown
Chairman of the Board

RB:hg

Enclosures:
1. Bee Allergy Free - Asthma Bee Gone 1/2" VHS copy of the video summary
2. Copy of the fax to the American Association of Retired Persons bulletin.
3. Copy of the 32 FDA IND's with more than 100 indications - the cures of all the major degenerative diseases.
4. Copy of the fax to Prudential Life Insurance Co.
5. CC Pollen Co. Axioms::: that are always true.

C C POLLER CO.

3627 East Indian School Road
Suite 209
Phoenix, Arizona 85018-5126

FAX: (602) 381-3130
Telex: 559-834
Cable: CCPOLLEN
Phone: (602) 957-0096

April 20, 1992
From: Royden Brown
Chairman of the Board

FAX: 501-682-1382
Robert Winters, President/CEO
Prudential Life Insurance Co.

Renaissance Laboratories has filed 32 Investigational New Drug Applications (IND) with the U.S. Food & Drug Administration (FDA) for more than 100 indications among which are the cure and permanent cure of all the major degenerative diseases. A summary of these filings is being sent to you by UPS Overnight separately.

We ask ourselves who in the United States would profit the most if a non-toxic, no side effect, food cure of the killer degenerative disease is found and brought forth?

The obvious answer is the giant life insurance companies. The cure of degenerative disease would eschew the mortality tables greatly in favor of the life insurance companies.

This is the reason we have contacted you.

You are the one in the Prudential Life Insurance Co. who would know how valuable the elimination of more than 1,600,000 annual American deaths from degenerative diseases would be to your bottom right-hand line.

We itemize the savings of American lives which would result if the Renaissance Laboratory safe cures of the following degenerative diseases were made available, listed in descending order of the causes of death in the United States (1989), as follows.

1.	Diseases of the heart	733,308
2.	Cancer	496,757
3.	Cerebrovascular Diseases	146,231
5.	Chronic Obstructive Pulmonary Diseases, Allergies Asthma, Hay Fever, Sinus and like conditions	88,868
6.	Pneumonia and Influenza	77,416
7.	Diabetes Mellitus	47,310
13.	Arteriosclerosis	19,354
	Total American lives that would be saved each year	1,604,224

Each one of these seven leading causes of death can be investigated in ten 100 patient clinical investigations for a total of 1,000 patients each for an approximate cost of $2 million each, or only $14 million in total.

In addition, Renaissance Laboratories has the cure for Alzheimer's Disease. There are over 4 million Americans now suffering from Alzheimer's Disease and Harvard University predicts there will be more than 14 million with Alzheimer's Disease by the year 2010 if a cure isn't found. We believe the same 1,000 patient clinical investigation would cost about $2 million.

Renaissance Laboratories realizes your head medical director will tell you that these degenerative diseases are incurable. We agree with him ---- these degenerative diseases are incurable by any M.D., by Harvard Medical School, by the FDA, or by Mayo Clinic, or by the 700,000 M.D.'s in the United States using their dangerous toxic poison drugs. However, the food cures from CC Pollen Co. originating out of the beehive that have no side effects and are GRAS, have been curing these degenerative diseases for decades.

GRAS is an acronym and an abbreviation of the phrase and definition . . . generally recog-nized as safe . . . found in the U.S. Code of Federal Regulations Section 21 Parts 170.30.

We realize your chief underwriter will say Prudential Life Insurance Co. has never done this before and you have no expertise to do this and you should not and cannot do it.

However, Renaissance Laboratories is just naive enough to believe you are first, last and always, as good a true blue, red-blooded, all-American as we are, and since $16 million to Prudential is a pittance -- you would make these funds available to save American lives - - if you could be assured Renaissance Laboratories does, indeed, have the absolute cures of degenerative diseases.

If yes, you could cause Prudential to either advance these funds or you could loan the funds to Renaissance Laboratories who would pay them back within a year of receiving a drug license from the FDA.

How do we assure the Prudential Life Insurance Co., Renaissance Laboratories are not a bunch of flakes and have nothing - - instead do have the absolute cure of degenerative diseases?

Renaissance Laboratories suggest an informal study at your home office in about the following manner will convince you for sure Renaissance Laboratories does have the absolute correction, elimination, cure, and permanent cure, of the fifth leading cause of death in the United States, Chronic Obstructive Pulmonary Disease, Allergies, Asthma, Hay Fever and like conditions, in the following manner:

1. Prudential Life Insurance Co. find in their company 20 people, 50, 100, or whatever number you wish, who are afflicted with these diseases of the fifth leading cause of death in the United States.

2. Have them assembled in the gymnasium, conference room, or auditorium, where they can be all in one room the first thing in the morning on some day under the following conditions.
   a. Their stomach must be empty not having eaten any food since the previous evening, at least 8 hours prior.
   b. They must be feeling their symptoms so they can tell if they are cured when their symptoms go away.
   c. Notify Renaissance Laboratories, and Royden Brown will fly to Newark the day before this informal test with the Bee Allergy Free, Asthma Bee Gone, products to effect the cure of the Prudential employees.
   d. On the appointed morning at the appointed time, all will be seated with a glass of water and a bottle of the tablets.
   e. They will be instructed to ingest 12 tablets with water every 15 minutes until their symptoms go away.
   f. Most will have their symptoms leave them with the ingestion of the first 12 tablets.
   g. When the symptoms go away, disappear, or are gone, they are cured, probably for the first time in their entire life.

h. Some will be required to take 24, perhaps even 36 or 48 tablets, to correct and eliminate their symptoms and for them to be cured.

i. All will be cured that first morning - most in just a few minutes.

3. When this informal study has proven 100% successful and all the Prudential employees have been cured of their symptoms whatever they were, Prudential will advance the $2 million to fund this clinical investigation either in the form of a donation or as a loan.

4. A similar investigation can be undertaken for each one of the cures of degenerative diseases listed.

5. In this manner, Prudential Life Insurance Co. would know in advance their funding of these various clinical investigations will be well spent and the cures of the conditions will be obtained.

6. If what Renaissance Laboratories says is true and Prudential will have the informal proof before the money is advanced, how could Prudential Life Insurance Co. spend their $14 million or $16 million more wisely than saving 1,600,000 lives, plus the 4 million Alzheimer's disease lives?

7. We do not believe the Prudential Life Insurance Co. could spend their money more wisely than eliminating the fifth leading cause of death in the United States.

8. When this study has been completed and the Prudential employees are 100% cured, Prudential Life Insurance Co. will know there is a strong possibility the rest of the statements made in this fax are also true. If these statements are true, Prudential Life Insurance Co. would usher in an absolute era of good health and prolong longevity like the world has never known.

9. All of the longevity tables, the actuarial tables, would be obsolete. totally useless.

10. All Renaissance Laboratories asks is the opportunity to prove to the Prudential Life Insurance Co. that CC Pollen Co., Bee Allergy Free, Asthma Bee Gone, is the absolute cure for the fifth leading cause of death in the United States.

11. September and October of 1990, CC Pollen Co. summoned 119 Americans off the street of Phoenix, ages 4 to 86 for the trial and demonstration of Bee Allergy Free, Asthma Bee Gone, tablets in the cure for the fifth leading cause of death in the United States.

12. Every one of the 119 were cured of their symptoms. No-one took more than 12 tablets. All 119 were photographed on SP Beta Cam broadcast quality video tapes to permit the absolute reproducibility of these results.

13. These people were cured ----- no-one could successfully dispute the cures of these 119 persons.

14. The youngest person cured in this trial and demonstration was a 4 year old chronic obstructive pulmonary baby born with asthmatic blockage and suffered with it all its 4 years of life. Since this 4 year old boy could not take the tablets we ground the tablets and put them in honey water. Surprisingly, this baby's symptoms left him at the second tablespoon of the Bee Allergy Free, Asthma Bee Gone honey water -- never to return to this day.

15. The most chronic case was a retired pharmacist from Philadelphia, Pennsylvania, who retired to Sun City. He and his wife came in. He said that he was born an asthmatic baby and developed pulmonary disease upon graduating from pharmacy school and has had it all his life. He said he had suffered 26 life-threatening seizures where he had to be hospitalized in order to breathe and 23 life-threatening seizures where he was either carried or wheeled into the doc-

tor's office in order to breathe. Before he finished taking the first 12 tablets his symptoms left him and they have not returned to this day.

16. As we said, these 119 cures are all on SP Beta Cam broadcast quality reproducible tapes for positive future proof.

17. A representative sampling of these cured 119 persons was made into a 23-minute video tape.

18. Renaissance Laboratories is also sending you that 23-minute video tape which is proof positive Renaissance Laboratories has the absolute cure for this fifth leading cause of death. This film could not have been made by anyone else in the world except CC Pollen Co. Why? Because CC Pollen Co. is the only company in the world that has the cure for the fifth leading cause of death in the United States - Pulmonary Disease, Allergies, Asthma, Hay Fever, Sinus and like conditions.

19. For the first time ever, this film will show you the following:

    1. A random selection of Americans brought in off the streets of Phoenix by display ads in the local newspaper.

    2. All these people have suffered from their Pulmonary Disease, Asthmatic blockage, etc. virtually all their lives.

    3. You will see these people sitting in front of the television cameras taking their first 12 tablets.

    4. You will see the startled look come over their face when they feel their symptoms starting to leave.

    5. You will see the look of disbelief when they realize their symptoms are gone, they are cured, for the first time in their life.

    6. You will see the exhilaration, the happiness, some cried they were so happy.

    7. You will also see in this film how these same people looked 6 months later.

    8. You will see how much happier they were in the after pictures.

    9. You will see how much more beautiful they appeared to be in the after pictures.

    10. You will see how much more energetic they appeared in the after pictures.

    11. You will see how much more self-satisfied they appeared to be in the after pictures.

    12. You will see how much younger they appeared in the after pictures.

    13. You will see a visual demonstration of how the Bee Allergy Free, Asthma Bee Gone tablets can actually reverse the aging process for people who have been life-time sufferers of these insidious diseases.

20. January 11th and 12th, 1992, a similar demonstration of 185 persons was conducted at the CC Pollen Co. office. Two Arizona allergist, Dr. Dave Smith and Dr. H.C. Romero were in attendance and observed the first day. Maurice Tinterow, M.D., Ph.D. from RECNAC Project, Wichita, Kansas, was in attendance and is in the process of publishing a report of these 185 patients in the American Journal of Clinical Nutrition. This test only had a success ratio of 98%. Dr. Tinterow speculates, and I agree, the reason the 2% were not cured is because they could not take sufficient tables to obtain the cure they were seeking. We are expected to have a copy of this report to be published any day. As soon as we receive it we will send you a copy.

21. All Renaissance Laboratories asks is the opportunity to prove to the Prudential Life Insurance Co. - CC Pollen Co's, Bee Allergy Free Asthma Bee Gone is the absolute cure of the fifth leading cause of death in the United States and the world.

22. Renaissance Laboratories is presenting Prudential Life Insurance Co. a sure winner!

C C POL L E N CO.
3627 East Indian School Road
Suite 209
Phoenix, Arizona 85018-5126

FAX: (602) 381-3130
Telex: 559-834
Cable: CCPOLLEN
Phone: (602) 957-0096

March 9, 1992
From: Royden Brown
Chairman of the Board

FAX: 202-434-2320
Horace B. Deets, Executive Director
AARP News Bulletin

Please include the following notice in your next newsletter.

Renaissance Laboratories is seeking a benefactor — a true philanthropist — a "do-gooder in the very best sense" — to contribute $2 million to fund the final 1,000 patient clinical investigations of the CC Pollen Co. new drug "Bee Allergies Free - Asthma Bee Gone" found in FDA IND 37318 to be presented to the FDA for a drug license to cure — not treat - yes, permanently cure chronic obstructive pulmonary disease, allergies, asthma, hay fever, sinus and like conditions - the fifth leading cause of death in the United States - with a non-toxic High Desert drug from the beehive that is GRAS safe.

Benefactor will be able to include whoever they choose in the clinical investigations.

The results are guaranteed to be either 100% effective, or with an effectiveness approaching 100% (better than 95% effective).

Renaissance Laboratories, 3627 E. Indian School Road, Suite 209, Phoenix, AZ 85018. Tel: 602-957-0096 - ask for Royden Brown. Fax: 602-381-3130.

Chronic obstructive pulmonary blockage takes 100,000 American lives every year, 225 every day, and the rate is increasing and accelerating.

Unfortunately, most of the persons who die from this insidious disease are our most valuable citizens, 2, 3, 4, 5 and 6 yr. old babies.

We realize most of your subscribers are senior citizens but they all have grandchildren, or great-grandchildren, they treasure very much. Your readers, at least some of them, could contribute $2 million and never miss the money. Who wouldn't contribute $2 million to eliminate the fifth leading cause of death in the United States if the party could afford it?

We want to thank you for your help and will certainly give you credit when this drug is made available to save American lives.

While I take the AARP News Bulletin, I would appreciate your sending me separate copies as you run this notice and call it to my attention. Otherwise, I am likely to overlook it. We are getting so busy you wouldn't believe it.

When I sold my banks in Colorado in 1956, I retired to Arizona. Now I am busier than I have ever been in my life and having more fun.

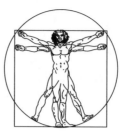

FDA Form 1571-10
Summary of the
Investigation New
Drug Applications (IND)
filed with the FDA

All of the Renaissance
Laboratories filed INDs
are for the CC Pollen Co.
formulated and
manufactured drugs

The many INDs/NDAs are listed by serial numbers in the same sequence filed with the FDA, including the FDA IND/NDA number, where appropriate, which additionally lists the indications <u>cured</u>, <u>not treated</u>, <u>but cured</u> by the products of the beehive as follows:

Remember – the following are <u>cures</u> – not treatments – <u>but cures</u>, <u>permanent cures</u> – for virtually all degenerative diseases with the CC Pollen Co. safe foods from the beehive!

1. IND 37318

    PRIMARY INDICATIONS: — (<u>See</u> Exhibit B attached for definitions).
    1. Chronic obstructive pulmonary disease and allied conditions.
    2. Allergies and like conditions.
    3. Asthma, all asthmatic conditions and like conditions.
    4. Hay fever and like conditions.
    5. Sinusitus and like conditions.

    SECONDARY INDICATIONS: — (<u>See</u> Exhibit B Attached for definitions).
    The <u>prevention</u> in all people of the following indications:
    1. Chronic obstructive pulmonary disease and allied conditions.
    2. Allergies and like conditions.
    3. Asthma, all asthmatic conditions and like conditions.
    4. Hay fever and like conditions.
    5. Sinusitus and like conditions.

    THIRD LEVEL OF INDICATIONS: — (<u>See</u> Exhibit B attached for definitions).
    1. Organ transplant allergic rejection
    2. Intravenous allergic shock.
    3. Thrombolysis, the dissolving of thrombi (blood clots), and a/k/a
    4. Allergic chock from the use of Streptokinase to dissolve blood clots.
    5. Allergic shock from the use of Urokinase.
    6. Allergic shock from the ingestion of bee pollen.
    7. Allergic shock from the ingestion of any and all food substances.
    8. Allergic shock from bee stings and the stings of all insects.
    9. Allergic shock from snake bites and the venom from all reptile bites.
    10. And all like conditions.

-2 -

RATIONALE FOR THIRD LEVEL OF INDICATIONS:

If the above 10 are truly allergic reactions, and

Since Food Product X66 is almost an instantaneous cure of allergic shock and all allergies, and

Since Food Product X66 will stop, correct, eliminate and cure allergic reactions and allergic shock.

It is only reasonable and logical to believe the above 10 indications will Bee stopped, corrected, eliminated and cured by Food Product X66.

2. IND 38158-1-003 — Severe, chronic, long-standing joint pain, inflammation, soreness, especially arthritis, bursitis and like conditions.

   1. IND 38158-2-001 — Pre-Menstrual Syndrome, Pre-Menstrual Tension, Pre-Menstrual Pains and like conditions.

   2. IND 38158-3-001 — Depression, anxiety, panic, fear, trauma, borderline behavior problems, deviate behavior problems and like conditions.

   3. IND 38158-4-001 — Headaches, migraine headaches, head pains and like conditions.

   4. IND 38158-5-001 — Mental diseases, psychiatric diseases, insanity, schizophrenia and like conditions.

   5. IND 38158-6-001 — Senility and like conditions

   6. IND 38158-7-001 — Back pain, skeleton pain and like conditions.

   7. IND 38158-8-001 — Dementia, diseases associated with old age and like conditions.

   8. IND 38158-9-001 — Alcoholism, alcohol addiction and like problems.

   9. IND 38158-10-001 — Drug addiction and like conditions.

   10. IND 38158-11-001 — Repetitive motion injury, repetitive stress injury, carpal tunnel syndrome and like conditions.

   11. IND 38158-12-001 — Motor Neuron diseases and like conditions.

   12. IND 38158-13-001 — Eating disorders, anorexia, bulimia and like conditions.

3. IND 37061 — Obesity, overweight and like conditions.

4. IND 37319 — Premature aging, especially when accompanied by sexual impotency and/or sexual dysfunction and like conditions.

5. 1. 37336-1-006 — Ulcers, bleeding ulcers and like conditions, pain from ulcers, pain from bleeding ulcers and like conditions.

   2. 37336-2-001 — Hoarseness, raspy voice, sore throat and mouth, mouth and throat infection and inflammation and like conditions, including lost voice.

   3. 37336-3-001 — Loose teeth, gingivitis, bleeding gums, pyorrhea and like conditions.

-3-

4. 37336-4-001 — Pneumonia, influenza, infections, inflammations, colds, localized infections and like conditions.

6. IND 37124 — Fatigue, lack of energy, lethargic, weariness, nervous exhaustion, lack of stamina, lack of endurance, chronic fatigue syndrome, Epstein-Barr Virus, and just being "pooped" and like conditions.

7. IND 37262 — Intense, high-level radiation, including cancer radiation treatments and all lower-level radiation treatments and like conditions.

8. IND 37426 — Hoarseness, raspy voice, sore throat and mouth; mouth and throat infection and inflammation and like conditions, including lost voice.

19. IND 37511 — Loose teeth, gingivitis, bleeding gums, pyorrhea and like conditions.

10. IND 37262-2 — Bee Chemotherapy Safe - When chemotherapy is recommended and like conditions.

11. IND 37515 — Heart disease, coronary artery disease, cerebral vascular accident, stroke, cholesterol above 150 mg/dl and like conditions.

12. IND 37516 — For those wishing to run faster and for those wishing to bee stronger.

13. IND 37517 — Memory loss, forgetfulness, senility and like conditions.

14. IND 37518 — Arthritis, bursitis and like conditions.

15. IND 37505 — Stiff joints, painful joints, joint inflammation, joint pain, arthritis, bursitis and like conditions.

16. IND 37550 — Wearing glasses, wearing spectacles, eye weakness, eye failure and like conditions.

17. IND 37158-14 — Bee PMS Free - Premenstrual syndrome, premenstrual tension, premenstrual pains and like conditions.

18. IND 37558 — Sunburning, to prevent sunburning, to prevent skin cancer and like conditions.

19. IND 37557 — Pimples, acne and like conditions.

20. IND 37158-15 — Bee depression free - depression, anxiety, panic, fear, trauma and like conditions.

21. IND 37124 — Blood pressure above 120/60 and like conditions.

22. IND 38348

1. IND 38348 — Chronic, obstructive, pulmonary disease and allied conditions and allergies, asthma, hay fever, sinus and like conditions

-4-

2. IND 38348 — Fatigue, lack of energy, lethargy, worriness, nervous exhaustion, lack of stamina, lack of endurance, chronic fatigue syndrome, Epstein-Barr virus, and just being "pooped" and like conditions.

3. IND 38348 — Wearing glasses, wearing spectacles, eye weakness, eye failure, including presbyopia — commonly called failing old-age sight — and myopia — commonly called nearsightedness and like conditions.

4. IND 38348 — Overweight and obesity and like conditions.

5. IND 38348 — Alzheimer's disease and like conditions.

6. IND 38348 — Mental disorders, psychiatric disorders, schizophrenia, senility, insanity and like conditions.

7. IND 38348 — Heart disease and like conditions.

8. IND 38348 — The Best Drink - The Drink of Life.

9. IND 38348 — Blood pressure above 120/60 mg/dl, hypertension and like conditions.

10. IND 38348 — Multiple sclerosis and like conditions.

11. IND 38348 — Diabetes mellitus, hypoglycemia an d like conditions.

12. IND 38348 — Hypoglycemia, diabetes mellitus and like conditions.

13. IND 38348 — Hyperactivity and hypertension and like conditions.

14. IND 38348 — Hypertension, hyperactivity and like conditions.

15. IND 38348 — Emphysema and like conditions.

16. IND 38348 — Atmospheric and ozone radiation protection and like conditions.

17. IND 38348 — Environmental toxins, pollutants and like conditions.

18. IND 38348 — Recidivism, criminality, criminal behavior and like conditions.

19. IND 38348 — For those wishing to Bee Taller — Gro-Taller.

20. IND 38348 — For those wishing to Bee Faster and for those wishing to Bee Stronger.

21. IND 38348 — Anemia, all forms of anemia including pernicious anemia and like conditions.

22. IND 38348 — Inflammation of the prostate gland, prostathelcosis, prostatic calculus, prostatism, prostatitis, prostatocystitis, prostatodynia, prostatomegaly, prostatorrhea, prostatosis, prostatovesiculitis and/or other prostate inflammations and abnormalities and like conditions. The High Desert® Bee Pollen is a specific for all prostate problems.

23. IND 38348 — Infertility in males and like conditions.

24. IND 38348 — Infertility in females and like conditions.

25. IND 38348 — Male failure to achieve an erection, failure to conceive and like conditions.

-5-

26. IND 38348 — Cancer - malignant neoplasms, including neoplasms of lymphatic and hematopoietic tissues - cancer and like conditions.
27. IND 38348 — Depression, anxiety, trauma, fear, panic and like conditions.
28. IND 38348 — Premenstrual syndrome, premenstrual tension, premenstrual pain, menstrual tension and like conditions.
29. IND 38348 — Migraine headaches, headaches and like conditions.
30. IND 38348 — Schizophrenia and like conditions.
31. IND 38348 — Deviate behavior, lifestyles and like conditions.
32. IND 38348 — Parkinson's disease and like conditions.
33. IND 38348 — Dementia, multi-infarct dementia and like conditions.
34. IND 38348 — Senility and like conditions.
35. IND 38348 — Coronary artery disease and like conditions.
36. IND 38348 — Headaches, migraine headaches and like conditions.
37. IND 38348 — Anxiety disorders, trauma, pain, fear and like conditions.
38. IND 38348 — Arterial sclerosis, atteroschlerosis and like conditions.
39. IND 38348 — Herpes simplex, esophagitis and like conditions.
40. IND 38348 — Impotence and like conditions.
41. IND 38348 — Growth disorders.
42. IND 38348 — Arthritis, bursitis, osteoporosis and like conditions.
43. IND 38348 — Osteoporosis, arthritis, bursitis and like conditions.
44. IND 38348 — Radiation protection and like conditions.
45. IND 38348 — Chemotherapy protection and like conditions.
46. IND 38348 — Those requiring increased intelligence quotients (I.Q.) and like conditions.
47. IND 38348 — Emphysema and like conditions.
48. IND 38348 — Motor neuron diseases and like conditions.
49. IND 38348 — Systemic detoxification of the entire body.
50. IND 38348 — Alcoholism and alcohol addiction and like conditions.
51. IND 38348 — Drug addictions and like conditions.
52. IND 38348 — Joint pain and back pain and like conditions.
53. IND 38348 — Senility and like conditions.
54. IND 38348 — Psychiatric disorders and like conditions.
55. IND 38348 — Insanity and like conditions.
56. IND 38348 — Inflammatory bowel diseases and like conditions.
57. IND 38348 — To elevate the red blood count (hemoglobin as a percentage of total blood volume) and like conditions.
58. IND 38348 — To lower the white blood count by driving infection from the body and like conditions.
59. IND 38348 — To assist in carrying a pregnancy to full term and like conditions.

-6-

60. IND 38348 — To increase the lactation of nursing females and like conditions.

61. IND 38348 — To make the prenatal conditions for birth normal or perfect and like conditions.

THE FOLLOWING ARE SECONDARY LEVEL INDICATIONS:

It has been the experience of Renaissance Laboratories that every one of the investigational new drug applications and new drug applications filed with the FDA will prevent the same symptoms they will cure and heal.

The prevention of the indications listed herein are the secondary level of indications for all of these investigational new drug applications.

THE FOLLOWING ARE THIRD LEVEL INDICATIONS: (SEE EXHIBIT B FOR DEFINITION):

1. Acquired Immune Deficiency syndrome, commonly called AIDS.
2. Crohn's disease and like conditions.
3. Leukemia, blood cancer diseases and like conditions.
4. Addison's disease and like conditions.
5. Parkinson's disease and like conditions.

23. IND 38348 — Cancer - malignant neoplasms, including neoplasms of lymphatic and hematopietic tissues - cancer and like conditions.

24. IND 38348 — Bleeding - both internal and external and like conditions.

25. IND 38348 — Acquired Immune Deficiency Syndrome - AIDS.

26. IND 38348 — Diabetes Mellitus, Hypoglycemia and like conditions.

27. IND 38348 — Cramps, cramps of the extremities, professional cramps, writer's cramps, telegrapher's cramps, watchmaker's cramps, seamstress cramps, heat cramps, and like conditions.

28. IND 38348 — Insomnia, sleeplessness, and like conditions; and stressfulness, nervousness, and like conditions.

29. IND 38348 — Digestion failure, stomach upsets, stomach discomfort, diarrhea and like conditions.

30. IND 38348 — For those persons wishing to have faster growing, longer and more beautiful hair and nails.

31. IND 38348 — Jet lag, lack of energy after long trip — principally by air and like conditions.

32. IND 38348 — Wrinkles acquired after the age of 18 and like conditions.

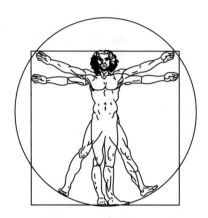

CC POLLEN CO. AXIOMS — THAT ARE ALWAYS TRUE — !

STATEMENT OF FACTS!

1. When a CC Pollen Co. High Desert bee pollen product cures any degener-
    ative disease and/or corrects a condition in one person:

    — that CC Pollen Co. High Desert® bee pollen product from the beehive
    will <u>always</u> continue <u>to cure</u> — not treat — <u>yes, always continues to per-
    manently cure</u> — that degenerative disease with either 100% effectiveness
    in all persons or <u>always</u> with an effectiveness approaching 100% (always
    better than 95% effective).

    <u>THERE ARE NO EXCEPTIONS!</u>

2. When a CC Pollen Co. High Desert® bee pollen product will not cure a
    degenerative disease or correct a condition in a few, say five randomly
    selected, that CC Pollen Co. High Desert® bee pollen cure from the bee-
    hive is always 100% ineffective for that particular degenerative disease or
    condition.

    <u>THERE ARE NO EXCEPTIONS!</u>

3. Therefore, when Renaissance Laboratories successfully does the informal
    study with a few persons (1-2-3-4- or 5-or whatever) Foundation has cho-
    sen — Foundation will know for certain the results will be exactly the
    same in the randomized, controlled, double-blind with placebo, cross-over
    study with 1,000-patients to be presented to the FDA.

4. If the informal study cured the degenerative disease or the condition, the
    1,000-patient clinical investigation can be funded with confidence, know-
    ing the results are going to be positive, favorable and the same in the

-2-

1,000-patient clinical investigation as they were in this informal study. The condition or degenerative disease is going to be cured in better than 95% of the participants in the 1,000-patient clinical investigation.

5. Surely the cost of this 1,000-patient clinical investigation must be the most wisely spent money the Foundation has ever spent. The Foundation will obtain the cures being sought.

6. This cure of a degenerative disease will be the first cure, the first permanent cure, for any degenerative disease in the entire recorded history of mankind and the first the FDA has ever licensed in its entire existence.

7. The cure of this degenerative disease will be acclaimed as the miracle medical breakthrough of all times.

8. This cure of a degenerative disease will be the greatest medical discovery of all times.

9. This cure of a degenerative disease will immediately bestow the greatest American public health benefit of all times.

10. The Foundation will be hailed as the greatest American public health benefactor of all times. The entire world will applaud and congratulate the Foundation for its humanitarian actions, great insight and greater wisdom. The acclaim the Fund will probably receive cannot be overstated.

FINAL COMMENT

What happened?

Nothing.

I believe Henry Ford is still turning in his grave angry as a cat on a tin roof at the failure of The Ford Foundation to at least risk the first $2 million to eliminate degenerative disease in the U.S.A.

UNBELIEVABLE.

As an exhibit to the letter going to the Ford Foundation and every other Foundation in the U.S.A., we have a summary of the 32 IND's we filed with the FDA having cures for virtually all the degenerative diseases and many of the conditions affecting mankind.

Any rational person would have thought that some of these giant Foundations with all this money to spend would have thought 1,600,000 American lives being saved every year was worth the investment of a one-time expenditure of $2 million to start these clinical investigations and a total expenditure of $16 million to save 1,600,000 American lives every year. But that is obviously not the case.

Not one favorable response. What conclusion do you make?

No-one gives a tinker.

No-one cares whether 1,600,000 Americans are dying or not.

No-one wants to make the effort to save 1,600,000 American lives.

What other conclusion can you possibly make?

Stupidity?

Disbelief?

Your guess is as good as mine.

The FDA wrote Renaissance Laboratories a letter, copy follows fax No. 1. The FDA, like they always do, hide behind legalistic language to prevent food cures from the beehive and other foods having medical properties from being released. Even though these food cures are safer than any drug the FDA has ever licensed, the FDA diabolically and clandestinely fight these safe cures from the beehive to the death.

Of course we want to remember that the primary cause of the diseased and dying Americans is the White House and Congress. They defined a drug which failed to exempt foods. This mistake has never been rectified.

You would think that the President and Congress have enough guts, enough courage, to admit their mistake and correct this definition to exempt foods from the definition of a drug. To do otherwise is absolutely ridiculous and ludicrous in the extreme.

Renaissance Laboratories received the typical response from the FDA the FDA makes to all communications about GRAS safe food products that have medical properties that someone is trying to get released to cure degenerative disease. These 15 responses to this August 5, 1992 letter from the FDA is spread herein with the hopes that somebody who reads this book will become outraged and incensed the FDA is keeping the GRAS safe cures from the beehive from saving American lives.

The FDA is sacrificing more than 1,600,000 lives every year because they have not released the CC Pollen Co. absolutely safe cures from the beehive for virtually all degenerative diseases.

Exact copies of these faxes which were sent to the FDA, the President, Vice President and other members of Congress follows:

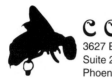

C C POLLER CO.

3627 East Indian School Road
Suite 209
Phoenix, Arizona 85018-5126

FAX: (602) 381-3130
Telex: 559-834
Cable: CCPOLLEN

Phone: (602) 957-0096

August 25, 1992   First Response to your August 5, 1992 letter.

From: Royden Brown
Chairman of the Board

cc: Senator Orrin G. Hatch
FAX: 202-224-6331
cc: Senator Edward G. Kennedy
FAX: 202-224-2417
cc: Representative John Dingle
FAX: 202-225-2525
cc: Senator Dennis DeConcini
FAX: 202-224-2302; 602-670-6831

FAX: 301-443-9282
Marc J. Scheineson, Assoc.
Commissioner for Legislative Affairs, FDA
cc: Sally Kelley, Agency Liason, Rm. 91
The White House, FAX: 202-456-2461
cc: President George Bush
FAX: 202-456-2461
cc: Vice President Dan Quayle
FAX: 202-456-6231
cc: Senator John McCain
FAX: 202-224-8938; 602-640-2576

We are sending the parties receiving the carbon copies of this fax a copy of your August 5, 1992 letter addressed to me to permit them to follow the trend of thought in response to your letter.

The last concluding sentence in the second paragraph, we quote, "Further, it has been determined that when special dietary foods are labeled with claims of disease prevention, treatment, mitigation, cure, or diagnosis, they must comply with the drug provisions of the Act."

This statement is contrary, counter-productive and very detrimental to the American public health and welfare. Making special dietary foods go through the same tests the FDA makes their dangerous, toxic, poison drugs go through to try to make them kill as few Americans as possible is ludicrous - assinine in the extreme.

Nevertheless, we realize the initial fault lies with Congress and the Executive Branch. Congress and the Executive Branch, in their great wisdom, mistakenly enacted legislation which permits the FDA to legally say, "When special dietary foods are labeled with claims of disease prevention, treatment, mitigation, cure or diagnosis, they (special dietary foods) must comply with the drug provisions of the Act."

Unless the FDA comes to their senses and finally realize the saving of more than 1,600,000 American lives every year and the saving of more than 4 million Alzheimer diseased Americans is more important to the FDA than a continual, strict, absolute compliance with the wrong, mistaken definition of a food, we shall never cure the first degenerative disease.

Renaissance Laboratories has submitted 32 IND"s to the FDA. The products in these IND's are the cures for all the killer degenerative diseases currently taking American Lives needlessly.

Doesn't that matter to the FDA? Doesn't the FDA give a damn whether Americans are dying needlessly or not? Should these 3, 4, 5 and 6 yr. old chronic obstructive pulmonary disease babies, the asthmatic blockage babies, continue to die from suffocation because the FDA refuses to release Food Product X66 which is the absolute, almost instantaneous cure, for these insidious diseases?

FDA IND 37318 contains Food Product X66 which is the absolute, almost instantaneous cure, for chronic obstructive pulmonary disease, allergies, asthma, hay fever, sinus and like conditions, which is the fifth leading cause of death in the USA and the world.

CC Pollen Co. has sold this product for more than a decade in every state in the nation to probably 50,000 Americans or more without the first report of any side effect of any kind except an almost instant cure of the conditions, and an efficiency approaching 100%, probably about 99.99% effective.

Food Product X66 by empirical evidence - the strongest evidence of all - Food Product X66 is absolutely safe and more effective than any drug the FDA has ever licensed. The risk benefit ratio of Food Product X66 is:

Risk ....Zero
Benefit 99.99%

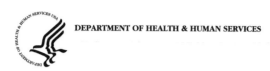

DEPARTMENT OF HEALTH & HUMAN SERVICES

Public Health Service

Food and Drug Administration
Washington DC 20204

Mr. Royden Brown
Renaissance Laboratories
3627 East Indian School Road, Suite 209
Phoenix, Arizona 85018-5126

Dear Mr. Brown:

This is in further response to your telefacsimile communication addressed to President Bush dated June 24, 1992, concerning the unapproved new drug, "Food Product X66."

Since you have again raised the question regarding the designation of this product as a drug, we would like to point out that the Federal Food, Drug, and Cosmetic (FDC) Act defines the term "drug" to be, among other thing, "articles intended for use in the diagnosis, cure, mitigation, treatment, or prevention of disease in man or other animals..." In other words, it is the labeling claim of intended medical or health-related use that makes an article a drug. Further, it has been determined that when special dietary foods are labeled with claims of disease prevention, treatment, mitigation, cure, or diagnosis, they must comply with the drug provisions of the Act.

Because the labeling for "Food Product X66" contains the statement "INDICATIONS: Allergies, Asthma, Hay Fever, Sinus and like conditions," which are drug claims, "GRAS" status (a food additive designation) is not relevant. Instead, the new drug requirement for submission of substantial scientific evidence of effectiveness must be met before interstate marketing in the United States is permissible.

We also refer to the October 17, 1991, meeting between representatives of the Agency and you and Mr. Bruce Brown in which we described and discussed the steps needed to lift the "clinical hold" on your IND for "Food Product X66" (IND 37,318) so that clinical studies could proceed.

We further refer to our communication dated March 16, 1992, responding to your letter dated December 27, 1991, to the Commissioner. That communication described in detail the reasons that your product is considered a drug and why it was placed on clinical hold.

We hope this information is helpful.

Sincerely yours,
Marc J. Scheineson
Associate Commissioner
for Legislative Affairs

cc: Sally Kelley
Agency Liaison
Room 91
The White House, 20500
September 9, 1992   Second Response to your August 5, 1992 letter.

C C POLLER CO.

3627 East Indian School Road
Suite 209
Phoenix, Arizona 85018-5126

FAX: (602) 381-3130
Telex: 559-834
Cable: CCPOLLEN

Phone: (602) 957-0096

From: Royden Brown
Chairman of the Board

cc: Senator Orrin G. Hatch
FAX: 202-224-6331
cc: Senator Edward G. Kennedy
FAX: 202-224-2417
cc: Representative John Dingle
FAX: 202-225-2525
cc: Senator Dennis DeConcini
FAX: 202-224-2302; 602-670-6831

FAX: 301-443-9282
Marc J. Scheineson, Assoc.
Commissioner for Legislative Affairs, FDA
cc: Sally Kelley, Agency Liason, Rm. 91
The White House, FAX: 202-456-2461
cc: President George Bush
FAX: 202-456-2461
cc: Vice President Dan Quayle
FAX: 202-456-6231
cc: Senator John McCain
FAX: 202-224-8938; 602-640-2576

Before proceeding in the definitive response to your August 5, 1992 letter, Renaissance Laboratories believes we should give fault and blame, call a spade a spade, to who, when, and where fault and blame truly rests for the disastrous, unhealthy, diseased, dying, carnage and massacre of innocent Americans.

When Congress passed the legislation and defined a drug 40 years ago, Congress created the greatest of all obstacles, the greatest of all detriments to better American public health. The definition was too broad and too inclusive. The definition of a drug should have excluded food, dietary and nutritional supplements.

Any time a law is passed by Congress making air and water drugs in any situation is wrong - totally wrong!

Any time a law is passed by Congress making someone guilty of a felony if they utter any harmless, well-meaning sentence - the law is wrong - 100% wrong.

For example:

We see a man dying of thirst on the desert of Arizona. President George Bush says this man is dying of thirst. Let's cure his thirst and give him some water. President George Bush is guilty of a felony and the FDA could incarcerate him because the senseless regulations of defining a drug above are invoked.

Example 2:

President George Bush is down in Miami, Florida and sees these hurricane sufferers dying of hunger. President George Bush says let's cure their hunger and give them some of this donated food.

President George Bush is guilty of a felony and the FDA could incarcerate him because of the above, senseless definition of a drug.

Renaissance Laboratories does not know how long Congress and The White

House is going to permit a great, perhaps the greatest of all legislative wrongs to continue - and continue to kill Americans. Perhaps the Congress and The White House have not been aware of the great wrong they have created. This wrong may go down in history as the greatest, most deadly, most unintentional, mass legislative execution, murder and massacre of humans in the history of the world.

How many millions have died needlessly because of the all inclusive, senselessness, wrong definition of a drug?

But if Congress and the Executive Branch had been wise enough to properly and correctly define a drug initially, degenerative disease, as we know degenerative disease today, would not exist - degenerative disease would be history - past history!

The food cures from the beehive and from others having medical properties would have been introduced in the mainstream of health and medicine and these food cures would be the common cure - not treatment - for the rare possible current occurrence of degenerative disease.

Using your hind sight - we can say Congress and the President are directly responsible for and the cause of more than 1.6 million Americans dying needlessly every year from preventable and curable degenerative diseases.

1,600,000 American lives, 1,600.000 dead Americans, lie on the doorsteps of Congress and The White House - every year!

4,000,000+ Alzheimers diseased Americans' future deaths will lie on the steps of Congress and The White House.

More than 60,000,000 deaths will lie on the doorsteps of Congress and The White House by the year 2010 unless - any 1 of 3 miracles occurs:

First Miracle:

Congress and the President immediately, in the current session of Congress, pass the Orrin G. Hatch Health Freedom Act of 1992, S2835 and make S2835 the law of the land, or

Second Miracle:

Congress and the President cause all 32 FDA INDs filed by Renaissance Laboratories to be immediately temporarily licensed for the cures of all degenerative diseases indicated therein, or

Third Miracle:

Congress and the President bravely and fearlessly correct the great mistake made in wrongly defining a drug in the first place.

If Congress and the President have the intelligence, the will, the courage, yes, the guts to right the wrong created 40 years ago - probably 20,00,000+ Americans lives ago - they could usher an era of best health, good fellowship and general prosperity for the U.S.A., the likes of which has never been known nor experienced in the entire history of the United States of America.

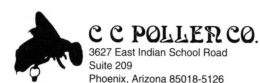

C C POLLER CO.
3627 East Indian School Road
Suite 209
Phoenix, Arizona 85018-5126

FAX: (602) 381-3130
Telex: 559-834
Cable: CCPOLLEN

Phone: (602) 957-0096

September 10, 1992   Third Response to your August 5, 1992 letter.

From: Royden Brown
Chairman of the Board

cc: Senator Orrin G. Hatch
FAX: 202-224-6331
cc: Senator Edward G. Kennedy
FAX: 202-224-2417
cc: Representative John Dingle
FAX: 202-225-2525
cc: Senator Dennis DeConcini
FAX: 202-224-2302; 602-670-6831

FAX: 301-443-9282
Marc J. Scheineson, Assoc.
Commissioner for Legislative Affairs, FDA
cc: Sally Kelley, Agency Liason, Rm. 91
The White House, FAX: 202-456-2461
cc: President George Bush
FAX: 202-456-2461
cc: Vice President Dan Quayle
FAX: 202-456-6231
cc: Senator John McCain
FAX: 202-224-8938; 602-640-2576

In the second paragraph of your August 5, 1992 letter, you quote the Federal Food, Drug and Cosmetic Act, which you say defines the term "drugs" to be, among other things, as follows:

"Articles intended for use in the diagnosis, cure, mitigation, treatment or prevention of disease in men or animals..."

This is the (B) paragraph in the Definition of a Drug. However, the (C) paragraph in the same Definition of a Drug reads as follows:

"...and (C) articles (other than foods) intended to affect the structure or any function of the body of man or other animals."

Why has the FDA totally ignored the (C) section of the Definition of a Drug for these 40 long years?

The FDA knows full well that all written laws are always construed or should be construed - against the maker, the FDA; therefore, if the FDA had been the agency whose true motto was:

Save American lives, if possible, at all cost, and sacrifice the regulations for the cures — the FDA would have stopped worshipping the holy, sacred, FDA regulations and, instead, would shepherd the food cures into the main-stream of food and health to save American lives.

Instead of the FDA continuing their obvious hatred and attempt to destroy and battle to the death against food cures from the beehive and other food cures - the FDA would look at these food cures and say they are GRAS safe - there has never been one death caused by these safe or safer than GRAS food cures from the beehive - and it is the intention of Congress and the President to save American lives at all costs — therefore, let us license all of these GRAS safe food cures because it is a great deal more important to save 5,600,000 American lives than it is to continue to worship our holy, sacred FDA regulations that weren't meant for food cures in the first place but were meant for the dangerous, toxic, poison drugs we licensed.

FDA IND 37318 filed by Renaissance Laboratories is the absolute cure for the fifth leading cause of death in the United States and the world, chronic obstructive pulmonary disease, allergies, asthma, hay fever, sinus and like conditions, and the other 31 IND's would cure, correct and eliminate the other killer degenerative diseases saving more than 1,600,000 American lives every year.

In addition, Renaissance Laboratories has filed the absolute, safe, cure of Alzheimer's disease which is affecting more than 4 million Americans.

Doesn't this mean anything to the FDA?

Doesn't the FDA give a damn that Americans are dying needlessly and yet the FDA continues their fight to destroy the food cures and say to Congress and the President that the holy, sacred regulations which were meant for the dangerous, toxic, poison drugs the FDA license has not been fulfilled?

Which is more important? The holy, sacred FDA regulations, or 5,600,000 American lives?

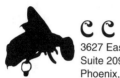

C C POLLEN CO.

3627 East Indian School Road
Suite 209
Phoenix, Arizona 85018-5126

FAX: (602) 381-3130
Telex: 559-834
Cable: CCPOLLEN

Phone: (602) 957-0096

September 13, 1992 sent 9/14/92 Fourth Response to your Aug. 5, 1992 letter.

From: Royden Brown
Chairman of the Board

cc: Senator Orrin G. Hatch
FAX: 202-224-6331
cc: Senator Edward G. Kennedy
FAX: 202-224-2417
cc: Representative John Dingle
FAX: 202-225-2525
cc: Senator Dennis DeConcini
FAX: 202-224-2302; 602-670-6831

FAX: 301-443-9282
Marc J. Scheineson, Assoc.
Commissioner for Legislative Affairs, FDA
cc: Sally Kelley, Agency Liason, Rm. 91
The White House, FAX: 202-456-2461
cc: President George Bush
FAX: 202-456-2461
cc: Vice President Dan Quayle
FAX: 202-456-6231
cc: Senator John McCain
FAX: 202-224-8938; 602-640-2576

Your reference to, "GRAS" status (a food additive designation) is not relevant" in the third paragraph of your August 5, 1992 letter is wrong. You have made a mistake. Apparently the FDA has misinterpreted this section of the Code of Federal Regulations.

If you will again review the definition of GRAS status, you will notice there is no mention whatsoever in the definition to a food additive. Granted, this definition is in the food additive section of the Code of REgulations, but Senator Carl Hayden told me years ago that Congress only defined GRAS once and that was in the food additive designation because it was the opinion of Congress that every food in some application could become an additive within the definition of food additives. That was the reason that GRAS does not refer to food additives in itself.

Renaissance Laboratories declared and notified the FDA last year every one of the products in the 32 IND's submitted to the FDA were GRAS by definition - an acronym or abbreviation for...generally recognized as safe...as found in the Code of Federal Regulations Section 21, paragraph 170.30.

Since all of the products found in these 32 IND's are nothing but foods - foods Americans and people in the world have been eating, most of them since the beginning, and no-one has ever experienced a toxic side effect, no-one has ever experienced permanent disability or damage, nor death, from ingesting any of these foods found in these 32 IND's, these food products exactly fit the definition of GRAS.

It is very strange that after Renaissance Laboratories declared these 32 IND's all GRAS - safer than any drug ever licensed by the FDA - the FDA has not seen fit to even respond to the declaration. They haven't even argued that some of these food products might kill some Americans or try to bring us some proof that they were dangerous toxic substances like the drugs they regulate.

As we know, foods, year in and year out, never caused the first death. They are GRAS. They are absolutely safe for all intents and purposes.

Therefore, your statement, "GRAS" status (a food additive designation) is not relevant" is exactly wrong.

The GRAS status of the product in these 32 IND's is the most relevant thing the FDA has ever received.

We venture these 32 IND's are the first ever cures that have been submitted to the FDA for degenerative diseases - and certainly the first ever for all of them.

If the FDA disagrees with the declarations in this fax, let the FDA point out the first toxic side effect, the first death ever caused by these products in the past three millenniums.

As we all know, empirical proof, in the final analysis, is the best, strongest proof of all.

The proof of the pudding is in the tasting thereof.

The proof of the GRAS substance is the actual eating of the GRAS substance by many, especially for 4, 5 and 6 yr. old babies.

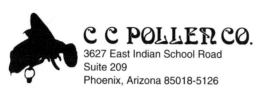

C C POLLEN CO.

3627 East Indian School Road
Suite 209
Phoenix, Arizona 85018-5126

FAX: (602) 381-3130
Telex: 559-834
Cable: CCPOLLEN

Phone: (602) 957-0096

September 16, 1992   Fifth Response to your August 5, 1992 letter.

From: Royden Brown
Chairman of the Board

cc: Senator Orrin G. Hatch
FAX: 202-224-6331
cc: Senator Edward G. Kennedy
FAX: 202-224-2417
cc: Representative John Dingle
FAX: 202-225-2525
cc: Senator Dennis DeConcini
FAX: 202-224-2302; 602-670-6831

FAX: 301-443-9282
Marc J. Scheineson, Assoc.
Commissioner for Legislative Affairs, FDA
cc: Sally Kelley, Agency Liason, Rm. 91
The White House, FAX: 202-456-2461
cc: President George Bush
FAX: 202-456-2461
cc: Vice President Dan Quayle
FAX: 202-456-6231
cc: Senator John McCain
FAX: 202-224-8938; 602-640-2576

In your August 5, 1992 letter, the second sentence in your third paragraph reads as follows:

"Instead, the new drug requirement for submission of substantial scientific evidence of effectiveness must be met before interstate marketing in the United States is permissible."

We agree with the FDA's requirement for "substantial scientific evidence of effectiveness" when you are dealing with the dangerous, toxic, poison drugs the FDA always licenses. The FDA cannot be too careful. These dangerous, toxic, poison drugs the FDA license may be the leading cause of death in the United States. You know for certain these FDA licensed dangerous, toxic, poison drugs kill many Americans every day.

Empirical evidence is the strongest evidence we have of effectiveness.

Food Product X66 has been fed to Americans for more than a decade, probably 13 years, sold in every state of the nation, taken successfully and effectively by probably 50,000 Americans or more with an effectiveness or efficiency of 99.99%. How can we say 99.99% effectiveness or efficiency? Because we believe these 50,000 plus Americans who bought this product and took it to cure their chronic obstructive pulmonary disease, allergies, asthma, hay fever, sinus and like conditions, would have complained immediately if they had not received the relief and cures they sought. CC Pollen Co., the manufacturer, would have been the first to have heard because the product is exactly guaranteed money back. Since I formulated this product and have always fielded all of the complaints about lack of effectiveness of Food Product X66, I speak from knowledge. In this past ten to thirteen years there has been less than ten people who have asked for and CC Pollen Co. refunded their money.

"Substantial scientific evidence of effectiveness."

There is no drug ever licensed by the FDA that has as high an effectiveness as Food Product X66.

Since Food Product X66 is safer than GRAS and has a 99.99% efficiency or effectiveness, why hasn't the FDA released and licensed this drug? Surely the FDA wants to save American lives as much as President George Bush, or as much as Renaissance Laboratories, or as much as Senator John McCain, or as much as Senator Orrin Hatch, or Edward G. Kennedy, or John Dingle, or Dennis DeConcini, or Vice President Dan Quayle?

Saving American lives must be the highest possible service the FDA can render to the American public health. Do you dispute that statement?

The FDA has the tool to by-pass the rigid, structured, onerous, clinical investigations for the dangerous, poison, toxic drugs the FDA licensed. We remind you of the FDA general considerations for the clinical evaluation of drugs and quote exactly therefrom as follows:

"The guidelines must not be used to force new compounds into their mold as the fruit of original ideas may be lost."

"History is replete with discovery that could not have been made if the investigation was constrained by established methods.

C C POLLEN CO.
3627 East Indian School Road
Suite 209
Phoenix, Arizona 85018-5126

FAX: (602) 381-3130
Telex: 559-834
Cable: CCPOLLEN

Phone: (602) 957-0096

September 21, 1992   Sixth Response to your August 5, 1992 letter.

From: Royden Brown
Chairman of the Board

cc: Senator Orrin G. Hatch
FAX: 202-224-6331
cc: Senator Edward G. Kennedy
FAX: 202-224-2417
cc: Representative John Dingle
FAX: 202-225-2525
cc: Senator Dennis DeConcini
FAX: 202-224-2302; 602-670-6831

FAX: 301-443-9282
Marc J. Scheineson, Assoc.
Commissioner for Legislative Affairs, FDA
cc: Sally Kelley, Agency Liason, Rm. 91
The White House, FAX: 202-456-2461
cc: President George Bush
FAX: 202-456-2461
cc: Vice President Dan Quayle
FAX: 202-456-6231
cc: Senator John McCain
FAX: 202-224-8938; 602-640-2576

We refer to your fourth paragraph in your August 5, 1992 letter which reads as follows:

"We also refer to the October 17, 1991, meeting between representatives of the Agency and you and Mr. Bruce Brown in which we described and discussed the steps needed to lift the "clinical hold" on your IND for "Food Product X66" (IND 37,318) so that clinical studies could proceed."

Did the FDA actually tell you what they wanted Renaissance Laboratories to do even before they licensed Food Product X66 to correct, eliminate, heal and cure the fifth leading cause of death in the United States — chronic obstructive pulmonary disease, allergies, asthma, hay fever, sinus and like conditions? And all those doctors sitting around that long table did this without a smile on their face.

Every person from the FDA was dead serious when they told my son and I the senseless, contra-productive, unbelievable request, yes, iron-clad compliance demand that was designed for the dangerous, toxic, poison drugs the FDA always licenses that kill Americans right and left and not designed, absolutely not designed, for GRAS safe substances such as every product from the beehive is classified.

John Short who was the chairman of this meeting between the leaders of the FDA and my son and myself, insisted, and stated there were no exceptions to this rule. We must do the following or they would not release IND 37318 containing Food Product X66 for clinical investigations until each and every clinical laboratory study was done - 33 possible clinical investigations taking 10 to 15 years.

Food Product X66 contains 34 different ingredients. Most of them are herbs that have been on earth and eaten by mankind since the days of Adam and Eve. Every one of the other ingredients were in commercial commerce before 1958 and have been eaten by Americans and people of the world safely for many decades.

That means, all 34 of the ingredients in Food Product X66 fit the definition of GRAS exactly - making Food Product X66 GRAS safe.

When these 34 ingredients are compressed together to make a tablet, none of them are extracted like drugs that become dangerous, toxic, poison substances. Instead, Food Product X66 contains the whole herb, the whole food, in that tablet. Therefore, Food Product X66 is safer than any drug ever licensed thus far in the entire existence of the FDA and is GRAS safe - there is not one FDA licensed drug out of the 40,000 plus FDA prescription drugs, nor one out of the 100,000 over-the-counter drugs that the FDA has licensed that is GRAS safe.

Yet, John Short, the FDA leader, insisted, Renaissance Laboratories conduct clinical investigations on animals, eliminating one ingredient at a time, until such time as we come to the place where we could not eliminate any more ingredients otherwise the product wouldn't work.

What is the purpose of these clinical investigations?

The announced purpose and the purpose in the regulations of doing these clinical investigations is to eliminate as many dangerous, toxic, poison drug ingredients in Food Product X66 as possible and still have it work so that the dangerous, toxic, poison drug would kill as few Americans as possible or would destroy as few Americans' health as possible, or would lessen the dangerous, toxic, poison side effects.

Isn't that rather ridiculous?

Here we have a food product that is safer than any drug ever licensed. Why would the FDA place themselves in such a compromised position where they are trying to force Renaissance Laboratories to do absolute ridiculous, ludicrous, senseless, contra-productive, clinical investigations to eliminate ingredients when it is impossible to improve the safety of Food Product X66?

After talking to Senator John McCain's office, it is very likely the FDA upon receipt of the Food Product X66 IND 37318, did not actually analyze the ingredients in Food Product X66. Instead, the FDA probably sent their standard form letter which they send on all IND's automatically because the FDA always in the past has received IND's that contain the usual dangerous, toxic, poison drug ingredients.

As Commissioner David A. Kessler, M.D., Ph.D. says:

"There are no safe drugs."

If that is the case, the fault lies with the FDA for not actually investigating the ingredients in Food Product X66 to see if there were any dangerous, toxic, poison drug ingredients in Food Product X66 that should be investigated to see if they can be eliminated to reduce the chances of damaging Americans who might take the Food Product X66 and/or eliminate the possibility Food Product X66 might kill Americans if taken.

In our next response we shall go into the 34 ingredients definitively.

The conclusion that will be reached is so obvious, no-one could possibly challenge the conclusion Food Product X66 is GRAS by definition found in the Code of U.S. Federal Regulations, Section 21, Part 170.30.

As we all know, GRAS is an acronym or abbreviation for the phrase found in the Code of Federal Regulations for "generally recognized as safe."

C C POLLEN CO.

3627 East Indian School Road
Suite 209
Phoenix, Arizona 85018-5126

FAX: (602) 381-3130
Telex: 559-834
Cable: CCPOLLEN
Phone: (602) 957-0096

September 22, 1992   Seventh Response to your August 5, 1992 letter.

From: Royden Brown
Chairman of the Board

cc: Senator Orrin G. Hatch
FAX: 202-224-6331
cc: Senator Edward G. Kennedy
FAX: 202-224-2417
cc: Representative John Dingle
FAX: 202-225-2525
cc: Senator Dennis DeConcini
FAX: 202-224-2302; 602-670-6831

FAX: 301-443-9282
Marc J. Scheineson, Assoc.
Commissioner for Legislative Affairs, FDA
cc: Sally Kelley, Agency Liason, Rm. 91
The White House, FAX: 202-456-2461
cc: President George Bush
FAX: 202-456-2461
cc: Vice President Dan Quayle
FAX: 202-456-6231
cc: Senator John McCain
FAX: 202-224-8938; 602-640-2576

We outlined the absurd request for possibly 33 different clinical ingredient investigations, requiring 10 to 15 years and costing $200 to $300 million, the FDA makes, yes demands and would force, Renaissance Laboratories to do on Food Product X66 to eliminate the dangerous, poison, toxic drug ingredients that are always present in the dangerous, toxic, poison drugs the FDA licenses. These dangerous, toxic, poison drug ingredients are never, absolutely never, present in the food cures from the beehive.

Unless we analyze the ingredients in Food Product X66, Marc, you and the other seven gentlemen receiving this fax will not really know how asinine the FDA is in trying to force Renaissance Laboratories to do these 33 clinical investigations. Here is a copy of the label submitted to the FDA that would be on Food Product X66:

FDA Form - 7

CHEMISTRY, MANUFACTURING AND CONTROL DATA OF
FOOD PRODUCT X66

The suggested label for Food Product X66 is detailed in the following typed label:

INDICATIONS:
Chronic Obstructive Pulmonary Disease, Allergies, Asthma, Hay Fever, Sinus, and like conditions

SUGGESTED USE:

First time: 12 tablets on empty stomach just before a meal. Look at your watch: if your symptoms are not gone, corrected or eliminated in 15 minutes, take 12 more tablets, keep taking 12 tablets every 15 minutes until your symptoms are gone. Thereafter; if symptoms start to reoccur take 12 tablets each 15 minutes until symptoms are gone for first 30 days. Each month reduce by 2 tablets.

INGREDIENTS:

Glutamic Acid HCL, Betaine HCL, High Desert® Bee Pollen, Pepsin, Potassium Chloride, Pyridoxine, Whole Pancreas, Extract of Ox, Cayenne, Niacinamide, Papain, Alfalfa, Golden Seal Root, Burdock Root, Skullcap, Slippery Elm Bark, Marshmallow Root, Horseradish Root, Queen of the Meadow, Shavegrass, Eyebright Herb, Parsley Leaf, Mulleinflower, Blessed Thistle Herb, Chickweed Herb, White Oak Bark, Chaparral Leaf, Black Walnut Leaf, Papaya Leaf, Passion Flower, Barberry Root, Oat Straw, Fenugreek Seed.

Manufactured for:

CC Pollen Co.
3627 East Indian School Road • Suite 209
Phoenix, AZ 85018
(602) 957-0096
FAX: (602) 381-3130

CABLE: CC POLLEN

You should try our other marvellous products from the beehive formulated under the High Desert® brand with:

Bee Pollen	Honey	Bee Bread	The President's Lunch Bar
Bee Propolis	Beeswax	Bee Venom	The First Lady's Lunch Bar
Royal Jelly	Pollenergy 520 Capsules and Tablets		

You will not be disappointed!

ALWAYS BUY THE BEST - YOUR HEALTH IS PRICELESS!

Marc, you have not seen the actual ingredients in Food Product X66 and we feel sure that the other seven most powerful men in Washington, D.C. do not know the specific ingredients in Food Product X66. We listed these GRAS safe ingredients with comments as follows:

1. Fenugreek Seed   GRAS
2. Oat Straw   GRAS
3. Barberry Root   GRAS
4. Passion Flower   GRAS
5. Papaya Leaf   GRAS
6. Black Walnut Leaf   GRAS
7. Chaparral Leaf   GRAS

8. White Oak Bark   GRAS
9. Chickweed Herb   GRAS
10. Blessed Thistle Herb   GRAS
11. Mulleinflower   GRAS
12. Parsley Leaf   GRAS
25. Papain
    Webster's Dictionary tells us papain is a proteinase in the juice of unripe papaya, surely the FDA with their super knowledge would agree that papain is GRAS by definition
26. Niacinamide
    The FDA has already declared niacinamide as GRAS
27. Extract of Ox Bile
    A food having been eaten by man since the days of discovery of fire and is certainly GRAS by definition
28. Whole Pancreas
    A gland of vertebrates, the pancreas of cattle is like eating the heart, liver, steak, roast. The pancreas is part of the animal and is GRAS by definition
29. Pyridoxine
    A vitamin that has been declared GRAS by the FDA
30. Potassium Chloride
    A crystalline salt occurring as a mineral and in natural waters - GRAS by definition
31. Pepsin
    A proteinase of the stomach - GRAS by definition
32. High Desert® bee pollen
    High Desert® bee pollen was the first food on earth and is certainly GRAS by definition
33. Betaine HCL
    A sweet crystalline quaternary ammonium salt occurring especially in beet juice - GRAS by definition
34. Glutamic Acid HCL
    A crystalline amino acid widely distributed in plant and animal proteins - GRAS by definition and declared GRAS by the FDA.

GRAS is an abbreviation and acronym for...Generally Recognized As Safe...found in the Code of Federal Regulations, Section 21, Part 170..30. This is the only place in all of the Federal Regulations the definition of GRAS appears. GRAS is applied, if applicable, to all substances, food products and otherwise, if they fit the definition of GRAS.

Generally speaking, if a food product was in general circulation, generally eaten, or in general commerce prior to 1958, with no reported toxicity, the food or substance is GRAS by virtue of The Grandfather Clause.

It is obvious that all of the first 24 ingredients are herbs that are GRAS safe, having been eaten by mankind since the days of Adam and Eve and so were the other 10 ingredients.

The FDA could hardly challenge the safety of any of these 34 ingredients.

If every ingredient in Food Product X66 is GRAS - and it is - why would the FDA make such a ludicrous request that Renaissance Laboratories do the 33 clinical investigations to eliminate the dangerous, poison, toxic drug ingredients in Food Product X66 when there were none?

It appears the FDA is reacting out of force of habit. They did not read and analyze the ingredients in this GRAS safe food product.

The FDA is operating from habit.

The hold up by the FDA these past two years for Renaissance Laboratories' clinical investigations is a shameful story.

Marc, you must contact Commissioner David A. Kessler. You must give him a copy of this fax immediately. Commissioner Kessler is the only person having the authority to bypass the clinical investigations and license Food Product X66.

Commissioner David A. Kessler must immediately temporarily license Food Product X66 to correct, eliminate, and cure the fifth leading cause of death in the United States and the world - chronic obstructive pulmonary disease, allergies, asthma, hay fever, sinus, and like conditions found in FDA IND 37318.

To the seven gentlemen receiving this fax:

If Commissioner David A. Kessler does not have this food product temporarily licensed one week from today, you must force Commissioner Kessler to temporarily license Food Product X66.

You have no choice. Now that you know the absolute absurdity of the FDA's clinical hold for Food Product X66, you must act to force the FDA to license this drug or you would be guilty of malfeasance.

We do not want any more Americans dying needlessly from these diseases when the cure is at hand especially when the GRAS safe cure is at hand.

The blood of millions of Americans has been shed needlessly too long.

Let's stop this unnecessary blood bath and massacre of Americans - today!

Everyday the FDA continues to procrastinate, or you continue to procrastinate, another 225 Americans die.

C C POLLEN CO.

3627 East Indian School Road
Suite 209
Phoenix, Arizona 85018-5126

FAX: (602) 381-3130
Telex: 559-834
Cable: CCPOLLEN

Phone: (602) 957-0096

September 23, 1992   Eighth Response to your August 5, 1992 letter.

From: Royden Brown
Chairman of the Board

cc: Senator Orrin G. Hatch
FAX: 202-224-6331
cc: Senator Edward G. Kennedy
FAX: 202-224-2417
cc: Representative John Dingle
FAX: 202-225-2525
cc: Senator Dennis DeConcini
FAX: 202-224-2302; 602-670-6831

FAX: 301-443-9282
Marc J. Scheineson, Assoc.
Commissioner for Legislative Affairs, FDA
cc: Sally Kelley, Agency Liason, Rm. 91
The White House, FAX: 202-456-2461
cc: President George Bush
FAX: 202-456-2461
cc: Vice President Dan Quayle
FAX: 202-456-6231
cc: Senator John McCain
FAX: 202-224-8938; 602-640-2576

Marc, in our seventh response we outlined the 34 ingredients in Food Product X66. As any fifth grader would know, every one of these ingredients in Food Product X66 is GRAS by definition. Food Product X66 is only a small portion of each one of these 34 ingredients gathered together and put in a capsule, or pressed together and made into a tablet. The assembling into a capsule or pressing into a tablet does not change the characteristics of the 34 ingredients. The resulting tablet or capsule is GRAS, just like the 34 ingredients in the tablet or capsule. Each one of these ingredients fits perfectly the definition of GRAS found in the Code of Federal Regulations, Section 21, Part 170.30.

This means the FDA cannot successfully dispute the fact Food Product X66 is GRAS and is not only safe for Americans to ingest, but Food Product X66 is safer than any drug the FDA has ever licensed thus far in its existence.

We know a GRAS substance will do no harm to the ingestor.

We also know the FDA has told Congress time and time again the FDA has only two duties - two responsibilities - with any drug:

      1. Safety
      2. Effectiveness

I will swear on a stack of Bibles that Food Product X66 has an effectiveness approaching 100% - more than 99% effective. I am not talking about a treatment that never cures like the antihistamines and other drugs the FDA has licensed for this fifth leading cause of death in the United States.

I am talking about the correction, elimination and cure and permanent cure of the fifth leading cause of death in the United States and the world, allergies, asthma, hay fever, sinus, chronic obstructive pulmonary disease and like conditions.

Referring to the fourth paragraph in your August 5, 1992 letter, it is obvious the FDA is making a fatal mistake - a 225 American lives lost every day mistake - in withholding Food Product X66 by virtue of a clinical hold for and because of the safety of Food Product X66.

Since the absolute GRAS safety of Food Product X66 has been indisputably established Marc, and since 225 Americans are dying every day for want of Food Product X66, and since the FDA can rely upon my sworn statement for any GRAS product without endangering American lives, and since we both know the President and Congress hold American lives a great deal more important than the FDA regulations, we are sending Commissioner David A. Kessler, M.D., Ph.D, a copy of this fax and a copy of our seventh response to enable the Commissioner to immediately temporarily release and license Food Product X66 found in FDA IND 37318.

Every day the FDA delays, 225 American lives are lost.

The FDA must act. They must end this unnecessary horrible blood bath of massacred Americans.

cc: David A. Kessler, M.D., Ph.D.
       Commissioner, FDA
       FAX: 301-443-5930

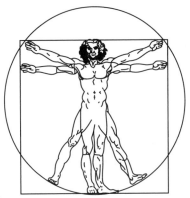

September 24, 1992

From: Royden Brown
Chairman of the Board

FAX: 202-224-4803
Senator Warren B. Rudman
U.S. Senate, Washington, D.C. 20510

Senator, you have your priorities wrong.

You said you were concerned about unsubstantiated health claims made in an industry "that has had problems with fraud."

The problems with fraud are all created by the FDA because - Congress was not wise enough to exclude foods when they defined the dangerous toxic poison drugs that are regulated and licensed by the FDA.

How many people have the unsubstantiated health claims killed - how many American lives have been taken?

If you will review the records you will find there has not been a single American life lost for a health food product in over a decade; so you concern is misplaced.

By the same token, how many American lives have been lost by those FDA licensed dangerous toxic poison drugs that are substantiated?

Probably 200,000 or more a year - the FDA admits 12,000 a year.

Which would you rather have in New Hampshire, Senator?

An unsubstantiated health claim that is harmless, or,

A dangerous toxic poison drug that has been licensed by the FDA because it was substantiated by tests, but does kill one in every 100 users and treats, never cures?

In fact, the Physicians Desk Reference, a 3,500 page small print large book is necessary just to list the toxic side effects of the drugs the FDA license.

What is the matter with Congress? Why would you permit such a thing to happen?

You have defined a drug so that if I say Vitamin C cures scurvy, that is a felony and the FDA could throw me in jail.

As I say, Senator, you had better get your priorities straight.

Do you know Senator, every time M.D's go on strike total mortality declines? If the strike lasts 85 days or longer, total mortality declines more than 50%. This is true in California, Connecticut, Saskatchewan, Colombia, Israel. It doesn't make any difference where it happens in the world, total mortality declines 50%.

There are no exceptions worldwide.

Does that send a message to you Senator?

Instead of being worried about unsubstantiated health claims which are probably true, but they don't have the scientific proof - ha, that's a laugh, too. All the FDA licensed drugs have the scientific proof and yet they are probably the third leading cause of death in the United States and the world, and,

If you put in the M.D's with the licensed drugs, the leading cause of death worldwide.

You should get your priorities straight, Senator.

C C POLLER CO.

3627 East Indian School Road
Suite 209
Phoenix, Arizona 85018-5126

FAX: (602) 381-3130
Telex: 559-834
Cable: CCPOLLEN

Phone: (602) 957-0096

September 24, 1992   Ninth Response to your August 5, 1992 letter.

From: Royden Brown
Chairman of the Board

cc: Senator Orrin G. Hatch
FAX: 202-224-6331
cc: Senator Edward G. Kennedy
FAX: 202-224-2417
cc: Representative John Dingle
FAX: 202-225-2525
cc: Senator Dennis DeConcini
FAX: 202-224-2302; 602-670-6831

FAX: 301-443-9282
Marc J. Scheineson, Assoc.
Commissioner for Legislative Affairs, FDA
cc: Sally Kelley, Agency Liason, Rm. 91
The White House, FAX: 202-456-2461
cc: President George Bush
FAX: 202-456-2461
cc: Vice President Dan Quayle
FAX: 202-456-6231
cc: Senator John McCain
FAX: 202-224-8938; 602-640-2576

Renaissance Laboratories decided it owed a duty to American public health and welfare to again call Congressional attention and the Executive Branch attention to the greatest mistake ever made in public health legislation.

The Federal Food, Drug and Cosmetic Act should have defined the word drug as follows:

"Articles, other than food, dietary and nutritional supplements, intended for use in the diagnosis, cure, litigation, treatment or prevention of disease in man or animal."

This failure of Congress and the President to insert the phrase underlined has probably cost 30 million American lives. Think of it - 30 million American Lives.

This mistake by Congress and the President is the direct cause of more than 1,600,000 Americans losing their life every year to degenerative disease and the direct cause of preventing a safe effective cure of the 4 million plus Alzheimer's diseased Americans.

Apparently, no-one before has had the awareness and the courage to call this mistake in legislation the greatest enemy of American public health of all time. Strong words? Actually, the understatement of the day.

When Congress and the President enacted legislation describing and defining a drug to include air and water under certain circumstances it is obvious and apparent the definition of a drug was wrong, absolutely wrong.

When someone is in the desert dying of thirst and a passer-by says if water is given to this man dying of thirst it would cure his dehydration - a felony.

When we have a man starving to death for lack of food and a passer-by says let's give this man some food and cure his hunger - a felony.

Both instances are felonies under the present law enacted by Congress and signed by the President.

Obviously a mistake of the greatest proportions.

If this is true, and you can rest assured it is true, why hasn't the FDA urged Congress to correct this mistake?

C C POLLEN CO.

3627 East Indian School Road
Suite 209
Phoenix, Arizona 85018-5126

FAX: (602) 381-3130
Telex: 559-834
Cable: CCPOLLEN

Phone: (602) 957-0096

September 25, 1992　　Tenth Response to your August 5, 1992 letter.

From: Royden Brown
Chairman of the Board

cc: Senator Orrin G. Hatch
FAX: 202-224-6331
cc: Senator Edward G. Kennedy
FAX: 202-224-2417
cc: Representative John Dingle
FAX: 202-225-2525
cc: Senator Dennis DeConcini
FAX: 202-224-2302; 602-670-6831

FAX: 301-443-9282
Marc J. Scheineson, Assoc.
Commissioner for Legislative Affairs, FDA
cc: Sally Kelley, Agency Liason, Rm. 91
The White House, FAX: 202-456-2461
cc: President George Bush
FAX: 202-456-2461
cc: Vice President Dan Quayle
FAX: 202-456-6231
cc: Senator John McCain
FAX: 202-224-8938; 602-640-2576

Marc, we do not believe you, the Congress nor the President actually is aware of the cures - not treatments but cures - of these 32 IND's filed by Renaissance Laboratories with the FDA have more than 100 indications. In these indications is the cure for virtually all degenerative disease and the absolute positive cures of all of the major killer degenerative diseases. These cures are cures, not treatments, but cures, and they have laid dormant for these past two years, while over 3 million Americans have died needlessly. Each one of these products found in the following IND's is GRAS safe - 3, 4, 5 and 6 yr. old babies eat them freely. Think what it would mean to American public health when the CC Pollen Co. cures from the beehive are made generally available to Americans. The products in these IND's correct, eliminate and cure - not treat, but cure - the following degenerative diseases:

1. FDA IND 37318, chronic obstructive pulmonary disease, allergies, asthmas, hay fever, sinus and like conditions - 5th leading cause of death in the USA and worldwide.

2. FDA IND 38158-1, joint pain, especially arthritis, bursitis and like conditions - estimated more than 50 million sufferers. President George Bush could cure his arthritic hip and go back to jogging again.

3. FDA IND 37319, premature aging, especially when accompanied by sexual impotency and sexual disfunction and like conditions.

4. FDA IND 37326-1, ulcers, bleeding ulcers and like conditions.

5. FDA IND 37336-4, pneumonia, influenza, infections, inflammations and like conditions - sixth leading cause of death in the United Stated and the world.

6. FDA IND 37124, fatigue, lack of energy, chronic fatigue syndrome, Epstein Barr virus and like conditions - cause of the most visits to M.D.'s office.

7. FDA IND 37262, intense high level radiation, including cancer radiation and like conditions - probably the most perfect protection for all radiation including ozone radiation.

8. FDA IND 37426, hoarseness, raspy voice, sore throat and mouth, infections and like conditions.

9. FDA IND 37511, loose teeth, gingivitis, bleeding gums, pyorrhea and like conditions - dentists will fight this to the death just like the M.D.'s.

10. FDA IND 38348, toxic side effects of chemotherapy - cancer patients love.

11. FDA IND 37515, heart disease, coronary artery disease, cerebral vascular accidents, atheroschlerosis, strokes, and cholesterol above 150 mg/dl and like conditions - cure of the first, third and thirteenth leading cause of death in the United States and the world and does so in most people in 90 days or less.

12. FDA IND 37517, memory loss, forgetfulness, senility and like conditions - how many people would benefit?

13. FDA IND 37557, pimples, acne and like conditions - virtually all teenagers would benefit.

14. FDA IND 37124, high blood pressure, blood pressure above 120/60 and like conditions - an absolute cure.

15. FDA IND 38348-1, Alzheimer's disease and like conditions - Harvard estimates more than 4 million now afflicted and more than 20 million by the year 2010 - presently the world's leading death to come disease, unless Bee Alzheimer's Disease Free is released.

16. FDA IND 38348-2, multiple-sclerosis and like conditions.

17. FDA IND 38348-3, diabetes, mellitus, hypoglycemia and like conditions - the seventh leading cause of death in the United States and the world.

18. FDA IND 38348-4, hypertension, hyperactivity and like conditions.

19. FDA IND 38348-5, emphysema and like conditions.

20. FDA IND 38348-8, all prostate gland problems and like conditions - affects nearly all senior males one time or another.

21. FDA IND 38348-9, male failure to achieve an erection, failure to conceive and like conditions - probably most of Congress could benefit and, perhaps, even the President.

22. FDA IND 38348-23, cancer - malignant neoplasms, etc. and like conditions - the second leading cause of death in the United States and the world.

23. FDA IND 37550, wearing glasses, eye weakness, eye failure   and like conditions - estimate nearly 50% of all Americans have this degenerative disease - weak eyes.

24. FDA IND 38348-25, AIDS - Acquired Immune Deficiency Syndrome - minor problem at the moment, might become epidemic.

25. FDA IND 38348-24, hemorrhaging, bleeding and like conditions - bleeding normally stops in a minute or two.

26. FDA IND 38348-27, cramps, cramps of the extremities and like conditions - millions have this problem.

27. FDA IND 38348-46, increased intelligence quotient (I.Q.) and like conditions - would be extremely beneficial for all American students and our competition with Japan and the world.

28. FDA IND 38348-29, diarrhea and like conditions - a blessing for foreign travellers.

29. FDA IND 38348-28, insomnia, sleeplessness, stress, nervousness and like conditions - President George Bush would not have fainted in Japan if he had been using Bee Sleepy® instead of the dangerous toxic poison Halcyon which doesn't work anyway.

Marc, there are more, many more, but the foregoing will give you and Congress and the President some idea of the FDA cover-up of these cures of degenerative diseases.

Every one of these cures is GRAS safe.

If nothing else, the FDA should challenge Renaissance Laboratories.

The FDA should immediately temporarily license Food Product X66 in IND 37318.

Have every M.D. that uses Food Product X66 to cure the fifth leading cause of death in the United States and the world to make a monthly report to the FDA.

If at the end of 90 days of use every M.D. using Food Product X66 reports Food Product X66 corrected and eliminated the symptoms of 95% or more of their patients with no toxic side effects, the FDA would release at least two more IND's without clinical investigation.

If the M.D.'s administering Food PRoduct X66 continued favorable reporting and the M.D's report favorably on the two additional releases, the FDA would release four more.

If the same sequence followed, the FDA would then release eight.

If the sequence is favorably reported, the FDA would release all the balance of the IND's and degenerative disease as we know it would be well on its way to being history - past history.

And the blood bath and massacre of Americans would stop once and for all time.

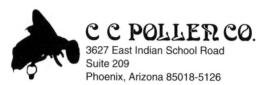

C C POLLEN CO.

3627 East Indian School Road
Suite 209
Phoenix, Arizona 85018-5126

FAX: (602) 381-3130
Telex: 559-834
Cable: CCPOLLEN

Phone: (602) 957-0096

September 28, 1992   Eleventh Response to your August 5, 1992 letter.

From: Royden Brown
Chairman of the Board

cc: Senator Orrin G. Hatch
FAX: 202-224-6331
cc: Senator Edward G. Kennedy
FAX: 202-224-2417
cc: Representative John Dingle
FAX: 202-225-2525
cc: Senator Dennis DeConcini
FAX: 202-224-2302; 602-670-6831

FAX: 301-443-9282
Marc J. Scheineson, Assoc.
Commissioner for Legislative Affairs, FDA
cc: Sally Kelley, Agency Liason, Rm. 91
The White House, FAX: 202-456-2461
cc: President George Bush
FAX: 202-456-2461
cc: Vice President Dan Quayle
FAX: 202-456-6231
cc: Senator John McCain
FAX: 202-224-8938;602-640-2576

Marc, we quote from your letter, the last sentence in the fifth paragraph in which you said, "That communication described in detail the reason that your product is considered a drug and why it was placed on clinical hold."

Again, I ask why did not the FDA read the rest of the definition of a drug Part C. which reads as follows, "Articles (other than food) intended to affect the structure or any function of the body of man or other animals."

Please inform me why the FDA did not say Food Product X66 belongs as an exception in the C. definition found in the definition of a drug - (other than food).

If Food Product X66 had been properly placed in the C. exception definition, the fifth leading cause of death in the United States and the world would be history today.

David A. Kessler, M.D., Ph.D. knows of his own knowledge, Food Product X66 is the absolute sure cure for the fifth leading cause of death in the United States. There is no question about it.

I make this statement knowing that if this statement is false it is a felony, a federal felony.

Since David A. Kessler knows of his own knowledge Food Product X66 is GRAS safe - safer than any drug the FDA has ever licensed - and I make this hard statement about the effectiveness of Food Produce X66, David A. Kessler can temporarily license Food Product X66 and start saving 225 American lives every day.

Surely the FDA cannot ignore Food Product X66 any longer, especially when the FDA knows for certain Food Product X66 is GRAS safe with an effectiveness approaching 100% and would save 225 lives today, tomorrow and every day of the year.

Marc, please take this up with Commissioner David A. Kessler, M.D., Ph.D. Commissioner Kessler must be as sensitive as anyone else is to needlessly dying Americans. He must act. we know he has the power to immediately temporarily license Food Product X66 to save American lives.

We also know that he has the power to take advantage of the exception already in place as found in the general considerations for the clinical evaluation of drugs, and I quote as follows:

1. "The guidelines must not be used to force new compounds into their mold else the fruit of original ideas may be lost."

2. "History is replete with discoveries that could not have been made if the investigation was constrained by established methods."

3. "A person may choose to use alternate procedures even though they are not provided for in the guidelines."

Surely the saving of 225 American lives every day is more important, a great deal more important than forcing Food Product X66 to strictly comply with the FDA regulations, compounded for the specific purpose of trying to guard Americans against the dangerous toxic poison drugs the FDA licenses and never conceived or meant for GRAS safe food cures from the beehive.

Conclusion:

We feel certain if we could gain the attention of President George Bush he would order Commissioner Kessler to immediately temporarily license Food Product X66 and release it to save 225 American lives every day.

Commissioner Kessler should release Food Product X66 of his own volition.

In the final analysis, Marc — which should be more important to the FDA?

Saving 100,000 American lives every year or the continued inviolate and unalterable holding of the FDA drug regulations?

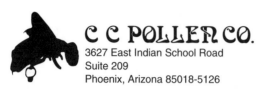

C C POLLEN CO.
3627 East Indian School Road
Suite 209
Phoenix, Arizona 85018-5126

FAX: (602) 381-3130
Telex: 559-834
Cable: CCPOLLEN

Phone: (602) 957-0096

September 29, 1992

From: Royden Brown
Chairman of the Board

Vice President Dan Quayle
cc: FAX: 202-224-6331

FAX: 202-456-2461
President George Bush
cc: FAX: 202-456-6231
Senator Orrin G. Hatch
cc. FAX: Senator John McCain

You must realize by now you are destined to bee a one term president. Americans are sick and tired of the way things are run in Washington, D.C. — and I cannot fault them.

I have sent you more than 20 faxes telling you CC Pollen Co. has the GRAS safe food cures for all the degenerative diseases.

Why can't we get your attention?

Are you so isolated from reality you are in a world of your own?

Or don't you give a hoot, want to be rid of the crime, drug-infested Washington, D.C. and get back to living?

In either event, the flame is about to be extinguished.

You do not have any choice — either you must chock the nation with the announcement you have found the GRAS safe cures from the beehive for all degenerative diseases, including Alzheimer's, heart disease, cancer, allergies, asthma, AIDS, etc. and have ordered Commissioner David A. Kessler to immediately temporarily license the Bee Allergy Free Asthma Bee Gone drug to save 100,000 American lives every year, to be followed with the release of each food cure from the beehive until all the GRAS safe food cures from the beehive are released, and be a re-elected president, or,

You will go down to a worse defeat than Senator McGovern.

YOU HAVE NO OTHER ALTERNATIVES!

If you wish, I will come to Washington, D.C. when requested.

Time is awasting!

Attention: whoever receives this fax!

THIS FAX MUST BEE DELIVERED TO THE PRESIDENT PERSONALLY.

ANYTHING SHORT OF IMMEDIATE PERSONAL DELIVERY IS TREASON!

C C POLLEN CO.
3627 East Indian School Road
Suite 209
Phoenix, Arizona 85018-5126

FAX: (602) 381-3130
Telex: 559-834
Cable: CCPOLLEN

Phone: (602) 957-0096

September 29, 1992   Twelfth Response to your August 5, 1992 letter.

From: Royden Brown
Chairman of the Board

cc: Senator Orrin G. Hatch
FAX: 202-224-6331
cc: Senator Edward G. Kennedy
FAX: 202-224-2417
cc: Representative John Dingle
FAX: 202-225-2525
cc: Senator Dennis DeConcini
FAX: 202-224-2302; 602-670-6831

FAX: 301-443-9282
Marc J. Scheineson, Assoc.
Commissioner for Legislative Affairs, FDA
cc: Sally Kelley, Agency Liason, Rm. 91
The White House, FAX: 202-456-2461
cc: President George Bush
FAX: 202-456-2461
cc: Vice President Dan Quayle
FAX: 202-456-6231
cc: Senator John McCain
FAX: 202-224-8938; 602-640-2576

Marc, we have presented the FDA the absolute cure of the first, second, third, fifth, sixth, seventh, eleventh, and thirteenth causes of death in the United States and hope to have your response before Congress adjourns. You haven't yet responded to a single fax. When you respond, we would expect you to send a copy to the seven people receiving these faxes.

In addition, Renaissance Laboratories has INDs pending with the FDA for the absolute positive cure of arthritis, bursitis, headache, back pain, PMS, and all of the other degenerative diseases except AIDS.

Renaissance Laboratories did present an IND covering the cure of AIDS, but Renaissance Laboratories has had no actual experience,neither has CC Pollen Co., with AIDS patients.

However, Renaissance Laboratories believes these strong cancer cures presented to the FDA, which re-establishes the immune system when medical science says the immune system is destroyed, will also cure AIDS.

Renaissance Laboratories believes the Bee Cancer Free cure from the beehive will re-establish the immune system of an AIDS patient just as well as it will with a cancer patient after chemotherapy and radiation.

Renaissance Laboratories has presented food cures for all degenerative diseases.

Renaissance Laboratories has presented INDs which will reduce the population of the federal and state hospitals, formerly called insane asylums, by 50 to 75 and perhaps even 90 percent.

Renaissance Laboratories has presented INDs to the FDA which would reduce recidivism in the state and federal penitentiaries by more than 50 percent.

Renaissance Laboratories has presented INDs to the FDA that will elevate intelligent quotient (I.Q.) of virtually all youngsters attending school.

Renaissance Laboratories has presented INDs to the FDA that will cure the pain of ulcers.

Renaissance Laboratories has presented INDs as previously mentioned having over 100 indications and what has the FDA done? Nothing.

Marc, please answer the question - which is more important to the FDA?

The FDA regulations or saving American lives?

C C POLLEN CO.

3627 East Indian School Road
Suite 209
Phoenix, Arizona 85018-5126

FAX: (602) 381-3130
Telex: 559-834
Cable: CCPOLLEN

Phone: (602) 957-0096

September 30, 1992   Thirteenth Response to your August 5, 1992 letter.

From: Royden Brown   FAX: 301-443-9282
Chairman of the Board   Marc J. Scheineson, Assoc.
                                  Commissioner for Legislative Affairs, FDA
cc: Senator Orrin G. Hatch   cc: Sally Kelley, Agency Liason, Rm. 91
FAX: 202-224-6331   The White House, FAX: 202-456-2461
cc: Senator Edward G. Kennedy   cc: President George Bush
FAX: 202-224-2417   FAX: 202-456-2461
cc: Representative John Dingle   cc: Vice President Dan Quayle
FAX: 202-225-2525   FAX: 202-456-6231
cc: Senator Dennis DeConcini   cc: Senator John McCain
FAX: 202-224-2302; 602-670-6831   FAX: 202-224-8938; 602-640-2576

Marc, we have presented the indisputable fact that Food Product X66 found in FDA IND 37318 is absolutely GRAS safe and I have guaranteed the commissioner, actually with my life in the balance, that Food Product X66 has an efficiency approaching 100% - more effective than any drug thus far ever licensed in the history of the FDA. As we have repeated over and over again, Food Product X66 is the absolute GRAS safe sure for the fifth leading cause of death in the United States and the world - chronic obstructive pulmonary disease, allergies, asthma, hay fever, sinus and like conditions.

Marc, if you or the FDA can dispute anything I have presented to the President and members of Congress, please do so within the next ten days. Surely with 18,000 employees that should not be a hardship for the FDA. Do not write but fax me your rebuttal with copies to the 7 men previously receiving faxed copies. If you have not faxed your rebuttal of anything and everything that you and the FDA dispute in the responses I have made by adjournment, October 5, 1992, we all will take for granted what I have said is the gospel truth and accepted as such by the FDA.

What about the leading cause of death in the United States and the world, heart disease?

Renaissance Laboratories submitted the CC Pollen Co. absolute cure for not only the leading cause of death in the world, heart disease, but the same product absolutely cures cerebrovascular diseases, the third leading cause of death in the United States and the world, and arteriosclerosis, the thirteenth leading cause of death in the United States and the world.

The Bee Heart Rite products found in FDA IND 37515 not only absolutely cure heart disease, coronary artery disease, cerebral vascular accident, stroke, cerebral vascular diseases and atheriosclerosis, but in doing so cleans out the veins and arteries as clean as a houndstooth and reverses these conditions when they exist. The Bee Heart Rite products normally reduce the total blood cholesterol by 50% in 90 days or less, or to 150 mg/dl in most if not all people. What does this mean?

This means Bee Heart Rite products would save 900,000 American lives every year.

What does the FDA say about this?

After this IND was submitted the FDA, Solomon Sobel, M.D. sent out the same form letter, put IND 37515 on clinical hold because of safety. No concern whatsoever was given to the fact 900,000 Americans were dying every year, 2500 every day, for want of Bee Heart Rite.

Was the FDA right in saying Bee Heart Rite was unsafe? Let's examine the facts:

We are faxing you hereinafter copies of the two labels given the FDA which make up Bee Heart Rite. Let us analyze these two products:

The first product is High Desert® bee pollen — High Desert® bee pollen was the first food on earth. Bee pollen has been eaten by an unknown number of millions and millions and millions of people since the beginning. It is obvious High Desert® bee pollen is the most GRAS of all GRAS substances probably on this earth.

The FDA could not successfully challenge the GRAS classification of High Desert® bee pollen.

The second product is Bee Heart Rite tablets. We list the ingredients as follows:

1. Gentian Root	6. Echinacea	11. Foti
2. Black Cohosh	7. Dandelion Root	12. Capsicum
3. Ginger Root	8. Myrrh	13. Papaya
4. Fenugreek	9. Golden Seal	14. Peppermint Leaves
5. Hawthorne Berries	10. GotuKola	15. Fennel Seed

All 15 of these herbs were eaten by Adam and Eve in the Garden of Eden. They are obviously GRAS.

14. Cyancobalamine

These 3 are vitamins and the FDA has declared them GRAS.

17. Lecithin
These 3 ingredients are GRAS and declared GRAS by the FDA.

20. Bee pollen
The first food on earth, obviously GRAS.

If every ingredient in Bee Heart Rite is GRAS, it is obvious to one and all, except to the FDA, that these 2 products are GRAS - safer than any drug the FDA has ever licensed.

The FDA has made a serious mistake in stating these Bee Heart Rite products are unsafe for humans to eat — this is especially true when 2500 Americans are losing their lives every day for want of these Bee Heart Rite products.

Since these products are GRAS and CC Pollen Co. has stated these products have an effectiveness approaching 100%, these products should have been released with a temporary license to save American lives - 900,000 Americans are dying every year needlessly.

Any casual observer would conclude the FDA is derelict in their duty to the American public.

How will those relatives of those 900,000 Americans dying every year from these deadly diseases react when they find out the FDA has been harboring, covering up, the absolute cure for these diseases?

Marc, let the FDA defend themselves.

I know the 7 most powerful men in Washington, D.C. receiving this fax are anxious to hear the FDA rebuttal to the information contained herein.

Either I have made mistakes in this presentation, or the FDA has the blood of 1,800,000 Americans on their doorstep.

If true - the FDA's behavior is inexcusable.

Bee Heart Rite should be temporarily licensed by the FDA immediately.

C C POLLEN CO.

3627 East Indian School Road
Suite 209
Phoenix, Arizona 85018-5126

FAX: (602) 381-3130
Telex: 559-834
Cable: CCPOLLEN

Phone: (602) 957-0096

October 1, 1992   Fourteenth Response to your August 5, 1992 letter.

From: Royden Brown
Chairman of the Board

cc: Senator Orrin G. Hatch
FAX: 202-224-6331
cc: Senator Edward G. Kennedy
FAX: 202-224-2417
cc: Representative John Dingle
FAX: 202-225-2525
cc: Senator Dennis DeConcini
FAX: 202-224-2302; 602-670-6831

FAX: 301-443-9282
Marc J. Scheineson, Assoc.
Commissioner for Legislative Affairs, FDA
cc: Sally Kelley, Agency Liason, Rm. 91
The White House, FAX: 202-456-2461
cc: President George Bush
FAX: 202-456-2461
cc: Vice President Dan Quayle
FAX: 202-456-6231
cc: Senator John McCain
FAX: 202-224-8938; 602-640-2576

In our 13th response discussing the inexcusable FDA behavior of placing a clinical hold on Bee Heart Right, an absolute GRAS substance that would save 900,000 Americans lives every year. The FDA behavior in this instance is indefensible - 2,500 American lives die everyday for want of GRAS safe Bee Heart Right.

Now we have Alzheimer's disease.

Harvard Medical School estimates there's more than 4 million Americans that are now Alzheimer's diseased and sure to die because there's no known drug that will cure Alzheimer's disease. Harvard estimates by the year 2010, there will be more than 16 million similarly situated.

However - there's a light at the end of the tunnel - Renaissance Laboratories is happy to report CC Pollen Co. has the absolute cure of Alzheimer's disease. This IND was submitted to the FDA a long time ago. Bee Alzheimer's Disease Free has not been temporarily licensed. How many Alzheimer's diseased Americans are dying everyday is an unknown figure, but no doubt thousands die everyday.

Let's see if we can find out why the FDA has not temporarily licensed Bee Alzheimer's Disease Free. We are following this fax with a copy of the two labels in Bee Alzheimer's Disease Free products.

Here are the facts from those labels:

Product No. 1 is simply the High Desert® bee pollen.

As we know from previous faxes, bee pollen was the first food on earth and probably the most GRAS of all foods.

Bee Alzheimer's Disease Free product no. 2 list of ingredients:

1. High Desert® apple cider vinegar
2. High Desert® bee pollen
3. High Desert® honey
4. High Desert® water

It is obvious these four ingredients are GRAS.

If the four ingredients in this drink are GRAS, it is obvious to anyone who can read this drink itself is GRAS. If this drink is GRAS, it's absolutely safe for Americans to ingest without problems.

If both of these products are GRAS, why hasn't the FDA temporarily licensed Bee Alzheimer's Disease Free to save American lives?

Marc, I am sure the President and members of Congress receiving this fax would like to have a response from the FDA in answer to the question:

Why hasn't the FDA temporarily licensed the GRAS safe Bee Alzheimer's Disease Free drug -The absolute GRAS safe sure for Alzheimer's Disease?

Marc, has the FDA ever in its entire existence sacrificed and bypassed the deadly drug regulations to bring forth one GRAS safe food cure?

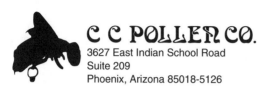

C C POLLEN CO.

3627 East Indian School Road
Suite 209
Phoenix, Arizona 85018-5126

FAX: (602) 381-3130
Telex: 559-834
Cable: CCPOLLEN

Phone: (602) 957-0096

October 5, 1992   Fifteenth Response to your August 5, 1992 letter.

From: Royden Brown
Chairman of the Board

cc: Senator Orrin G. Hatch
FAX: 202-224-6331
cc: Senator Edward G. Kennedy
FAX: 202-224-2417
cc: Representative John Dingle
FAX: 202-225-2525
cc: Senator Dennis DeConcini
FAX: 202-224-2302; 602-670-6831

FAX: 301-443-9282
Marc J. Scheineson, Assoc.
Commissioner for Legislative Affairs, FDA
cc: Sally Kelley, Agency Liason, Rm. 91
The White House, FAX: 202-456-2461
cc: President George Bush
FAX: 202-456-2461
cc: Vice President Dan Quayle
FAX: 202-456-6231
cc: Senator John McCain
FAX: 202-224-8938; 602-640-2576

Marc, we have sent you fourteen separate responses, thus far, to your August 5, 1992 letter.

You have ignored them all.

You have not seen fit to reply to a single response.

Nor have you answered a single question.

What is your problem?…What is the FDA's problem?

We think the President and the Vice President of the United States and the 5 Congressmen receiving these faxes deserve the attention of the FDA. The FDA has more than 18,000 employees and yet the FDA has completely ignored our responses.

We are talking about saving American lives. We are talking about the cures of degenerative diseases. We realize the FDA has had no experience whatsoever with the cures of anything only treatments that never cure.

Under the circumstances, we believe the President and Vice PResident of the United STates and the 5 Congressmen need to get basic and fundamental with the FDA. We need some basic questions answered.

Marc, please have the FDA answer the following most fundamental and basic questions:

1. Does the FDA believe the saving of one American life every day is more important than any and all the FDA regulations?

2. If not, does the FDA believe the saving of 10 American lives every single day is more important than any and all the FDA regulations?

3. If not, does the FDA believe the saving of 100 American lives every single day is more important than any and all the FDA regulations?

4. If not, does the FDA believe the saving of 200 American Lives every single day is more important than any and all the FDA regulations?

5. If not, does the FDA believe the saving of 225 American lives every single day is more important than any and all the FDA regulations?

6. If not, at what point does the saving of American lives become more important than the FDA regulations?

7. At what point does the saving of American lives become more important than the FDA regulations and would cause the FDA to take advantage of the definition of a drug found in the C. Section of the definition and the provisions found in the General Considerations for Clinical Evaluation of Drugs?

Marc, if American lives are meaningless to the FDA, the regulations are paramount, supreme, and cannot be violated — there is no need for any further communication between us.

We wish to know. We do not want to waste any more time if our efforts to save millions of American lives are hopeless and impossible of achieving because of the inviolate American FDA regulations.

EXHIBIT B

Exhibit B is attached to and made a part of that FDA Form 1571, Investigational New Drug Application, which is a part of every IND filed with the FDA, defining the levels of indications for any and every food product and drug product submitted to the FDA by Renaissance Laboratories, as follows:

1. PRIMARY INDICATIONS:

    Renaissance Laboratories defines primary indications as those indications Renaissance Laboratories knows and will guarantee for certain their food product or their drug will stop, correct, eliminate and cure, in all people with a GRAS safety and an effectiveness approaching 100% – and will absolutely, unconditionally, irrevocably guarantee 100% effectiveness.

2. SECONDARY INDICATIONS:

    Renaissance Laboratories defines secondary indications as those indications Renaissance Laboratories knows the food product or the drug will stop, correct, eliminate and *cure*, but as yet has not done the experimental work to be able to say for certain the food product or the drug will *prevent* and, as a result, does not make any statements concerning effectiveness of the food product of the drug in the prevention of the indications.

3. THIRD INDICATIONS:

    Renaissance Laboratories defines the third indications or the third level of indications as those indications espoused, stated, indicated or reported by others, primarily licensed M.D.'s, stating an indication will be or can be cured by one of Renaissance Laboratories' drugs, but Renaissance Laboratories has had no previous experience.

STATED EFFECTIVENESS:

Renaissance Laboratories reports C C Pollen Co. informs Renaissance Laboratories in every instance thus far, there are no exceptions, when a food product from C C Pollen Co. or a drug product from C C Pollen Co. stops, corrects, eliminates and *cures* a degenerative disease in one person, that food product or drug from C C Pollen Co. will stop, correct, eliminate and *cure* that degenerative disease in nearly all persons with an effectiveness approaching 100%.

Renaissance Laboratories reports that C C Pollen Co. states when a C C Pollen Co. food product or drug fails to stop, correct, eliminate and *cure* a degenerative disease in a few, that food product or drug is 100% ineffective in all.

ACTUAL SAFETY:

Empirical evidence, the strongest evidence, from the past many years, proves all the C C Pollen Co. products could not be safer and are safer than the FDA GRAS substances – there has *never* been one instance of a C C Pollen Co. food product, nor a C C Pollen Co. drug product, causing any adverse, permanent damage of any kind to any one and,

C C Pollen Co. reports there has never, ever been a single product liability claim ever paid in the long, long existence of the company.

The C C Pollen Co. products could not bee safer or more effective!

C C Pollen Co. and Winners Bee Pollen Co. informs Renaissance Laboratories and guarantees to the FDA, both companies will notify the Physician's Desk Reference publishers of both the PDRs for M.D.'s and the veterinarian pharmaceuticals and biologicals and all similar and like publications to list all drugs licensed by the FDA for both companies as follows:

1. PRECAUTIONS: Fresh food – treated as fresh food.

2. ANECDOTE: None necessary – poisoning never occurs.

3. CAUTION: No restrictions on use. *See* usage below.

4. WARNING: Probably the strongest food of all. Beginning intake for the bee pollen should be gradual and in accordance with instructions on the label.

CONDITIONS	BEE POLLEN CURES
1. Indications treated	Never treated; always cured
2. Indications cured	Always
3. Indications always cured	Always
4. Indications healed	Always
5. Contraindications	Never
6. Action	Never any problems. Action is never detrimental. Action of the drug heals the indications and eliminates the symptoms completely.
7. Adverse reactions	None when ingested properly
8. Side effects	Never
9. Side effects – temporary	Never
10. Side effects – permanent	Never
11. Destructive to body	Never
12. Lethal	Never
13. Warnings	Never
14. Upper limits of ingestion	Never. No reasonable upper limits.
15. Cautions	Never
16. Interreactions	Never
17. Cumulative in the soft tissue	Never
18. Cumulative in the fatty tissue	Never
19. Residue	Never
20. Addictive	Never
21. Overdosage	Never; no reasonable upper limits of ingestion.
22. Possibility of manufacturing mistakes	Never a danger
23. Stability	Fresh food
24. Precautions	Never

25. Safe for seniors	Always
26. Safe for babies	Always
27. Safe for children	Always
28. Safe during pregnancy	Always
29. Safe during breeding	Always
30. Safe during lactation	Always
31. Fresh food	Always
32. Cooked or heated above 105°F	Never
33. Contains enzymes	Always
34. Contains life force	Always
35. Effectiveness	Approaches 100%. Manufacturer will absolutely, unconditionally, irrevocably guarantee 100% effectiveness.

CONCLUSION

Any American who is concerned with unnecessary loss of American lives, after reading these 15 faxes, will be horrified, outraged and should become militant.

The cures for virtually all degenerative diseases have been filed with the FDA for 2 years and not one has been released.

Exhibit A to the CC Pollen FSC LTD Export Agreements lists the cures of all degenerative diseases available from CC Pollen Co. and filed with the USA FDA.

This means there are more than 3,200,000 American lives on the doorstep of the FDA.

But the FDA doesn't care if all Americans die.

If the American people only knew the FDA, the FDA licensed drugs, and the allopathic M.D.'s administering these FDA licensed drugs are the number one killer, the number one cause of death in the United States and the world — I think a great groundswell would visit Washington and Rockville, Maryland, and eliminate the FDA and their offices.

What a wonderful country the USA would bee – if the FDA would disappear – forever!

Giving the FDA jurisdiction over foods, dietary and nutritonal supplements and is like having the fox guard the hen house.

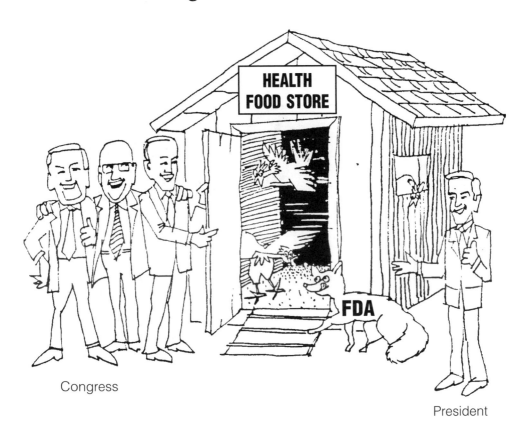

Congress

President

What was the original sin?

Drug definition.

Who is to blame?

Congress and the President.

Giving the FDA jurisdiction over foods, dietary and nutritonal supplements – is like having the fox guard the hen house.

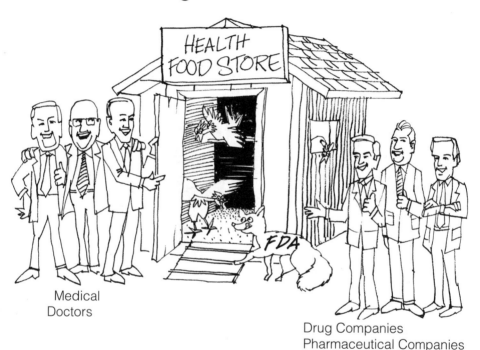

Medical Doctors

Drug Companies
Pharmaceutical Companies

What was the original sin?

Drug definition.

Who is to blame?

Congress and the President.

Latest development just before this book went to press:

Royden Brown had cured the lifelong allergies of Berkeley Bedell, a former long-term congressman from Iowa. Berkeley Bedell's wife's asthma was also cured by Royden Brown with the Aller Bee Gone tablets. Berkeley Bedell told U.S. Senator Tom Harkin from Iowa about the cure of his allergies, asthma, hay fever, sinusitis and chronic obstructive pulmonary diseases ... the five degenerative diseases he has had virtually all his life that were getting worse and worse every year and interfering with his work as U.S. Senator.

Berkeley Bedell asked Royden Brown to go to Washington, D.C. and cure Tom Harkin. Royden Brown left Arizona and arrived in Washington, D.C. on Tuesday, April 19, 1993. Wednesday, April 20, 1993 at 8:30 that morning, Royden Brown gave U.S. Senator Tom Harkin 12 of the Aller Bee Gone tablets and then 15 minutes later gave him another 12 of the Aller Bee Gone tablets on an empty stomache. After the passage of 40 minutes, U.S. Senator Tom Harkin was free of his symptoms of allergies, asthma, hay fever, sinusitis and chronic obstructive pulmonary - the fifth leading cause of death in the United States and the world - for the first time in his entire life.

That day Senator Tom Harkin was symptom free until just before retiring when his symptoms started to re-occur. Senator Tom Harkin immediately took 12 more Aller Bee Gone tablets and his symptoms disappeared. Senator Tom Harkin reports he slept clear through the night for the first time in his memory, symptom free.

The next morning he got up and felt his symptoms start to re-occur. He took 12 tablets, waited 15 minutes, took 12 more, waited another 15 minutes and took an additional 12 tablets. He took 36 tablets the morning upon arising on April 21st. He took no more tablets because his symptoms did not re-occur until the following day. April 22nd Senator Tom Harkin took 12 additional tablets and his symptoms disappeared again.

U.S. Senator Tom Harkin reports he is taking the Dynamic Trio every morning and he believes the Dynamic Trio is keeping him symptom free.

Senator Tom Harkin now says he is cured of his allergies and has reported so in a press conference, May 7th, in the U.S. Senate Press Room.

Reports of his cure were carried in the Cedar Rapids Gazette, the Des Moines Register, Omaha World Herald and on Associated Press wires everywhere.

U.S. Senator Tom Harkin told Royden Brown if he was symptom free for the next week he would have Royden Brown back to cure President Bill Clinton's allergies, asthma, hay fever, sinusitis, chronic obstructive pulmonary disease and his throat and voice problems.

It is a shame anyone in the United States continues to suffer from any degenerative diseases when the cures for virtually all degenerative diseases had been filed with the U.S. Food and Drug Administration over two years ago.

As reported earlier, this cover-up of the food cures from the beehive from CC Pollen Co. by the FDA is the greatest cover-up of all time, costing over 1,600,000 American lives every year and a trillion dollars in unnecessary medical expense.

Senator Harkin reported June 1, 1993 he is still symptom free.